50 LANDMARK PAPERS

every

Acute Care Surgeon Should Know

50 LANDMARK PAPERS

every

Acute Care Surgeon Should Know

EDITORS

Stephen M. Cohn, MD, FACS

Hackensack Meridian School of Medicine
Seton Hall University
Nutley, New Jersey, USA

Peter Rhee, MD, MPH

New York Medical College
Westchester Medical Center
Valhalla, New York, USA

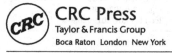

CRC Press
Taylor & Francis Group
Boca Raton London New York

CRC Press is an imprint of the
Taylor & Francis Group, an **informa** business

CRC Press
Taylor & Francis Group
6000 Broken Sound Parkway NW, Suite 300
Boca Raton, FL 33487-2742

Printed on acid-free paper

International Standard Book Number-13: 978-0-367-32140-6 (Hardback)
                                        978-1-138-62444-3 (Paperback)

Library of Congress Cataloging-in-Publication Data

Title: 50 landmark papers every acute care surgeon should know / [edited by] Stephen M. Cohn, Peter Rhee.
Other titles: Fifty landmark papers every acute care surgeon should know
Description: Boca : CRC Press, [2020] | Includes bibliographical references and index. | Summary: "This book identifies the 50 key scientific articles in the field of acute and emergency surgery and explains, via expert reflections and editorial perspectives, why these papers are important. Identifying those influential contributors who have shaped the practice of modern acute surgery, the book covers surgical emergencies in the areas of esophageal, gastric, duodenal, intestinal, biliary, pancreatic, anorectal, and general surgery. This an invaluable reference for trainees, fellows, and surgeons studying for exams, as well as for seasoned surgeons who want to stay current in this field."--Provided by publisher.
Identifiers: LCCN 2019026899 (print) | ISBN 9781138624443 (paperback ; alk. paper) | ISBN 9780367321406 (hardback ; alk. paper) | ISBN 9780429316944 (ebook)
Subjects: MESH: Critical Care--methods | Surgical Procedures, Operative--methods | Emergency Treatment--methods | Review
Classification: LCC RD51.5 (print) | LCC RD51.5 (ebook) | NLM WO 700 | DDC 617/.026--dc23
LC record available at https://lccn.loc.gov/2019026899
LC ebook record available at https://lccn.loc.gov/2019026900

Visit the Taylor & Francis Web site at
http://www.taylorandfrancis.com

and the CRC Press Web site at
http://www.crcpress.com

Contents

Section Two   Intestinal

Section Three   Hepatobiliary and Pancreatic

Section Six   Miscellaneous

Section Seven   Surgical Intensive Care Unit

Preface

The questions never change ... just the answers

Owen Wangensteen

Surgery is an innovative and rapidly changing discipline. As busy clinicians, we all strive to provide optimal care for our patients based on available evidence, but rarely do we have time to keep up with the multitude of developments in the field. In this text we have asked a surgical colleague to summarize the current status of essential topics in acute care surgery and select key annotated references that would be of particular interest to the reader. Working with the editors, a "landmark" high-quality manuscript from the twenty-first century was chosen from the available literature. An editorial note (or original author commentary when available) is provided to highlight key aspects of these monographs. As many of these topics have a plethora of critical papers, this process was naturally somewhat subjective. The goals of the editors were to provide helpful information on a wide variety of subject matter concerning emergency general surgical issues in a concise, logical, and hopefully enjoyable format.

Stephen M. Cohn and Peter Rhee

Contributors

Suresh Agarwal
Duke University
Durham, North Carolina

Hasan B. Alam
University of Michigan
Ann Arbor, Michigan

Abdul Q. Alarhayem
The Cleveland Clinic Foundation
Cleveland, Ohio

Chad G. Ball
University of Calgary
Calgary, Alberta, Canada

Jessica Barton
Philadelphia College of Osteopathic Medicine
Philadelphia, Pennsylvania

Jaime Benarroch-Gampel
Emory University
Atlanta, Georgia

Elizabeth R. Benjamin
University of Southern California
Los Angeles, California

Umar F. Bhatti
University of Michigan
Ann Arbor, Michigan

John K. Bini
Wright State University
Dayton, Ohio

Daniel J. Bonville
Methodist Hospital
Houston, Texas

Carlos V.R. Brown
University of Texas
Austin, Texas

Julie Bruce
University of Warwick
Coventry, United Kingdom

Eileen M. Bulger
University of Washington
Seattle, Washington

Michael P. Casaer
University Hospitals and Catholic
    University
Leuven, Belgium

Manuel Castillo-Angeles
Brigham and Women's Hospital
Boston, Massachusetts

James Middleton Chang
Emory University
Atlanta, Georgia

Jean Chastre
Service de Réanimation Médicale
Groupe Hospitalier Pitié–Salpêtrière
Assistance Publique–Hôpitaux de Paris
Université Pierre et Marie Curie
Paris, France

Michael L. Cheatham
Orlando Regional Medical Center
Orlando, Florida

Vishwanath Chegireddy
Methodist Hospital
Houston, Texas

Clarence E. Clark, III
Morehouse School of Medicine
Atlanta, Georgia

Christine S. Cocanour
University of California Davis
Sacramento, California

Jazmín M. Cole
Methodist Hospital
Houston, Texas

Mary Condron
St. Charles Medical Center
Bend, Oregon

Zara Cooper
Harvard Medical School
Boston, Massachusetts

Craig M. Coopersmith
Emory University
Atlanta, Georgia

Bruce Crookes
Medical University of South Carolina
Charleston, South Carolina

Pamela Daher-Tobia
University of Texas
Austin, Texas

Mark G. Davies
University of Texas Health Sciences
    Center
San Antonio, Texas

Marc de Moya
Medical College of Wisconsin
Milwaukee, Wisconsin

James C. Doherty
University of Illinois
Chicago, Illinois

Matt Dolich
University of California
Irvine, California

Juan C. Duchesne
Tulane School of Medicine
New Orleans, Louisiana

Akpofure Peter Ekeh
Miami Valley Hospital
Dayton, Ohio

Eric D. Endean
University of Kentucky
Lexington, Kentucky

Ara Feinstein
University of Arizona
Phoenix, Arizona

Matthew J. Forestiere
University of Southern California
Los Angeles, California

Rondi B. Gelbard
Emory University
Atlanta, Georgia

Larry M. Gentilello
University of Texas
Dallas, Texas

Fahim Habib
Allegheny Health Network
Pittsburgh, Pennsylvania

Morad Hameed
University of British Columbia
Vancouver, British Columbia, Canada

Samuel Hawkins
Staten Island University
Staten Island, New York

Stephen O. Heard
University of Massachusetts
Worcester, Massachusetts

James Holmes
Wake Forest University
Winston-Salem, North Carolina

Nathaniel Holmes
Staten Island University Hospital
Staten Island, New York

Kenji Inaba
University of Southern California
Los Angeles, California

Atif Jastaniah
University of British Columbia
Vancouver, British Columbia, Canada

Laura Johnson
Georgetown University
Washington, DC

Andrew Kamien
Medical College of Wisconsin
Milwaukee, Wisconsin

Krista L. Kaups
UCSF Medical School
Fresno, California

Natasha Keric
University of Arizona
Phoenix, Arizona

Leslie Kobayashi
University of California
San Diego, California

Narong Kulvatunyou
University of Arizona
Tucson, Arizona

Lydia Lam
University of Southern California
Los Angeles, California

Eric J. Lavonas
University of Colorado
Denver, Colorado

Eric J. Ley
Cedars-Sinai Medical Center
Los Angeles, California

Edward Lineen
Michigan State University College of
    Osteopathic Medicine
East Lansing, Michigan

Peter Lopez
Michigan State University College of
    Osteopathic Medicine
East Lansing, Michigan

Joseph Love
University of Houston
Houston, Texas

Matthew J. Martin
Scripps Mercy Medical Center
San Diego, California

Sarah Mathew
University of Pennsylvania
Philadelphia, Pennsylvania

Addison K. May
Carolinas Medical Center
Charlotte, North Carolina

Anchit Mehrotra
University of Arizona
Phoenix, Arizona

Andrew J. Michaels
Medicins Sans Frontières
Portland, Oregon

Joseph L. Mills
Baylor College of Medicine
Houston, Texas

Jonathan Nguyen
Morehouse School of Medicine
Atlanta, Georgia

David M. Notrica
Phoenix Children's Hospital
Phoenix, Arizona

Adrian W. Ong
University of Pennsylvania
Philadelphia, Pennsylvania

Raphael Parrado
Phoenix Children's Hospital
Phoenix, Arizona

Janet Powell
Imperial College London
London, United Kingdom

Christopher Reed
Duke University
Durham, North Carolina

Anne Rizzo
INOVA Fairfax Medical Campus
Fairfax, Virginia

Ali Salim
Brigham and Women's Hospital
Boston, Massachusetts

Paulina Salminen
Turku University Hospital
Turku, Finland

Mark Sawyer
Mayo Clinic
Rochester, Minnesota

Mark L. Shapiro
Portsmouth Regional Hospital
Portsmouth, New Hampshire

Vasiliy Sim
Staten Island University
Staten Island, New York

David A. Talan
Olive View—UCLA Medical Center
Los Angeles, California

Nabil Tariq
Methodist Hospital
Houston, Texas

Jacquelyn Seymour Turner
Morehouse School of Medicine
Atlanta, Georgia

Greet Van den Berghe
University Hospitals and Catholic University
Leuven, Belgium

Hjalmar C. van Santvoort
University Medical Center
Utrecht, the Netherlands

Esteban Varela
Florida State University
Tallahassee, Florida

Gary A. Vercruysse
University of Michigan
Ann Arbor, Michigan

Keneeshia Williams
Emory University
Atlanta, Georgia

CHAPTER 1

Perforated Peptic Ulcer

Review by Contributor: Matt Dolich

"Less is more." "Just treat the problem in front of you; don't make it more complicated than it needs to be." "Keep it simple" were the words of my mentors during surgical residency. Except that in many circumstances, we did exactly the opposite. As a resident, I remember watching meticulous, time-consuming dissection being performed during proximal gastric vagotomy while an anesthesiologist tensely focused on resuscitating our patient with a duodenal perforation and peritonitis. Fortunately, as our understanding of the pathophysiology of peptic ulcer disease has improved over the last quarter century, our management has become both more streamlined and more effective.

Though historians differ in their accounts, many believe that Princess Henrietta of England, youngest daughter of King Charles I, died of a perforated ulcer in 1670, after several years of abdominal pain and gastrointestinal complaints. Though she believed she was poisoned, an autopsy revealed a perforation that was likely related to ulcer disease. Almost 175 years later, Crisp reported 50 cases of perforated ulcer disease and is often quoted as saying that, "the symptoms are so typical, I hardly believe it possible that anyone can fail to make the correct diagnosis." Simple surgical closure of perforated peptic ulcers was first reported by the Polish surgeon Jan Mikulicz-Radecki in 1885. In many ways, he opened the door to modern surgical management of this disease process, stating, "every doctor who is faced with a perforated ulcer of the stomach or intestine must consider opening the abdomen, sewing up the hole and averting a possible inflammation by a careful cleansing of the abdominal cavity." Subsequently the omentum was recognized as a useful adjunct for repair of friable gastric and duodenal perforations and its use was advocated in the first part of the twentieth century by Graham and Cellan-Jones. Though commonly called "Graham's patch," Graham originally detailed the use of a free omental flap to plug the perforation. It was Cellan-Jones, eight years earlier in 1929, who described the use of a pedicle of omentum secured under an "archway" of full-thickness sutures placed across a perforated duodenal ulcer. This procedure, as described by Cellan-Jones, remains the workhorse of surgeons around the world when dealing with perforated peptic ulcer disease.

While surgical management of ulcer-related complications such as bleeding, perforation, and obstruction continued, several important breakthroughs in our understanding of the pathophysiology and treatment of ulcer disease transpired. It had long been recognized that a significant fraction of peptic ulcer disease was related to an imbalance of acid secretion and mucosal protection. In the 1960s, it was discovered that blockade of the H_2 receptor suppressed gastric acid secretion, leading to a new class of drugs called H_2-receptor antagonists. Another major breakthrough in the management of peptic ulcer disease occurred in 1982 with the recognition that an infection was causative (or at least involved) in the vast majority of cases. Australian researchers Barry J. Marshall and John Robin Warren demonstrated that a bacterium, *Helicobacter pylori*, played a major role in the causation of peptic ulcers, and that utilization of antibiotic regimens in conjunction with bismuth salts eliminated *H. pylori* infection and cured the majority of duodenal ulcers. In 2005, the pair was awarded the Nobel Prize in Physiology or Medicine for their work, which has improved the lives of millions throughout the world. In 1989, proton pump inhibitors received approval in the United States and largely superseded H_2-receptor antagonists. Last, the relationship between nonsteroidal anti-inflammatory drug (NSAID) use and peptic ulcer disease has become well established, and discontinuation or moderation of these medications is advised in all patients with evidence of peptic disease. Currently, the vast majority of patients with peptic ulcer disease are managed medically with NSAID discontinuation and proton pump inhibition, and subsequently undergo testing for the presence of *H. pylori* in the stomach. Those patients that test positive for *H. pylori* are treated with one of a variety of effective oral regimens designed to eradicate the microorganism.

The effectiveness of medical management of peptic ulcer disease has changed the face of gastrointestinal surgery over the last few decades. Once a mainstay of surgical residency training, ulcer operations are now relatively rare. Operations for recalcitrant, recurrent, or obstructive ulcers are so infrequent that most residents may never perform one. Indeed, even perforated ulcer, once thought to be a clear-cut indication for immediate laparotomy, is no longer so straightforward. We've discovered that the omentum, which we so artfully secure to perforated ulcers, frequently ends up plugging the hole spontaneously with no surgical intervention at all. In patients with contained perforations without diffuse peritonitis or septic shock, nonoperative management with nasogastric decompression, intravenous fluids, antibiotics, proton pump inhibitors, NSAID discontinuation, and *H. pylori* eradication is safe and effective. In cases of diffuse peritonitis or uncontained perforation, early surgery remains the most effective treatment. Options include standard open repair via upper midline laparotomy as well as laparoscopic and hybrid endoscopic/laparoscopic approaches. Irrespective of the operative approach, pedicled omental flap repair in the manner of Cellan-Jones is advised. In the past, more definitive anti-ulcer procedures including vagotomy and antrectomy and highly selective vagotomy were included during index procedures for initial perforations, out of desire to minimize the risk of recurrence. Unfortunately, these procedures add time and physiologic insult to patients with marginal hemodynamic parameters. Given the safety and efficacy of postoperative medical management with *H. pylori* eradication, less aggressive surgery appears to be the most prudent course of action in most instances of perforated peptic ulcer. Acid-reducing surgical procedures may have a limited role in recurrent perforations in those patients who are acid hypersecretors but repeatedly test negative for *H. pylori*, or more unusual causes of ulcer disease such as Zollinger-Ellison syndrome.

ANNOTATED REFERENCES FOR PERFORATED PEPTIC ULCER

1. Ng EK, Lam YW, Sung JJ, et al. Recurrence of ulcer after simple closure of duodenal ulcer perforation: Randomized controlled trial. *Ann Surg.* 2000;231(2):153–158.

   In this randomized controlled trial of patients with perforated duodenal ulcers, the authors found an 81% incidence of H. pylori *infection. Patients randomized to* H. pylori *eradication had a significantly lower rate of ulcer recurrence at 1 year than those receiving PPI alone (4.8% vs. 38.1%), leading the authors to conclude that more aggressive acid-reducing procedures are unnecessary.*

2. Bertleff MJ, Lange JF. Perforated peptic ulcer disease: A review of history and treatment. *Dig Surg.* 2010;27(3):161–169.

   Good historical overview of management including detailed descriptions of the techniques described by Graham and Cellan-Jones.

3. Sanabria A, Villegas MI, Morales Uribe CH. Laparoscopic repair for perforated peptic ulcer disease. *Cochrane Database Syst Rev.* 2013;28(2).

   The authors conducted a systematic review including three randomized controlled trials of laparoscopic versus open repair of perforated peptic ulcer, and found no statistically significant difference in septic complications, pulmonary complications, or length of stay.

4. Bose AC, Kate V, Ananthakrishnan N, et al. *Helicobacter pylori* eradication prevents recurrence after simple closure of perforated duodenal ulcer. *J Gastroenterol Hepatol.* 2007;22(3):345–348.

   The authors performed a single-center study of H. pylori *eradication therapy after simple closure of perforated duodenal ulcer. Ulcer recurrence was 18.6% in the eradicated group versus 70% in the non-eradicated group, leading them to recommend eradication therapy for all* H. pylori–positive patients.*

5. Gutiérrez de la Peña C, Márquez R, Fakih F, et al. Simple closure or vagotomy and pyloroplasty for the treatment of a perforated duodenal ulcer: Comparison of results. *Dig Surg.* 2000;17(3):225–228.

   Prospective randomized study of simple closure of perforated duodenal ulcer versus truncal vagotomy with pyloroplasty. The authors found no statistically significant differences between groups, leading them to conclude that simple closure is the treatment of choice.

6. Crofts TJ, Park KG, Steele RJ, et al. A randomized trial of nonoperative treatment for perforated peptic ulcer. *N Engl J Med.* 1989;320(15):970–973.

   Prospective randomized study of conservative management (including nasogastric suction, intravenous fluids and antibiotics, and H_2 blockade) versus emergency surgery. More than 70% of patients were able to avoid surgery with no difference in morbidity and mortality. Of note, the conservative approach had a higher likelihood of failure in patients older than age 70.

7. Berne TV, Donovan AJ. Nonoperative treatment of perforated duodenal ulcer. *Arch Surg.* 1989;124(7):830–832.

   Early case series describing successful nonoperative management of patients with sealed duodenal perforations demonstrated on upper GI series. Mortality was 3% for patients treated nonoperatively versus 6.2% for a larger group of patients treated operatively during the same time period.

8. Kumar A, Muir MT, Cohn SM, et al. The etiology of pneumoperitoneum in the 21st century. *J Trauma.* 2012;73(3):542–548.

Retrospective study of 114 patients with pneumoperitoneum who were found to have visceral perforation at operation. Interestingly, patients with massive pneumoperitoneum were equally likely to have gastroduodenal, small bowel, or colonic perforation, in contrast to earlier studies showing higher rates of perforated ulcer disease.

ERADICATION OF *HELICOBACTER PYLORI* PREVENTS RECURRENCE OF ULCER AFTER SIMPLE CLOSURE OF DUODENAL ULCER PERFORATION: RANDOMIZED CONTROLLED TRIAL

Ng EKW, Lam YH, Sung JJY, Yung MY, To KF, Chan ACW, Lee DWH, Law BKB, Lau JYW, Ling TKW, Lau WY, and Chung SCS, *Ann Surg.* 2000;231(2):153–158

ABSTRACT

Objective   In this randomized trial, the authors sought to determine whether eradication of *Helicobacter pylori* could reduce the risk of ulcer recurrence after simple closure of perforated duodenal ulcer.

Background   Immediate acid-reduction surgery has been strongly advocated for perforated duodenal ulcers because of the high incidence of ulcer relapse after simple patch repair. Although *H. pylori* eradication is now the standard treatment of uncomplicated and bleeding peptic ulcers, its role in perforation remains controversial. Recently a high prevalence of *H. pylori* infection has been reported in patients with perforations of duodenal ulcer. It is unclear whether eradication of the bacterium confers prolonged ulcer remission after simple repair and hence obviates the need for an immediate definitive operation.

Methods   Of 129 patients with perforated duodenal ulcers, 104 (81%) were shown to be infected with *H. pylori*. Ninety-nine *H. pylori*–positive patients were randomized to receive either a course of quadruple anti-*Helicobacter* therapy or a 4-week course of omeprazole alone. Follow-up endoscopy was performed 8 weeks, 16 weeks (if the ulcer did not heal at 8 weeks), and 1 year after hospital discharge for surveillance of ulcer healing and determination of *H. pylori* status. The endpoints were initial ulcer healing and ulcer relapse rate after 1 year.

Results   Fifty-one patients were assigned to the anti-*Helicobacter* therapy and 48 to omeprazole alone. Nine patients did not undergo the first follow-up endoscopy. Of the 90 patients who did undergo follow-up endoscopy, 43 of the 44 patients in the anti-*Helicobacter* group and 8 of the 46 in the omeprazole alone group had *H. pylori* eradicated; initial ulcer healing rates were similar in the two groups (82% vs. 87%). After 1 year, ulcer relapse was significantly less common in patients treated with anti-*Helicobacter* therapy than in those who received omeprazole alone (4.8% vs. 38.1%).

Conclusions Eradication of *H. pylori* prevents ulcer recurrence in patients with *H. pylori*–associated perforated duodenal ulcers. Immediate acid-reduction surgery in the presence of generalized peritonitis is unnecessary.

Editor Notes

Assessment: This was a small, single-center, randomized study performed at the Chinese University of Hong Kong. Patients who underwent open or laparoscopic surgery for perforated peptic ulcer were randomized to either 1 week of oral antibiotics (bismuth subcitrate 120 mg, tetracycline 500 mg, and metronidazole 400 mg four times daily) plus 4 weeks of omeprazole (20 mg twice daily) or just 4 weeks of omeprazole alone without antibiotics. Only patients who tested positive for *Helicobacter pylori* were eligible for the study. Primary outcome was ulcer healing by endoscopy. As expected, the group treated with antibiotics had a significantly higher rate of *H. pylori* eradication (84% vs. 17%) but the initial rates of complete ulcer healing were similar between the two groups (82% vs. 88%). However, the long-term (1 year) ulcer recurrence rate was significantly lower in the group that was treated with antibiotics to eradicate *H. pylori* (5% vs. 38%).

Limitations: Although the sample size was small, the study was able to adeptly demonstrate that antibiotic treatment plus acid suppression was better than acid suppression alone in patients with perforated peptic ulcer disease (PUD) requiring surgery. The control group did not receive placebo medications instead of antibiotics, but this omission is probably not a major limitation. There were subject dropouts in this study and long-term follow-up was not always possible, but the intention-to-treat analysis appeared adequate.

Conclusions: This study demonstrated how to optimize medical treatment of PUD utilizing antibiotics for eradication of *H. pylori*.

CHAPTER 2

Paraesophageal Hernia

Review by Contributor: Fahim Habib

In 1853, Henry Bowditch was the first to describe paraesophageal hernias. In a post-mortem analysis of diaphragmatic hernias he noted that in some cases, "it [the esophagus] descended through the diaphragm as usual but turned back toward the left to enter the abnormal aperture caused by the hernia and to join the stomach in the chest." In 1926, Ake Åkerlund analyzed contrast studies of a series of cases and proposed the term *hiatus hernia* to describe the protrusion of abdominal viscera, most commonly the stomach and occasionally other organs, into the mediastinum through an enlarged esophageal hiatus of the diaphragm.

The relationship of the gastroesophageal junction to the herniated fundus of the stomach, and presence of other herniated abdominal viscera, classifies hiatal hernias into four types. In *type 1 (sliding hiatal hernia)* the gastroesophageal junction along with a variable portion of the proximal stomach migrates into the mediastinum, the stomach remains below the gastroesophageal junction, and their longitudinal relationship is maintained. In *type 2 (true paraesophageal hernia)* the gastroesophageal junction remains in its normal position, and the fundus of the stomach herniates alongside the esophagus through disruptions in the phrenoesophageal membrane. In *type 3 (combined paraesophageal hernia)* the gastroesophageal junction herniates into the chest, as does the stomach, with its fundus lying above the gastroesophageal junction. In *type 4 (paraesophageal hernias)* there is the herniation of abdominal viscera into the mediastinum including the colon, small bowel, omentum, and spleen. A *giant paraesophageal hernia* is one in which either at least 50% of the stomach is herniated into the chest or the hernia is ≥6 cm. Over 90% of hiatal hernias are type 1; paraesophageal hernias (type 2 to type 4) comprise about 5%. The remainder have a congenital (Morgagni hernia and Bochdalek hernia) or traumatic basis.

Etiology of paraesophageal hernias remains unknown, likely a combination of acquired and genetic factors. Familial clustering suggests a possible autosomal dominant mode. In addition, mutations of a collagen-encoding gene and altered collagen remodeling due to increased matrix metalloproteinase activity have been suggested. The central acquired factor is chronically increased intra-abdominal pressure that results in disruption of the phrenoesophageal membrane with enlargement of the hiatus and ultimate herniation.

True prevalence remains unknown because many remain asymptomatic or are associated with nonspecific gastrointestinal complaints. When symptomatic, the clinical features vary with the size of the hernia. Small hernias, due to loss of barrier function of the lower esophageal sphincter, present most commonly with reflux-related symptoms, including heartburn and regurgitation. Medium-sized hernias often present with anemia resulting from linear erosions (*Cameron ulcers*) in the gastric mucosa at the level of the diaphragmatic hiatus. Large paraesophageal hernias present with dyspnea, chest pain, or epigastric discomfort, which are more pronounced after eating. Early satiety occurs due to distension of the herniated portion with food. On occasion, patients present with an abdominal emergency due to acute gastric volvulus with *Borchardt's triad* (severe epigastric pain, retching without the ability to vomit, and the inability to pass a nasogastric tube).

Diagnostic modalities include: Plain x-ray of the chest (retrocardiac air–fluid level, vertically oriented loops of bowel, upward displacement of the transverse colon, nasogastric tube coiled above the diaphragm), contrast esophagrams (size and reducibility of the hiatal hernia, relationship of gastroesophageal junction to hiatus, presence of a foreshortened esophagus, or esophageal diverticula), esophagogastroduodenoscopy (presence of esophagitis, biopsies for Barrett esophagus, gastric viability, size and type of paraesophageal hernia), computed tomography (gastric volvulus, intestinal obstruction, presence of additional organs besides stomach, location of gastroesophageal junction, and type of paraesophageal hernia). pH testing to demonstrate abnormal proximal acid exposure (DeMeester score >14.7) identifies sliding-type hiatal hernias that would benefit from operative intervention but is not critical in patients with paraesophageal hernias. Esophageal manometry is critical in selecting the optimal anti-reflux procedure.

While there are proponents of watchful waiting in patients with asymptomatic or minimally symptomatic paraesophageal hernias (Stylopoulos, 2002), the current consensus is to electively operate on patients who are acceptable candidates for surgery. This approach is supported by the fact that outcomes are significantly worse when emergent repair is needed. Similarly, there is general agreement that these hernias are best approached using minimally invasive laparoscopic techniques, and the operative approach is progressively becoming more defined (DeMeester, 2013). Critical operative steps include complete excision of the hernia sac, adequate mediastinal mobilization of the esophagus often up to the level of the inferior pulmonary ligament to gain approximately 3 centimeters of intra-abdominal esophagus, the use of a Collis gastroplasty when an adequate intra-abdominal length cannot be achieved, primary repair of the crura with relaxing incisions if needed to achieve a tension-free closure, reinforcement of the primary crural closure with an absorbable mesh, and performance of a fundoplication to both prevent reflux as well as to place stomach between the mesh and the esophagus. While the laparoscopic approach results in less pain, shorter hospital stays, and faster recovery, it comes at the expense of increased recurrences when compared to open surgery. Hence, there continues to be the search for alternative operative strategies. One promising option is a hybrid approach that combines features of both the Nissen fundoplication and the Hill repair. Here, in addition to performing a traditional Nissen fundoplication over an appropriately sized bougie (56F in the majority, and 54F in smaller individuals), two additional sutures are placed between the anterior collar sling musculature, the posterior Collis sling musculature, and the preaortic fascia. These sutures tether the fundoplication to the preaortic fascia, and on long-term follow-up (mean follow-up 60 months) were associated with anatomic recurrence rates of 5% versus 45% for patients undergoing a Nissen fundoplication alone (Shemmeri and Aye, 2019).

The most controversial issue regarding the operative management of paraesophageal hernias relates to mesh reinforcement of the crural repair. Concerns for erosion of synthetic mesh led to an interest in the use of biologic prosthesis as a means to reduce recurrence. In a prospective randomized multicenter trial, Oeschlager et al. (2006) utilized porcine small intestinal submucosa to reinforce the crural repair in 108 patients. At 6 months, there was a significantly lower rate of recurrence among the patients in whom a biologic prosthesis was used (9% vs. 24% where no prosthesis was used, p = 0.04). However, in the long term these results did not hold out. Recurrence was identified in 54% of patients with biologic prosthesis reinforcement, and 59% in those with the primary repair alone (p = 0.7). The issue currently remains unresolved.

Despite best efforts, a sizeable proportion of hernias will recur. Radiologic recurrence must be distinguished from clinical recurrence. The majority of these patients can undergo a redo fundoplication with hiatal hernia repair, performed laparoscopically. A small number may require conversion to a Roux-en-Y esophagojejunostomy. In the patients with multiple recurrences and disabling symptoms, esophagectomy may be needed as a last resort.

ANNOTATED REFERENCES FOR PARAESOPHAGEAL HERNIA

1. Stylopoulos N, Rattner DW. The history of hiatal hernia surgery: From Bowditch to laparoscopy. *Ann Surg.* 2005;241(1):185–193.

   This comprehensive review traces the fascinating history of paraesophageal hernias from their original recognition as a disease entity by Bowditch in 1853 to the development of open operative strategies for their repair, and the subsequent transition to minimally invasive techniques.

2. Stylopoulos N, Gazelle GS, Rattner DW. Paraesophageal hernias: Operation or observation? *Ann Surg.* 2002;236(4):492–501.

   The authors developed a Markov Monte Carlo analytical model to track a hypothetical cohort of patients who were either asymptomatic or had minimal symptoms, comparing elective laparoscopic hernia repair versus watchful waiting. Based on this model, development of acute symptoms requiring emergency surgery was 1.1%, with an attendant mortality of 5.4%. The model predicted that watchful waiting was the optimal strategy in 83% of patients. However, the model only assessed the development of acute symptoms requiring emergency surgery and did not take into account the reduced quality of life due to symptoms of chronic gastroesophageal reflux disease, the risk for Barrett esophagus, the risks for esophageal adenocarcinoma, and the cost and side effects of long-term acid-suppression therapy, particularly proton pump inhibitors.

3. Tam V, Luketich JD, Winger DG et al. Non-elective paraesophageal hernia repair portends worse outcomes in comparable patients: A propensity-adjusted analysis. *J Gastrointest Surg.* 2017;21(1):137–145.

The authors retrospectively compared outcomes in patients undergoing elective versus nonelective repair of paraesophageal hernias. Patients undergoing nonelective repair were older, more often female, and had lower BMI and a higher age-adjusted Charlson comorbidity index score. Patients undergoing nonelective repair were two times more likely to suffer a major complication (OR 1.7, CI 1.07–2.61) and nearly three times more likely to die (OR 2.74, CI 0.9308.1).

4. Zehetner J, DeMeester SR, Ayazi S et al. Laparoscopic versus open repair of paraesophageal hernia: The second decade. *J Am Coll Surg.* 2011;212(5):813–820.

This retrospective study was undertaken to determine if the high recurrence rates of laparoscopic repair (45% vs. 15% after open repair) persisted as experience increased, and the tenets of laparoscopic paraesophageal hernia repair became more established. Recurrence as diagnosed by esophagram was identified in 9 of 73 (12.3%) of laparoscopic and 18 of 73 (24.7%) with open repair (p = 0.09).

5. DeMeester SR. Laparoscopic paraesophageal hernia repair: Critical steps and adjunct techniques to minimize recurrence. *Surg Laparosc Endosc Percutan Tech.* 2013;23(5):429–435.

This review describes the current surgical approach to the laparoscopic management of paraesophageal hernias, emphasizing the importance of complete excision of the hernia sac, mediastinal esophageal mobilization, crural repair, and fundoplication with use of a Collis gastroplasty, and relaxing incisions in select cases.

6. Qureshi AP, Aye RW, Buduhan G et al. The laparoscopic Nissen-Hill hybrid: Pilot study of a combined anti-reflux procedure. *Surg Endosc.* 2013;27(6):1945–1952.

The group from Swedish Medical Center, Seattle, previously demonstrated equivalency for laparoscopic Nissen fundoplication and laparoscopic Hill repair for gastroesophageal reflux disease. In this pilot study the authors described a hybrid procedure that incorporates components of both operations and appears to suggest lower recurrence rates.

7. Oelschlager BK, Pellegrini CA, Hunter J et al. Biologic prosthesis reduces recurrence after laparoscopic paraesophageal hernia repair. A multicenter, prospective, randomized trial. *Ann Surg.* 2006;244(4):481–490.

This prospective randomized multicenter study was undertaken to evaluate the value of a biologic prosthesis, porcine small intestinal submucosa, as a reinforcement for crural repair. It was hypothesized that the biologic prosthesis would serve as a scaffold, providing additional strength initially on the basis of its inherent structure, and subsequently continuing to provide additional strength as there was in growth of native tissue into the extracellular matrix. The two groups were comparable in all respects; at 6 months a recurrent hernia (defined as a greater than 2-cm hernia on esophagram) occurred in 9% of patients in whom a biologic prosthesis was used, versus 24% in those where it was not (p = 0.04).

8. Luketich JD, Nason KS, Christie NA et al. Outcomes after a decade of laparoscopic giant paraesophageal hernia repair. *J Thorac Cardiovasc Surg.* 2010;139:395–404.

The authors report their experience with the laparoscopic repair of giant paraesophageal hernias performed non-emergently. Over time, the need for a Collis gastroplasty decreased from 86% to 53%, and use of mesh reinforcement for the crura also dropped from 17% to 12%. The 30-day mortality was 1.7%. Good to excellent results on GERD Health Related Quality of Life (HRQL) were noted in 90%. Radiographic recurrence was evident in 15.7%. Reoperation was required in 3.2%. These results suggest that favorable long-term outcomes are possible with the laparoscopic repair of giant paraesophageal hernias.

9. Kao AM, Otero J, Schlosser KA et al. One more time: Redo paraesophageal hernia repair results in safe, durable outcomes compared with primary repairs. *Am Surg.* 2018;84(7):1138–1145.

   In a retrospective review of a prospectively maintained institutional hernia, specific database outcomes were compared between patients undergoing primary versus redo paraesophageal hernia repair. While operative time was longer and conversion to open more frequent, there was no difference in postoperative complications, hernia recurrence, or mortality between the groups. This suggests that while redo minimally invasive para-esophageal hernia repair is technically more challenging, it is feasible and can be safely performed.

10. Shemmeri E, Aye RW. The role of laparoscopic Nissen, Hill, and Nissen-Hill hybrid repairs for uncomplicated gastroesophageal reflux disease. *Minerva Chir.* 2019;74(4):320–325.

    Based on an assessment of the causes of failure of the laparoscopic Nissen fundoplica-tion and laparoscopic Hill repairs identified during a multicenter randomized control trial the authors combined the essential components of the two procedures to create the Nissen-Hill hybrid repair. Here, two Hill sutures are placed through the anterior, then the posterior collar sling musculature and then through the preaortic fascia and left untied. A standard Nissen fundoplication is then performed over a bougie (56–58 Fr), the Hill sutures are then tied with the bougie still in place. In the comparative study with a mean follow-up of 60 months, recurrence rate was significantly lower in the hybrid group that the Nissen group (5% vs. 45%), suggesting that the Hill sutures not only pexy the fundoplication to the strong preaortic fascia keeping it in the abdomen but also take axial stresses off the Nissen fundoplication preserving its integrity.

Landmark Article of the 21st Century

BIOLOGIC PROSTHESIS TO PREVENT RECURRENCE AFTER LAPAROSCOPIC PARAESOPHAGEAL HERNIA REPAIR: LONG-TERM FOLLOW-UP FROM A MULTICENTER, PROSPECTIVE, RANDOMIZED TRIAL

Oelschlager BK, Pellegrini CA, Hunter JG, Brunt ML, Soper NJ, Sheppard BC, Polissar NL, Neradilek MB, Mitsumori LM, Rohrmann CA, and Swanstrom LL, *J Am Coll Surg.* 2011;213(4):461–468

ABSTRACT

Background In 2006, we reported results of a randomized trial of laparoscopic paraesophageal hernia repair (LPEHR), comparing primary repair (PR) of the diaphragm with primary repair buttressed with a biologic prosthesis (small intestinal submucosa [SIS]). The primary endpoint, radiologic hiatal hernia (HH) recurrence, was higher with PR (24%) than with SIS-buttressed repair (9%) after 6 months. The second phase of this trial was designed to determine the long-term durability of biologic mesh-buttressed repair.

Methods   We systematically searched for the 108 patients in phase I of this study to assess current clinical symptoms, quality of life (QOL), and determine ongoing durability of the repair by obtaining a follow-up upper gastrointestinal (UGI) series read by two radiologists blinded to treatment received. HH recurrence was defined as the greatest measured vertical height of stomach being at least 2 cm above the diaphragm.

Results   At median follow-up of 58 months (range 42–78 months), 10 patients had died, 26 patients were not found, 72 completed clinical follow-up (PR, n = 39; SIS, n = 33), and 60 repeated a UGI (PR, n = 34; SIS, n = 26). There were 20 patients (59%) with recurrent HH in the PR group and 14 patients (54%) with recurrent HH in the SIS group (p = 0.7). There was no statistically significant difference in relevant symptoms or QOL between patients undergoing PR and SIS-buttressed repair. There were no strictures, erosions, dysphagia, or other complications related to the use of SIS mesh.

Conclusions   LPEHR results in long and durable relief of symptoms and improvement in QOL with PR or SIS. There does not appear to be a higher rate of complications or side effects with biologic mesh, but its benefit in reducing HH recurrence diminishes at long-term follow-up (more than 5 years postoperatively) or earlier.

Editor Notes

Assessment: This study was a long-term follow-up of a multicenter, prospective randomized trial of laparoscopic paraesophageal hernia repair (LPEHR) compared to primary diaphragm repair. The initial study included only a 6-month follow-up. Seventy-two of 108 patients were evaluated with a median follow-up time of 58 months. Sixty patients underwent a repeat upper gastrointestinal radiographic series. There was a 59% recurrence in the primary repair group compared to 54% in the laparoscopic group. (Initially the report at 6-month follow-up showed that laparoscopic repair was better, with a 9% recurrence compared to 24% primary repair group).

Limitations: The lack of follow-up in 36 of the 108 patients in the initial study is concerning. Ten of these patients died, and 26 could not be found. Many of the study coauthors had financial agreements with Cook medical, the manufacturer of the biological mesh used in this study.

Conclusions: The study showed that laparoscopic repair with biological mesh was no different than repair without mesh when evaluated long term. This study demonstrates the importance of long-term follow-up.

CHAPTER 3

Esophageal Perforation

Review by Contributor: John K. Bini

Esophageal perforation has been and remains a significant diagnostic and clinical management dilemma. This challenging problem is significant and pertinent when one takes into account the potential extensive morbidity and reported mortality rates as high as 25%. Compounding the diagnostic and clinical management challenge is the number of potential causes and presenting environment in which these injuries are discovered. The causes of these perforations range from iatrogenic to trauma to Boerhaave syndrome as well as complications of preexisting esophageal pathology. Historically, the factor most often associated with a high mortality is a delay in diagnosis. Unless temporally related to esophageal instrumentation, perforation of the thoracic esophagus may be easily confused with myocardial infarction, aortic dissection, pancreatitis, or other chest or abdominal emergencies.

Esophageal injuries, although morbid, are in fact not that common. A recent multi-center retrospective study only found 199 esophageal perforations from 10 institutions in the United States and Canada over a 10-year period (Ali et al., 2017). To date, there have been no trials comparing treatment strategies head to head in a controlled manner. The body of literature relied upon is therefore limited to case series and some meta-analysis, and treatment protocols are often not specifically defined or controlled and there is a paucity of long-term follow-up data.

Historically, key decisions regarding the management of esophageal perforation relied upon several anatomic, physiologic, and temporal findings. Regardless of the diagnostic modality chosen, a high index of suspicion was usually required. Computed tomography was the most commonly employed diagnostic imaging method (Ali et al., 2017). Contrast esophagram and endoscopy were the other main diagnostic modalities (Ali et al., 2017).

Once these injuries were identified, management has historically been driven by the time from presumed injury until diagnosis. The time from injury was and still is used to decide whether operative intervention is warranted versus nonoperative techniques (Vogel et al., 2005). Classically, injuries that were identified early, usually within the first 24–48 hours, underwent operative and definitive intervention. Injuries diagnosed more than 24–48 hours after the index event often underwent nonoperative management or non-reconstructive operative management, and typically relied on the concept of wide drainage plus or minus diversion (Vogel et al., 2005).

With the advent of new advanced endoscopic techniques and the ready availability of stents, both covered and uncovered, recent attention has turned to the use of stenting with or without drainage versus definitive operative repair of benign esophageal perforations. Freeman and colleagues propensity matched 60 patients undergoing stent repair or surgical repair and found no differences in mortality but the stent group had shorter hospital stays, shorter times until taking an oral diet, and markedly reduced costs (Freeman et al., 2007, 2015). Freeman also conducted a study looking at only iatrogenic perforations and reported a 94% leak occlusion rate with stent graft placement. Biancari conducted a systematic review and meta-analysis of 75 studies with 2971 patients and found that stent grafting was associated with lower mortality when compared to primary repair, T-tube repair, or esophagectomy (Biancari et al., 2013).

Madhan and associates reported an increase in nonsurgical management over a 20-year period, with a concurrent decline in complication rates suggesting a similar decrease in morbidity associated with nonoperative management (Kuppusamy et al., 2011). As a follow-up to their meta-analysis, Biancari's group conducted a multicenter study that looked at 194 patients and found a significantly higher survival with a salvaged esophagus in patients undergoing stent grafting (Biancari et al., 2014). Likewise, Ali and colleagues conducted a multicenter study looking at 199 patients with esophageal perforations but only 29 patients were treated with stents (Ali et al., 2017).

Ben-David's group in Florida has an algorithm in place for the management of esophageal perforations. They conducted a retrospective review of 76 patients with acute esophageal perforation and confirmed leak occlusion in 68 patients within 48 hours of esophageal stent placement. Although they do not have a comparison to other management options such as definitive reconstruction, they do show that with a strict algorithm, stenting is feasible with minimal mortality, and perhaps most interestingly, none of the patients in this study required conversion to operative management (Ben-David et al., 2014).

In 2013, Gubler published a landmark paper presenting the largest single series of patients with benign esophageal perforations that were treated with stents where there is long-term follow-up data. They analyzed data on 85 patients collected over 12 years for sustained success, complications, time to stenting, lesion size, number of stents used, and need for percutaneous drainage. The primary endpoint was treatment success per stent and per patient. Stents were left in place for an average of 15 days, which made re-stenting necessary in some cases. The success rate of stent treatment, with an average of 1.3 stents per patient, was 79%. Immediate stent insertion upon endoscopic diagnosis of the perforation led to a 100% success score; delayed stent placement was less successful (71%). Use of multiple stents sequentially placed was necessary in 23% of the cases. Percutaneous drainage was necessary in 25% of all cases. In this series, 30-day mortality was 5.8%; however, there were no reported stent-related deaths. What is unique about this study is that the authors had a fairly strict protocol for early stent removal and/or exchange to minimize the morbidity associated with prolonged stent placement. They also look at different types of injuries/perforations and compare success rates for endoscopic management (Gubler and Bauerfeind, 2013).

There is no standardized treatment for esophageal perforations caused by benign processes and thus the debate rages on as to whether surgical or nonsurgical management is preferable. The pendulum of treatment has swung from early aggressive operative management to early aggressive conservative management. Neither of these is optimal, and both have significant morbidity and mortality. Endoscopic management may provide a nice bridge between early aggressive operative and early aggressive nonoperative management. Stent placement in the setting of early conservative management may reduce the need for surgery and improve outcomes in conservatively managed appropriately selected patients.

ANNOTATED REFERENCES FOR ESOPHAGEAL PERFORATION

1. Freeman RK, Herrera A, Ascioti AJ, Dake M, Mahidhara RS. A propensity-matched comparison of cost and outcomes after esophageal stent placement or primary surgical repair for iatrogenic esophageal perforation. *Thorac Cardiovasc Surg*. 2015;149(6):1550–1555.

   Study of 60 patients, stent versus surgery. Reduced morbidity, length of stay, time to oral intake, and cost in stent group. Operative mortality did not differ significantly.

2. Port J, Kent MS, Korst RJ, Bacchetta M, Altorki NK. Thoracic esophageal perforations: A decade of experience. *Ann Thorac Surg*. 2003;75:1071–1074.

   A retrospective chart review of 26 patients looked at early versus late management. All patients selected for conservative management successfully healed their perforation. Concluded that primary repair can be carried out in most cases of thoracic esophageal perforation regardless of time to presentation, with a low mortality rate.

3. Biancari F, D'Andrea V, Paone R et al. Current treatment and outcome of esophageal perforations in adults: Systematic review and meta-analysis of 75 studies. *World J Surg*. 2013;37:1051–1059.

   The authors conducted a systematic review and meta-analysis. Primary repair was associated with a pooled mortality of 9.5%, and stent grafting 7.3%. Stent grafting may be associated with somewhat lower mortality rates.

4. Vogel SB, Rout WR, Martin TD, Abbitt PL. Esophageal perforation in adults: Aggressive, conservative treatment lowers morbidity and mortality. *Ann Surg*. 2005;241:1016–1023.

   Single-center retrospective review of 47 patients (10 cervical, 37 thoracic) with esophageal perforations looked at early and late (>24 hr) presentation. They concluded that, contradictory to widely held beliefs, early nonoperative management lowers mortality.

5. Ben-David K, Behrns K, Hochwald S et al. Esophageal perforation management using a multidisciplinary minimally invasive treatment algorithm. *J Am Coll Surg*. 2014;218:768–775.

   Retrospective review of 76 patients with acute esophageal perforation. All patients were treated within 24 hours of initial presentation with a removable covered esophageal stent. Authors do have a standardized protocol for management of suspected esophageal perforations. Interestingly none of the patients in this study required conversion to operative management. It does show that with a strict algorithm stenting is feasible with minimal mortality.

6. Swinnen J, Eisendrath P, Rigaux J et al. Self-expandable metal stents for the treatment of benign upper GI leaks and perforations. *Gastrointest Endosc*. 2011;73:890–899.

A total of 153 SEMSs were placed in 88 patients; all placements were successful. Resolution of leaks and perforations was achieved in 59 patients (67%) with standard endoscopic treatment and in 64 patients (77.3%) after prolonged, repeated endoscopic treatment. Excellent report of experience, but 46 (52%) patients were gastric perforations associated with bariatric surgery.

7. Hasimoto C, Cataneo D, Eldib R et al. Efficacy of surgical versus conservative treatment in esophageal perforation. A systematic review of case series studies. *Acta Cirurgica Brasileira*. 2013;28(4).

Systematic review of literature revealed 33 case series including 1417 patients. Sixty-five percent of patients underwent initial surgical therapy while 34% underwent initial conservative management. The surgical group had a significantly lower mortality, 16.3% versus 21.3% (p < 0.05). The authors concluded that surgical management was more effective and safer than conservative therapy. The authors did not delineate cases where stents were used or even if they were used in any of the conservative groups.

8. Freeman RK, Van Woerkom JM, Ascioti AJ. Esophageal stent placement for the treatment of iatrogenic intrathoracic esophageal perforation. *Ann Thorac Surg*. 2007;83:2003–2008.

Patients found to have an iatrogenic intrathoracic esophageal perforation were offered endoluminal esophageal stent placement instead of operative repair of the esophagus as initial therapy. Patients were followed until their stents were removed. Leak occlusion occurred in 16 patients (94%). Fourteen patients (82%) were able to initiate oral nutrition within 72 hours of stent placement. The authors concluded that esophageal stent placement is an effective method for the treatment of acute, iatrogenic perforations of the intrathoracic esophagus.

9. Kuppusamy MK, Hubka M, Felisky CD et al. Evolving management strategies in esophageal perforation: Surgeons using nonoperative techniques to improve outcomes. *J Am Coll Surg*. 2011;213:164–172.

Eighty-one consecutive patients presented with acute esophageal perforation and were entered into a database prospectively over a 20-year period. Authors looked at timing and type of treatment, length of stay, complications, and mortality. Forty-eight patients (59%) were managed operatively, 33 (41%) nonoperatively, and 10 patients with hybrid approaches involving a combination of surgical and interventional techniques. There was an increase in nonoperative management over the study period. Shows current trend toward more aggressive nonoperative management with good outcomes in a tertiary referral center, but only 11 patients in entire series received endoluminal stents.

10. Brinster CJ, Singhal S, Lee L et al. Evolving options in the management of esophageal perforation. *Ann Thorac Surg*. 2004;77:1475–1483.

Review of literature where they looked at 726 patients. The authors concluded that surgical primary repair, with or without reinforcement, is the most successful treatment option in the management of esophageal perforation and reduces mortality by 50%–70% compared with other interventional therapies, although they did not specifically address endoscopic stent placement.

11. Dai Y, Chopra SS, Kneif S, Hünerbein M. Management of esophageal anastomotic leaks, perforations, and fistulae with self-expanding plastic stents. *J Thorac Cardiovasc Surg*. 2011;141:1213–1217.

This is a single-center retrospective review of patients treated with self-expanding stents for esophageal perforations or postoperative esophageal leaks. They reported successful treatment of all 41 patients with no procedure-related complications. They reported the mean time to healing with anastomotic leaks was 30 days, and 15 days for esophageal perforations. The average time to feeding was 3.9 days after stenting. They had an in-hospital mortality rate of 10% in their series.

12. Ali JT, Rice RD, David EA et al. Perforated esophageal intervention focus (PERF) study: A multi-center examination of contemporary treatment. *Diseases of the Esophagus.* 2017;30:1–8.

    A five-year (2009–2013) multicenter retrospective review of management and outcomes for patients with thoracic or abdominal esophageal perforation. The authors identified 199 patients from 10 centers. Observation was selected as initial management in 65 (32.7%), with only two failures. Direct operative intervention was initial management in 65 patients (32.7%), while 29 (14.6%) underwent esophageal stent coverage. The patients who were stented were older and more likely to have an iatrogenic mechanism. Secondary intervention requirement for patients with perforation was 33.7% overall. This is a large retrospective descriptive study that gives broad insight to current practice patterns.

13. Biancari F, Saarnio J, Mennander A et al. Outcome of patients with esophageal perforations: A multicenter study. *World J Surg.* 2014;38(4):902–909.

    Retrospective study that collected data on 194 patients from 9 centers who underwent conservative (43 patients), endoclip (4 patients), stent grafting (63 patients), or surgical treatment (84 patients) for esophageal perforation. Propensity-matched analysis showed that stent grafting achieved similar early mortality but significantly higher survival with salvaged esophagus than with surgical treatment.

14. Gubler C, Bauerfeind P. Self-expandable stents for benign esophageal leakages and perforations: Long-term single-center experience. *Scand J Gastroenterol.* 2013;49(1):23–29.

    This is the largest single series of patients with benign esophageal perforations that were treated with stents where there are long-term follow-up data. Eighty-five patients were analyzed for sustained success, complications, time to stenting, lesion size, number of stents used, and need for percutaneous drainage. The primary endpoint was treatment success per stent and per patient. Stents were left in place for an average of 15 days, which made re-stenting necessary in some cases. Immediate stent insertion upon endoscopic diagnosis of the perforation led to a 100% success score; delayed stent placement was less successful (71%). Success was highest (94%, n = 30 of 32, no complications or mortality) in iatrogenic lesions that were immediately diagnosed and treated. Use of multiple stents sequentially placed was necessary in 23% of the cases. In this series, 30-day mortality was 5.8%. There were no reported stent-related deaths. The authors advocated short-term stenting with removal and re-evaluation of the lesion, as this may minimize the long-term concerns of ingrowth and inability to remove the stents. The authors also go into great detail about the various types of stents and benefits of each based on the data from this study.

SELF-EXPANDABLE STENTS FOR BENIGN ESOPHAGEAL LEAKAGES AND PERFORATIONS: LONG-TERM SINGLE-CENTER EXPERIENCE

Gubler C and Bauerfeind P, *Scand J Gastroenterol.* 2014;49(1):23–29

ABSTRACT

Objective To date, there is no standardized treatment for esophageal perforations and leakages caused by underlying benign diseases, and it is still debated whether a conservative, endoscopic treatment or a surgical approach is preferable. However, some case series have successfully demonstrated the feasibility of temporary placement of self-expanding stents.

Design   All patients with benign leakages of the esophagus or gastroesophageal junction or fistulas at gastroesophageal anastomosis were collected during the past 12 years and analyzed retrospectively. The patients treated with endoscopic stenting were analyzed for sustained success, complications, time to stenting, lesion size, number of stents used, and need for percutaneous drainage.

Results   Eighty-five of 88 patients were included in this analysis. Three patients were conservatively managed only. The success rate of stent treatment with an average of 1.3 stents was 79%. Success was highest (94%, n = 30 of 32, no complications or mortality) in iatrogenic lesions that were immediately diagnosed and treated. Spontaneous lesions, including lesions due to Boerhaave syndrome, were healed in 73% and anastomotic leakages were closed in 71%. Fistula had a lower success rate of 43%. Use of multiple stents sequentially placed was necessary in 23% of the cases. Percutaneous drainage was necessary in 25% of all cases.

Conclusion   Temporary stent placement for benign leakages of the esophagus is safe and seems to improve treatment success. Adjacent fluid collections should be drained percutaneously.

Editor Notes

Assessment: This is a case series of 85 patients who had a self-expandable stent placed for benign esophageal leaks from a single institution in Zurich over a 12-year period. The etiologies of the perforations were iatrogenic, post-anastomotic insufficiency, Boerhaave syndrome, and fistulas. The stents were placed by four endoscopists and the stent types included a variety of fully or partially covered stents. The highest success rate (94%, n = 30/32) was in the iatrogenic lesions, and there were no complications or deaths in this group. The least successful group was the fistula group, with only the esophago-tracheal fistulas closing with the use of the stents. Fistulas to the pericardium, aorta, and pleura were not successfully closed with stenting alone. Perforations were anatomically located in the upper (30%), middle (23%), and lower third (48%), but the fistulas occurred in all areas of the esophagus; the spontaneous and iatrogenic perforations were in the middle and distal third. There were 31 patients with post-surgical leaks after esophagectomy and bariatric surgery; the success rate of stenting for these leaks was 74%.

Limitations: Esophageal perforations are not common, but there is another large case series that supports the findings of this study. Stenting is contrary to historical surgical literature, which favors repair and resection. The patients in this series were discussed with surgeons and managed collaboratively with endoscopy and stenting when possible. Thus the recognition of selection bias is important. The consequences of treating these perforations (costs involved or discomfort of the stents) were not discussed. The paper also does not address problems in the 22% of the patients who were unsuccessfully treated with stents.

Conclusions: Temporary stent placement for leakages of the esophagus from benign lesions seems to improve treatment success. The highest success rate is in patients with perforations from iatrogenic causes particularly if they are treated as soon as diagnosed.

CHAPTER 4

Small Bowel Obstruction

Review by Contributors: Marc de Moya and Andrew Kamien

Small bowel obstruction is a common admitting surgical diagnosis and results in over 300,000 operations in the United States per year. Although not all patients admitted with this diagnosis require operative intervention, both the operative and non-operative management of patients incur a significant cost to the health care industry (Krielen et al., 2016). Its history dates to the third and fourth centuries, and although there is now a variety of laboratory studies, imaging technologies, and decades of literature, it remains a challenge to manage and to prevent recurrence.

The most common cause of small bowel obstruction (SBO) in the developed countries is adhesive in nature, with the second most common cause being hernias. The adhesions are usually due to previous operation, although other inflammatory conditions may account for the development of adhesions as well. In addition, other pathologic states (ileus, vascular occlusion, pseudo-obstruction, and large bowel obstruction) may mimic the same nonspecific symptoms of pain, nausea, vomiting, distension, and lack of distal output of gas and stool. Symptomatology may be predicted by the location of the obstruction—proximal versus distal—as well as the degree of obstruction. If only a portion of the intestinal lumen is occluded, this is classified as a partial SBO, whereas if the entire lumen is occluded, this is classified as a complete SBO; however, this dichotomy of classification has become less important. A strangulated SBO is a more pathologic process in which some of the bowel is compromised due to increased intraluminal pressure to the point that microvascular circulation has been compromised, resulting in bowel ischemia.

A thorough history and physical is of utmost importance in a patient presenting with findings consistent with obstruction, paying close attention to history of intra-abdominal surgery. In the absence of prior operation, the physician needs to have a high index of suspicion that symptoms are due to a hernia or, less commonly, a bowel-obstructing tumor.

Physical exam should focus on assessment for hernias, and the presence of abdominal distension, tympany, pain out of proportion to exam, and peritonitis. Auscultation for bowel sounds is an art that was heralded in an era without plain films, let alone CT scans, and has been demonstrated to be poorly predictive. In the modern era, physicians have difficulty distinguishing normal bowel sounds from that of a patient with obstruction (Felder et al., 2014). Lack of palpable pulses in the lower extremities serves as an indicator for peripheral vascular disease and whether mesenteric pathology is the etiology.

In the patient who is nontoxic, without a rigid abdomen that prompts urgent exploration, plain films should be obtained next (upright and supine). Their accuracy can be as high as 93% and can be done quickly, and are portable, with limited radiation to the patient. Findings of small bowel diameter >3 cm with decompressed distal loops, lack of air in the colon, and air–fluid levels are consistent with small bowel obstruction. CT scans may be considered if bowel ischemia is a concern. CT scan has sensitivity and specificity that are both over 90% and can be 100% predictive for bowel ischemia. Additional information can be ascertained including pneumatosis of the bowel, portal venous air, closed loop obstruction, presence of masses or tumors, and the presence of hernia in an obese, otherwise non-examinable abdomen. The American Association for the Surgery of Trauma (AAST) CT-based grading system has been validated regarding severity of disease and can help predict course and outcomes for patients (Hernandez et al., 2018). Lab studies can serve as adjuncts to guide resuscitation and have been described to indicate the severity of pathology; however, analysis of white blood cell count and lactate have recently been demonstrated to not correlate with degree of obstruction. Normal lactate values should be interpreted with caution, as dead or dying bowel may not manifest a lactic acidosis if the mesenteric venous outflow is blocked, such as in a closed loop obstruction.

Initial treatment for these patients (without an absolute need for operative exploration) should be a trial of nonoperative management with nasogastric decompression, resuscitation with intravenous fluids, and electrolyte optimization. The previous dictum of "the sun shall not rise or set on a bowel obstruction" has been challenged in more recent decades, as only approximately one-third of these patients require an operation. Therefore, in the absence of overt signs requiring an urgent laparotomy, most bowel obstructions will be observed, which suggests that the classification of partial versus complete is no longer necessary. A trial of initial decompression followed by Gastrografin instillation can be predictive of nonoperative success. Gastrografin is a high-osmolar contrast agent that is felt to be potentially diagnostic and therapeutic, as the high osmolar content is believed to draw edema from the intestine intraluminally, relieving bowel congestion, and as it will show on plain films, its presence in the distal colon is indicative of a resolving obstruction. The positive predictive value of successful Gastrografin trial is over 90% in some series, and those treated with a Gastrografin trial are less likely to require operation and have shorter hospital stays (Zielinski et al., 2017).

Miller et al. (2000) investigated a group of 410 patients over a 10-year period and accounted for nearly 700 admissions. They separated patients into cohorts of those having had previous colorectal surgery, gynecological surgery, herniorrhaphy, and appendectomy. Adhesive disease was classified as being either matted or single band adhesive disease. Patients admitted for bowel obstruction more commonly had larger, more extensive operations (colorectal procedures), compared to smaller, more focused ones (hernia, appendectomy). They identified patients as having either matted, extensive adhesions or a single band responsible for obstruction. Overall, it was nearly evenly split regarding etiology; however, patients with prior colorectal surgery were more likely to have matted adhesions. Patients with dense or matted adhesions were statistically significantly more likely to require multiple readmissions but had no greater risk of additional surgery or bowel death. Of those patients operated on, the bowel resection rate was approximately 20%. Adhesiolysis with resection was associated with a lower rate of SBO, which may infer that diseased but viable bowel may continue to cause problems if not lysed; however, this was not statistically significant. Most patients do not require operative management, and the readmission rate is similar regardless of treatment strategy (approximately one-third of patients treated operatively or nonoperatively); however, the interval to readmission is shorter for the nonoperative group.

As the disease is persistent and seemingly unavoidable, there may be hope for a decreased burden of disease in an increasingly minimally invasive era. Operative technique and handling of the bowel has been attributed to the formation of adhesions. This thought process can be inferred from the results from Miller: colorectal procedures being more causative for obstruction than appendectomy, where there is a more focused exploration of the abdomen. Laparoscopic surgery has been demonstrated to be four times less likely to cause adhesive bowel obstruction requiring hospital admission (Angenete et al., 2012). Although minimally invasive procedures have higher index costs, the scales tend to balance at time of discharge. If minimally invasive surgery induces less tissue trauma and therefore causes fewer adhesions, this should be considered when planning operative needs, especially knowing the long-term consequences and recurrence of adhesive small bowel disease. If adhesive disease is inevitable, one should attempt to obviate or at least diminish that risk.

ANNOTATED REFERENCES FOR SMALL BOWEL OBSTRUCTION

1. Diaz JJ, Bokhari F, Mowery NT et al. Guidelines for the management of small bowel obstruction. *J Trauma*. 2008;64:1651–1664.

   General guidelines for decision making regarding SBO.

2. Krielen P, van den Beukel BA, Stommel MWJ, van Goor H, Strik C, Ten Broek RPG. In-hospital costs of an admission for adhesive small bowel obstruction. *World J Emerg Surg*. 2016;11:49.

   This Dutch study investigated the institution costs of patients managed both operatively and nonoperatively between 2013–2015. Those patients managed nonoperatively were cared for at a fraction of the cost (€2,277 vs. €16,305). Cost analysis was attributed to the increased length of stay (16 ± 11 days vs. 4 ± 2 days), and micro-costing analysis demonstrated statistically significant differences in costs of medication, feeding, blood products, and ICU utilization as well as radiology, laboratory, and microbiology resources.

3. Felder S, Margel D, Murrell Z, Fleshner P. Usefulness of bowel sound auscultation: A prospective evaluation. *J Surg Educ*. 2014;71(5):768–773.

   The authors utilized electronic stethoscopes to record bowel sounds of healthy volunteers, patients with small bowel obstruction, and patients with postoperative ileus, and replayed these recordings to a group of both internists and surgeons. The sensitivity and positive predictive values were both low for all three categories (range 22%–32% and 23%–44%, respectively). Surgeons did not perform better than the internists, and attending physicians did not perform better than medical students.

4. Hernandez MC, Haddad NN, Cullinane DC et al.; EAST SBO Workgroup. The American Association for the Surgery of Trauma Severity Grade is valid and generalizable in adhesive small bowel obstruction. *J Trauma Acute Care Surg.* 2018;84:372–378.

Another multicenter study in which patients (n = 635) admitted with adhesive small bowel obstruction were classified according to the imaging-based AAST gradings first published in 2016. Analysis of outcomes was then followed according to grade and correlated with other clinical findings. Low-grade obstructions were, as one could predict, less sick overall and more likely to be treated nonoperatively. Higher-grade obstructions were more likely to have the presence of peritonitis and meet sepsis criteria, have higher complications, and require operations. The presence of a small bowel feces sign and a transition point were more predictive in the low-grade patients. The presence of mesenteric edema or free fluid was not statistically significant among the various gradings.

5. Kulvatunyou N, Pandit V, Moutamn S et al. A multi-institution prospective observational study of small bowel obstruction: Clinical and computerized tomography predictors of which patients may require early surgery. *J Trauma Acute Care Surg.* 2015:79(3):393–398.

This multi-institutional clinical study tried to identify clinical and CT findings to predict who will need early surgery. This study focused on adhesive causes of SBO and excluded patients with other etiologies hernias, small bowel tumor, intussusception, or inflammatory bowel disease such as Crohn's disease. Two thousand patients were in the study and 50% underwent surgery. The median duration of nonoperative management before surgery was 1.5 days. Regression model identified lack of flatus and two CT findings of free fluid and high-grade obstruction to be significant predictors of SBO.

6. Zielinski MD, Haddad NN, Cullinane DC et al. Multi-institutional, prospective, observational study comparing the Gastrografin challenge versus standard treatment in adhesive small bowel obstruction. *J Trauma Acute Care Surg.* 2017;83:47–54.

This multi-institutional clinical study followed patients admitted with adhesion-related bowel obstruction; approximately half underwent a standardized Gastrograffin (GG) challenge, while the other half underwent standard treatment. This was observationally based, and treatment was at the discretion of the surgeon. Patients passed the GG challenge if they had a bowel movement after instillation of GG or if it was visualized in the colon on plain films at 8 hours after administration. Passing of a GG challenge was predictive of success of nonoperative management; hospital length of stay was shorter in the GG group, and the rate of operative need was half of that in the non-GG group. This study helps affirm the hypothesis that GG administration is both diagnostic and therapeutic in the management of bowel obstruction.

7. Morcos SK. Effects of radiographic contrast media on the lung. *Br J Radiol.* 2003;76:290–295.

This review article details the multitude of effects of contrast media on the lung; however, for the purposes of our review, highlights the risk of high osmolar contrast in the setting of aspiration, which can result in bronchial irritation, pulmonary edema, and even death. Low osmotic agents do not have that same effect and are considered safe in both clinical scenarios and on histologic analysis in animal models.

8. Kumar S, Wong PF, Leaper DJ. Intra-peritoneal prophylactic agents for preventing adhesions and adhesive intestinal obstruction after non-gynecological abdominal surgery. *Cochrane Database Syst Rev.* 2009 Jan 21;(1).

A Cochrane Review in 2009 examined Medline and Embase databases for articles investigating the use of intra-abdominal agents for adhesion prophylaxis. A total of seven randomized control trials were included comparing an intra-abdominal agent (hyaluronic acid/carboxymethyl cellulose membrane [Seprafilm] was used in six of the trials, 0.5% ferric hyaluronate gel used in the seventh) versus control (no intervention or distilled water in the ferric hyaluronate gel trial). Pooling that data, there was a statistically significant reduction in the presence of adhesions [OR 0.15 (95% CI: 0.05,0.43); p = 0.0005] and statistically significant reduction in the severity of adhesions (based upon grading scales as determined by the authors). There was, however, no statistically significant difference in long-term (follow-up of approximately 3.5 years) incidence of intestinal obstruction [OR 0.84 (95% CI: 0.34, 2.08)] or need for surgical intervention [OR 0.84 (95% CI: 0.24, 2.7)]. In addition, there was a trend toward but no statistically significant difference in the rate of anastomotic leaks [OR 1.61 (95% CI: 0.69, 3.71); p = 0.27].

9. Angenete E, Jacobsen A, Gellerstedt M, Haglind E. Effect of laparoscopy on the risk of small-bowel obstruction: A population-based register study. *Arch Surg.* 2012;147(4):359–365.

This Swedish study followed patients that underwent a variety of operations (cholecystectomy, hysterectomy, bilateral salpingo-oophorectomy, bowel resection, anterior resection, abdominoperineal resection, rectopexy, appendectomy, and bariatric surgery), done both open and laparoscopically. This investigated over 100,000 patients during a 5-year period. Open surgery increased the odds ratio of risk of admission for small bowel obstruction fourfold.

Landmark Article of 21st Century

NATURAL HISTORY OF PATIENTS WITH ADHESIVE SMALL BOWEL OBSTRUCTION

Miller G, Boman J, Shrier I, and Gordon PH, *Br J Surg.* 2000;87(9):1240–1247

ABSTRACT

Background   Small bowel obstruction (SBO) is a major cause of morbidity and financial expenditure. The goals of this study were to determine factors predisposing to adhesive SBO, to note the long-term prognosis and recurrence rates for operative and nonoperative treatment, to elicit the complication rate of operations, and to highlight factors predictive of recurrence.

Methods   The medical records of all patients admitted to one hospital between 1986 and 1996 with the diagnosis of SBO were reviewed retrospectively. This included 410 patients accounting for 675 admissions.

Results   The frequency of previous operations by procedure type was colorectal surgery (24%), followed by gynecological surgery (22%), herniorrhaphy (15%), and appendicectomy (14%). A history of colorectal surgery (odds 2.7) and vertical incisions (odds 2.5) tended to predispose to multiple matted adhesions rather than an obstructive band. At initial admission, 36% of patients were treated by means of operation. As the number of admissions increased, the recurrence rate increased while the time interval between admissions decreased. Patients with an adhesive band had a 25% readmission rate, compared with a 49% rate for patients with matted adhesions (P < 0.004). At the initial admission, 36% of patients were treated surgically. Patients treated without operation had a 34% readmission rate, compared with 32% for those treated surgically (P not significant), a shorter time to readmission (median 0.7 vs. 2.0 years; P < 0.05), no difference in reoperation rate (14 vs. 11%; P not significant) and fewer inpatient days over all admissions (4 vs. 12 days; P < 0.0001).

Conclusion   The likelihood of reobstruction increases and the time to reobstruction decreases with increasing number of previous episodes of obstruction. Patients with matted adhesions have a greater recurrence rate than those with band adhesions. Nonoperative treatment for adhesions in stable patients results in a shorter hospital stay and similar recurrence and reoperation rates, but a reduced interval to reobstruction when compared with operative treatment.

Editor Notes

Assessment: This was a secondary analysis of the Eastern Association for the Surgery of Trauma (EAST) multi-institutional prospective, observational study for adhesive small bowel obstruction (SBO). The aim of this study was to validate the American Association for the Surgery of Trauma (AAST) anatomic severity grading system for adhesive SBO. Fifteen centers contributed a total of 635 patients. Initial management of SBO in this data set was nonoperative in 61%. The AAST SBO grade was associated with the need for conversion to an open procedure, small bowel resection, postoperative temporary abdominal closure, and stoma creation. It was also predictive of longer duration of hospital stay, the need for ICU care, and development of complications.

Limitations: There is a correlation with higher scores with worse complications and use of hospital resources. These findings appear intuitive.

Conclusions: The higher the AAST SBO score, the worse the outcome from adhesive small bowel obstruction.

CHAPTER 5

Upper Gastrointestinal Bleeding

Review by Contributor: Bruce Crookes

Upper gastrointestinal bleeding (UGIB) is defined as intraluminal hemorrhage from a source proximal to the ligament of Treitz. UGIB accounts for over 300,000 hospital admissions per year in the United States and is a common cause for admission to the intensive care unit (ICU). The most recent data available suggest that UGIB occurs at a rate of 40–150 episodes per 100,000 persons per year.

Optimal outcomes are dependent upon prevention, rapid identification of the etiology of the hemorrhage, and the subsequent implementation of appropriate pharmacologic and procedural therapies. While only 2.5%–5% of UGIBs require surgical intervention, surgical consultation remains one of the cornerstones of management, making it imperative that surgeons are aware of both the medical and surgical options for management. Surgical intensivists must be familiar with the disease processes as well as potential therapeutic options. Fortunately, over 85% of UGI bleeds stop spontaneously, but when bleeding continues or when the bleed occurs in a high-risk patient, prompt decisive management is required.

The majority (80%–90%) of episodes of UGIB are due to nonvariceal causes, with ulcer disease accounting for the majority of these nonvariceal cases. Aside from ulcer disease, other etiologies of UGI bleeding include varices, Mallory-Weiss syndrome, vascular lesions, and inflammatory states of the upper GI tract.

Initial guidelines for the management of UGIB were published almost 20 years ago. In the last two decades, significant advancements in treatment and prophylaxis have been developed through multiple landmark studies. The subsequent advances in pharmacologic, endoscopic, and radiographic therapies have helped UGIB mortality rates to significantly decrease in the last three decades, most significantly in patients >65 years of age. Surgery, while once the mainstay of treatment, has become a rarity.

Prevention of UGIB has become a cornerstone of management, particularly in the ICU: pharmacologic prophylaxis may be the primary means of prevention in some cases, while in other cases, the prevention of secondary ulcers is the objective. Patients who are critically ill have a number of causes for ulcer formation, including decreased mucous secretion, altered GI motility, and mucosal ischemia. These factors are especially prevalent in patients with large burns, head injury, coagulopathy, or those patients who require mechanical ventilation. While acid suppression is the hallmark of prevention for ulcer-related bleeding, reduction of portal venous pressure is most effective for preventing esophageal bleeding. Beta-blockers are the main class of drugs used to accomplish this goal, having first been used in the 1980s.

As previously stated, most UGI bleeds stop spontaneously. Clinicians, however, can optimize patient outcomes through both pharmacologic and procedural interventions. As ulcer disease is the primary cause of the majority UGIB, providers must first identify the etiology of the ulceration, with three causes being the most prevalent: stress-related mucosal damage (SRMD), NSAID use, and *Helicobacter pylori* infection. UGIB caused by ulcer disease is treated with acid suppression, just as in prevention. The introduction of H_2RA drugs in the 1980s resulted in decreased rates of surgery and death in certain populations of patients with UGIB, marking the dawn of a new era in the treatment of what was then a common problem. The identification of *H. pylori* as a contributing factor to peptic ulcer disease revolutionized care, and treatment paradigms were rapidly established. Over the next decade, protein pump inhibitors (PPIs) were introduced, and they were generally found to be superior to H_2RA agents.

Medical treatment of variceal bleeding differs from that of the bleeding ulcer in that the therapeutic agents used are different in their mechanisms of action: the mainstays of the pharmacologic treatment of active variceal bleeding are vasoconstrictive and vasoactive drugs. Vasopressin and terlipressin are vasoconstrictive agents that have been shown to decrease active variceal bleeding. Octreotide, a hormone analog of somatostatin that alters GI hormone signaling, is currently the main vasoactive drug used to treat variceal bleeding. It decreases gastric and pancreatic secretions and alters splanchnic blood flow. Multiple studies have demonstrated the superior efficacy of octreotide over vasopressin for stopping active bleeding and preventing rebleeds. It should be kept in mind, however, that banding ligation is the most effective therapy for variceal bleeding and should be the primary intervention for stopping variceal bleeding.

Endoscopy is beneficial in UGI bleeds because it can be simultaneously diagnostic and therapeutic, particularly in patients with no prior history of bleeding. Ulcer bleeding can be stopped or reduced with medical treatment, as discussed previously, but multiple studies have shown that endoscopy confers further prevention of rebleeding. Endoscopic findings of active bleeding or a visible vessel require treatment due to their high rates of rebleeding.

While endoscopy is used solely for the treatment of ulcer disease, this intervention can be used for both the treatment of active bleeding and prophylaxis in patients with varices. Options for endoscopic management of varices include injection sclerotherapy and banding ligation. Both techniques have been used for the control of acute hemorrhage. Multiple studies, however, have found that ligation is superior to sclerotherapy.

Angiography has been established as the primary therapy for many lower GI bleeds, but its role in UGIB is not as well defined. While there are many case reports on the use of angiography for the identification and control of bleeding from more obscure bleeding sources (such as small bowel diverticula or mesenteric aneurysms), the data for its use in the control of typical UGI hemorrhage is far from robust. The advent of "super selective" angioembolization for UGIB seems to show a fairly high immediate success rate, but the intervention suffers from a high recurrence rate of clinically significant bleeding. Most studies indicate that embolization should be used in patients with massive ongoing hemorrhage who cannot tolerate surgery due to medical comorbidities.

Clearly, over the course of the last two decades there has been a revolution in the management of UGIB, much to the benefit of patients. The studies included below are a cross-section of the seminal papers that have served as a foundation for the treatment of UGIB.

ANNOTATED REFERENCES FOR UPPER GASTROINTESTINAL BLEEDING

1. Cook D, Guyatt G, Marshall J et al. A comparison of sucralfate and ranitidine for the prevention of upper gastrointestinal bleeding in patients requiring mechanical ventilation. Canadian Critical Care Trials Group. *N Engl J Med*. 1998;338:791–797.

   In this multicenter, randomized, blinded, placebo-controlled trial, members of the Canadian Critical Care Trials Group compared sucralfate with the H_2-receptor antagonist ranitidine for the prevention of UGIB. Twelve hundred critically ill patients on mechanical ventilation were enrolled, and those who received ranitidine had a significantly lower rate of clinically relevant gastrointestinal bleeding. There were no significant differences in the rates of ventilator-associated pneumonia, the duration of the stay in the ICU, or mortality.

2. Graham DY, Lew GM, Evans DG, Evans DJ, Klein PD. Effect of triple therapy (antibiotics plus bismuth) on duodenal ulcer healing. A randomized controlled trial. *Ann Intern Med*. 1991;115(4):266–269.

   In this study of 105 VA patients with UGI ulcers, patients were randomized to receive either ranitidine or ranitidine plus "triple therapy" (tetracycline, metronidazole, bismuth subsalicylate). Triple therapy was administered for the first 2 weeks of ulcer treatment only. Patients then underwent endoscopy after 2, 4, 8, 12, and 16 weeks of therapy. Triple therapy was superior to ranitidine alone for duodenal ulcer healing, as evidenced by more rapid ulcer healing on endoscopy.

3. Chan FK, Wong VW, Suen BY et al. Combination of a cyclo-oxygenase-2 inhibitor and a proton-pump inhibitor for prevention of recurrent ulcer bleeding in patients at very high risk: A double-blind, randomised trial. *Lancet*. 2007;369:1621–1626.

   Four hundred and forty-one patients who were taking nonselective NSAIDs and had a history of hospital admission for upper gastrointestinal bleeding (H. pylori negative) were randomized to receive either celecoxib and placebo or celecoxib and esomeprazol. Patients were then followed for 12 months, with the primary endpoint being recurrent ulcer bleeding. Combination treatment was more effective than celecoxib alone for prevention of ulcer bleeding in patients at high risk.

4. Groszmann RJ, Garcia-Tsao G, Bosch J et al. Beta-blockers to prevent gastroesophageal varices in patients with cirrhosis. *N Engl J Med*. 2005;353:2254–2261.

Nonselective beta-adrenergic blockers are known to decrease portal pressure, but their effectiveness in preventing varices was unknown at the time of this study. Two hundred and thirteen patients with cirrhosis and portal hypertension were randomly assigned to beta-blocker or placebo, with the primary endpoint being the development of gastroesophageal varices or variceal hemorrhage. There were no significant differences in the rates of variceal bleeds, and there were no significant differences in the rates of ascites, encephalopathy, liver transplantation, or death. Adverse events were more common among patients in the beta-blocker group than among those in the placebo group.

5. Khuroo MS, Yattoo GN, Javid G et al. A comparison of omeprazole and placebo for bleeding peptic ulcer. *N Engl J Med*. 1997;336:1054–1058.

The role of medical treatment for patients with bleeding peptic ulcers was uncertain at the time of this double-blind, placebo-controlled trial. Two hundred and twenty patients with duodenal, gastric, or stomal ulcers and signs of recent bleeding, confirmed by endoscopy, were enrolled and randomly assigned to receive 5 days of omeprazole or placebo. The outcome measures studied were further bleeding, surgery, and death. Treatment with omeprazole decreased the rate of further bleeding and the need for surgery.

6. Hwang SJ, Lin HC, Chang CF et al. A randomized controlled trial comparing octreotide and vasopressin in the control of acute esophageal variceal bleeding. *J Hepatol*. 1992;16:320–325.

This randomized controlled trial was conducted to compare the efficacy of intravenous infusion of octreotide with vasopressin. Forty-eight cirrhotic patients with endoscopically proven bleeding esophageal varices were randomized to one of the two treatment arms. Octreotide infusion was more effective and had fewer side effects than vasopressin in initially controlling acute esophageal variceal bleeding until definitive treatment (endoscopic sclerotherapy) could be performed.

7. Lau JY, Sung JJ, Lam YH et al. Endoscopic retreatment compared with surgery in patients with recurrent bleeding after initial endoscopic control of bleeding ulcers. *N Engl J Med*. 1999;340:751–756.

In this prospective, randomized study, the authors compared endoscopic retreatment with surgery after initial endoscopy for control of bleeding peptic ulcers. Endoscopic retreatment reduced the need for surgery without increasing the risk of death. Endoscopic therapy was also associated with fewer complications than surgery.

8. Sarin SK, Lamba GS, Kumar M, Misra A, Murthy NS. Comparison of endoscopic ligation and propranolol for the primary prevention of variceal bleeding. *N Engl J Med*. 1999;340:988–993.

The authors compared propranolol therapy and endoscopic ligation for the primary prevention of bleeding from esophageal varices. This prospective, controlled trial enrolled patients who had large varices (>5 mm in diameter) that were considered to be at high risk for bleeding. The patients were assigned to either propranolol therapy or weekly variceal ligation. After 18 months, the probability of bleeding was 43% in the propranolol group and 15% in the ligation group. Endoscopic ligation of the varices was proven to be safe and more effective than propranolol for the primary prevention of variceal bleeding.

9. Villanueva C, Minana J, Ortiz J et al. Endoscopic ligation compared with combined treatment with nadolol and isosorbide mononitrate to prevent recurrent variceal bleeding. *N Engl J Med.* 2001;345:647–655.

One hundred and forty-four patients with cirrhosis who were hospitalized with esophageal variceal bleeding were randomized to receive treatment with endoscopic ligation or medical therapy with nadolol and isosorbide mononitrate. Ligation sessions were repeated every 2−3 weeks until the varices were eradicated. The primary endpoints were recurrent bleeding, complications, and death. Combined therapy with nadolol and isosorbide mononitrate was more effective in preventing recurrent hemorrhage than endoscopic ligation and was associated with a lower rate of major complications.

10. Poultsides GA, Kim CJ, Orlando R 3rd, Peros G, Hallisey MJ, Vignati PV. Angiographic embolization for gastroduodenal hemorrhage: Safety, efficacy, and predictors of outcome. *Arch Surg.* 2008;143:457–461.

Fifty-seven patients were referred to a tertiary referral center for management after failed endoscopic treatment of UGIB. Surgery was not immediately considered in these patients because of poor surgical risk, patient refusal to consent, or endoscopist's decision. Angiographic embolization for gastroduodenal hemorrhage was associated with in-hospital rebleeding in almost half of these patients. Angiographic failure was associated with delay to embolization, blood transfusion of more than six units of packed red blood cells, or re-hemorrhage from a previously suture-ligated duodenal ulcer.

TRANSFUSION STRATEGIES FOR ACUTE UPPER GASTROINTESTINAL BLEEDING

Villanueva C, Colomo A, Bosch A, Concepción M, Hernandez-Gea V, Aracil C, Graupera I, Poca M, Alvarez-Urturi C, Gordillo J, Guarner-Argente C, Santaló M, Muñiz E, and Guarner C, *N Engl J Med.* 2013;368:11–21

ABSTRACT

Background The hemoglobin threshold for transfusion of red cells in patients with acute gastrointestinal bleeding is controversial. We compared the efficacy and safety of a restrictive transfusion strategy with those of a liberal transfusion strategy.

Methods We enrolled 921 patients with severe acute upper gastrointestinal bleeding and randomly assigned 461 of them to a restrictive strategy (transfusion when the hemoglobin level fell below 7 g per deciliter) and 460 to a liberal strategy (transfusion when the hemoglobin fell below 9 g per deciliter). Randomization was stratified according to the presence or absence of liver cirrhosis.

Results A total of 225 patients assigned to the restrictive strategy (48.8%), as compared with 61 assigned to the liberal strategy (13.3%), did not receive transfusions (P < 0.001). The probability of survival at 6 weeks was higher in the restrictive-strategy group than in the liberal-strategy group (95% vs. 91%; hazard ratio for death with restrictive strategy, 0.55; 95% confidence interval [CI], 0.33−0.92; P = 0.02).

Further bleeding occurred in 10% of the patients in the restrictive-strategy group as compared with 16% of the patients in the liberal-strategy group (P = 0.01), and adverse events occurred in 40% as compared with 48% (P = 0.02). The probability of survival was slightly higher with the restrictive strategy than with the liberal strategy in the subgroup of patients who had bleeding associated with a peptic ulcer (hazard ratio, 0.70; 95% CI, 0.26−1.25) and was significantly higher in the subgroup of patients with cirrhosis and Child-Pugh class A or B disease (hazard ratio, 0.30; 95% CI, 0.11−0.85), but not in those with cirrhosis and Child-Pugh class C disease (hazard ratio, 1.04; 95% CI, 0.45−2.37). Within the first 5 days, the portal-pressure gradient increased significantly in patients assigned to the liberal strategy (P = 0.03) but not in those assigned to the restrictive strategy.

Conclusions As compared with a liberal transfusion strategy, a restrictive strategy significantly improved outcomes in patients with acute upper gastrointestinal bleeding. (Funded by Fundació D'Investigació Sant Pau; ClinicalTrials.gov number NCT00414713.)

Editor Notes

Assessment: This prospective randomized study from Barcelona demonstrated that restrictive blood transfusion strategy significantly improved outcomes in patients with acute upper gastrointestinal (GI) bleeding. Prior work demonstrating the superiority or equivalence of a restricted blood transfusion strategy in critically ill populations (both adults and children [including neonates]) had excluded the patient with active GI hemorrhage. In this trial, 921 patients were enrolled in either a restrictive transfusion group (hemoglobin below 7 g/dL) or a liberal transfusion group (hemoglobin below 9 g/dL). Approximately 31% of the study population bled related to underlying cirrhosis, and peptic ulcer disease was the etiology of bleeding in 49%. In the restrictive group, 51% did not receive any transfusions, whereas only 14% in the liberal strategy avoided transfusion. At 6 weeks, the survival rate for the restrictive group was 95% versus 91% in the liberal group, which was statistically significantly different. In subgroup analysis, the patients who bled from peptic ulcer disease did not have a mortality benefit and only the group with Child-Pugh class A or B cirrhosis had a survival advantage.

Limitations: This study excluded patients with acute coronary syndrome, symptomatic peripheral vasculopathy, stroke, transient ischemic attack, or transfusion in the previous 90 days. Essentially, anemia was treated but not hypovolemia. The mean number of units of blood received was 1.5 versus 3.7, implying that the patients were probably not bleeding excessively. Minimal physiologic data was provided (such as hemodynamic status before and after the transfusions). Obviously, this study was not blinded as to the intervention. Finally, results of this investigation cannot be applied to the patient with massive GI exsanguination.

Conclusions: In patients with upper GI bleeding, a restrictive blood transfusion strategy appears safe and leads to improved survival.

CHAPTER 6

Adult Intussusception

Review by Contributors: Raphael Parrado and David M. Notrica

Intussusception is defined as the telescoping or invagination of one segment of bowel into an adjacent segment. It was first described by Paul Barbette in 1674 as an *intussusceptum* telescoping into an *intussuscipiens*. Later in 1789, John Hunter described a series of three patients using the term "intussusception," and in 1871, Sir Jonathan Hutchinson first described reduction as a successful treatment in a child.

In adults, intussusception is a rare entity that composes about 1% of all bowel obstructions, with a mean age of 50 years and no gender difference (Azar and Berger, 1997). It differs from its pediatric counterpart, as the vast majority of cases of pediatric intussusception are idiopathic versus in adults where about 90% of the cases have an identifiable cause. Neoplasms comprise about two-thirds of the identifiable causes, followed by infections, postoperative adhesions, Crohn granulomas, intestinal ulcers (*Yersinia*) and congenital abnormalities (such as Meckel diverticulum and cystic fibrosis). From the neoplastic cases, about 50% have been reported to be malignant (Wang et al., 2007).

The mechanism for primary intussusception in adults is unknown. For the cases of secondary intussusception, it is believed that the lesion (located on the bowel wall or the lumen) alters the normal peristalsis of these segments, promoting invagination or "intestinal prolapse." This process can be progressive, causing obstruction of the passage of intestinal contents and compromising blood flow, leading to ischemia and necrosis.

Most adult intussusceptions occur in the small intestine, comprising about 50%–75% of the cases. Common benign causes include Meckel diverticulum, adhesions, lymphoid hyperplasia, lipomas, or polyps. Chronic conditions such as anorexia nervosa and malabsorption states can predispose to intussusception, as a flaccid bowel wall may facilitate telescoping. Other predisposing conditions that have been reported include AIDS, blunt abdominal trauma, and previous Roux-en-Y anastomosis, which all have been related to lymphoid hyperplasia, submucosal edema, or hematomas. From the malignant causes, metastatic melanoma tops the list, followed by leiomyosarcoma, adenocarcinoma, GIST tumors, carcinoid tumors, neuroendocrine tumors, and lymphomas.

Colonic intussusception has been reported to occur in 20%–25% of the cases. The most common malignant cause is adenocarcinoma and the most common benign cause is colonic lipoma. It is unclear which one is more common, as literature has been conflictive; some series report that as many as 66% of colonic intussusception is caused by adenocarcinoma while other report suggest that the incidence of malignancy is similar to that found in small bowel intussusception (30%). Special concern must be taken in the setting of ileocolic intussusception, where the likelihood of malignancy may be as high as 100%, resulting from cecal adenocarcinoma involving the ileocecal valve.

Clinical presentation in adults can be nonspecific, with a wide array of symptoms, as opposed to the classic triad in children of pain, palpable mass, and bloody stools. It presents with symptoms of bowel obstruction, namely abdominal pain, nausea, vomiting, obstipation, gastrointestinal bleeding, constipation, or bloating (Nagorney et al., 1981). Physical exam can reveal a distended abdomen with focal or generalized tenderness, decreased or absent bowel sounds, or a palpable mass (less than 50% of the cases). As obstruction processes, peritonitis from bowel ischemia with hypotension or tachycardia may be present. Depending on the cause and course of disease, laboratory findings may include leukocytosis, thrombocytosis. and elevated C-reactive protein (Marsicovetere et al., 2017).

With multiple differential diagnoses, the most common tool used to diagnose intussusception is the CT scan. Multiple studies have reported a diagnostic accuracy of about 58%–100%, followed by ultrasound, enema, and colonoscopy. CT has predominantly been the best imaging study, with mixed results from other studies (Barussaud et al., 2006). Ultrasound has been used; however, it is less reliable than in the pediatric counterpart due to air levels, patient size, and nonspecific findings. CT findings include the "target," sausage-shaped and reniform patterns that reflect the severity and duration of the process. Target-like appearance is seen in early stages when the beam is perpendicular. A sausage-shaped lesion has areas of low and high attenuation that represent bowel mesentery, intestinal fluid, or contrast agents. Finally, the reniform pattern represents edema, mural thickening. and vascular compromise (Baleato-Gonzalez et al., 2012).

One of the pitfalls occurs with the recent development of high-resolution and 65 cut CT scans where nonpathologic and transient short-segment small bowel intussusceptions can be commonly seen. These cases always have to be put in clinical context as they can usually be ignored. In cases of colic or ileocolic intussusception, water-soluble enemas have been used for diagnostic and therapeutic effects (with a decreased efficacy rate, as there is commonly a lead point) as well as colonoscopy, more commonly used in subacute or chronic cases, which in the correct scenario may also help in obtaining tissue for biopsy on any identified lesion.

As adult intussusception has a different set of causes, the majority of adult cases will require definitive treatment (most commonly surgical resection) versus pneumatic or hydrostatic enema in the pediatric population. Surgical treatment has historically been the most common. However, with the introduction of higher-resolution CT scans and MRI there has been reported resolution with nonoperative management in up to 82% of cases with "radiographic intussusceptions." For this entero-enteric intussusception without a lead point, several series have reported that expectant management can be done for segments less than 3.8 cm. This can occur in healthy individuals but has been also associated with Crohn's disease and celiac disease. (Lvoff et al. 2003; Rea et al. 2007).

Surgical exploration is recommended in the setting of (1) signs of obstruction, (2) lead point mass appreciated, and (3) colocolonic or ileocolic intussusception because of high risk of malignancy. When indicated, this exploration can be performed either laparoscopically or open. If intraoperative malignancy or ischemia is suspected, resection without reduction is recommended following the usual oncologic principles based on location and patient characteristics. In this scenario a perforation can cause seeding of malignant cells, both intraluminal and in the peritoneum. Procedures may include exploration with bowel resection and primary anastomosis, Hartmann procedure, or bowel resection with primary anastomosis with proximal diverting loop ileostomy. For benign causes, attempts can be made to slowly reduce the affected segments with or without resection. Follow-up should be performed depending on the cause.

ANNOTATED REFERENCES FOR ADULT INTUSSUSCEPTION

1. Azar T, Berger DL. Adult intussusception. *Ann Surg*. 1997;226:134–138.

   One of the most important historic case series, a 29-year retrospective review of 58 cases of surgically proven adult intussusception.

2. Wang LT, Wu CC, Yu JC, Hsiao CW, Hsu CC, Jao SW. Clinical entity and treatment strategies for adult intussusceptions: 20 years' experience. *Dis Colon Rectum*. 2007;50(11):1941–1949.

   A 20-year retrospective review of 24 cases of adult intussusception from a cohort of 292 patients with intussusception, with focus on the interventions performed.

3. Nagorney DM, Sarr MG, McIlrath DC. Surgical management of intussusception in the adult. *Ann Surg*. 1981;193:230–236.

   A 20-year retrospective review of 48 cases of adult intussusception summed with a previous review of 96 patients is one of the largest cohorts that gives insight on clinical characteristics, treatment, and prognosis of the disease.

4. Marsicovetere P, Joga Ivatury S, White B, Holubar S. Intestinal intussusception: Etiology, diagnosis and treatment. *Clin Colon Rectal Surg*. 2017;30:30–39.

   One of the most comprehensive literature reviews of intussusception, it compares and contrasts it with the pediatric counterpart and has a visual comparison from some of the previously reported case series.

5. Barussaud M, Regenet N, Briennon X, et al. Clinical spectrum and surgical approach of adult intussusceptions: A multicentric study. *Int J Color Dis*. 2006;21(8):834–839.

   A 25-year retrospective review of 41 cases of adult intussusception with focus on diagnostic tool performance and treatment.

6. Baleato-Gonzalez S, Villanova J, Garcia-Figueiras R, Barral Juez I, Martinez de Alegria A. Intussusception in adults: What radiologists should know. *Emerg Radiol*. 2012;19:89–101.

This is an interesting literature review that is focused on each of the causes of intussusception, with an emphasis on radiological findings.

7. Lvoff N, Breiman RS, Coakley FV, Lu Y, Warren RS. Distinguishing features of self-limiting adult small-bowel. *Radiology.* 2003;227(1):68–72.

A retrospective review of 37 CT scans showing small-bowel intussusception over a 4-year period. In this cohort, 16% underwent surgical intervention. With a mean follow up of 5.2 months, a multivariate analysis showed that a length of 3.5 cm or less was more likely to be self-limiting.

Landmark Article of 21st Century

APPROACH TO MANAGEMENT OF INTUSSUSCEPTION IN ADULTS: A NEW PARADIGM IN THE COMPUTED TOMOGRAPHY ERA

Rea JD, Lockhart ME, Yarbrough DE, Leeth RR, Bledsoe SE, and Clements RH, *Am Surg.* 2007;73(11):1098–1105

ABSTRACT

Background   Intussusception has been considered an operative indication in adults as a result of the risk of ischemia and the possibility of a malignant lead point. Computed tomographic (CT) scans can reveal unsuspected intussusception.

Methods   All CT reports from July 1999 to December 2005 were scanned electronically for letter strings to include the keyword intussusception. Identified CT scans were analyzed to characterize the intussusception and associated findings. Clinical, laboratory, pathological, and follow-up variables were gleaned from medical records. Findings were analyzed by treatment and findings at operation.

A review of 380,999 CT reports yielded 170 (0.04%) adult patients (mean age, 41 years) with intussusceptions described as enteroenteric in 149 (87.6%), ileocecal in 8 (4.7%), colocolonic in 10 (5.9%), and gastroenteric in 3 (1.8%). Radiological features included mean length of 4.4 cm (range, 0.8–20.5 cm) and diameter of 3.2 cm (range, 1.6–11.5 cm). Twenty-nine (17.1%) had a lead point and 12 (7.1%) had bowel obstruction. Clinically, 88 (51.8%) patients reported abdominal pain, 52 (30.6%) had nausea and/or vomiting, and 74 (43.5%) had objective findings on abdominal examination.

Results   Thirty of 170 (17.6%) patients underwent operation, but only 15 (8.8%) patients had pathologic findings that correlated with CT findings. Seven had enteroenteric intussusceptions from benign neoplasms (two), adhesions (one), local inflammation (one), previous anastomosis (one), Crohn's disease (one), and idiopathic (one). Three had ileocolic disease, including cecal cancer (one), metastatic melanoma (one) and idiopathic (one); whereas five patients had colocolonic intussusception from colon cancer (three), tubulovillous adenoma (one), and local inflammation (one). Of the 15 without intussusception at exploration, 5 had pathology related to trauma, 4 had nonincarcerated internal hernia after Roux-en-Y gastric bypass, 4 had negative explorations, 1 had adhesions, and 1 had appendicitis that did not correlate with CT findings. No patient in the observation group required subsequent operative exploration for intussusception at mean 14.1 months (range, 0.25–67.5 months) follow-up. All operative patients demonstrated gastrointestinal symptoms versus 55.3% of the observation group (P < 0.006).

Analysis of CT features demonstrated differences among patients observed without operation, those without intussusception at exploration, and confirmed intussusception with regard to mean intussusception length 3.8 versus 3.8 versus 9.6 cm, diameter 3.0 versus 3.2 versus 4.8 cm, lead point 12.1% versus 30% versus 53.3%, and proximal obstruction 3.8% versus 0% versus 46.7%, respectively. Intussusceptions in adults discovered by CT scanning do not always mandate exploration.

Conclusion   Most cases can be treated expectantly despite the presence of gastrointestinal symptoms. Close follow-up is recommended with imaging and/or endoscopic surveillance. Length and diameter of the intussusception, presence of a lead point, or bowel obstruction on CT are predictive of findings that warrant exploration.

Editor Notes

Assessment: This study evaluated 170 adult patients with the CT diagnosis of intussusception among almost 381,000 abdominal CT scans performed. Just 30 of 170 intussusception patients (17.6%) required surgical exploration. The authors concluded that most cases of intussusception in adults can be treated expectantly despite gastrointestinal symptoms, as only a small percentage of patients were found to have a lesion that required excision. The length and diameter of the intussusception, the presence of a lead point, or associated bowel obstruction appeared predictive findings for mandatory exploration.

Limitations: The relative rarity of this entity makes accumulation of a large patient experience extremely difficult. The results therefore are dependent upon the attitudes of the operating teams. For the study, 170 patients were accrued over 6 years at a single center, but the methodology—initial diagnosis by CT imaging alone—ensured that a large percentage of the patients would be asymptomatic (over half were without abdominal findings on physical examination). No inter- or intra-rater variability was determined, so the diagnostic accuracy and consistency of the radiologists to determine intussusception was not established. Despite its limitations, this study permits us to make certain generalizations regarding this entity which is dealt with typically in small case series in the literature.

Conclusions: This relatively large experience regarding a fairly unusual lesion informs the clinician on the relative benignity of intussusception in the majority of instances and gives us some clues as to what factors predict the need for exploration.

CHAPTER 7

Enterocutaneous Fistulas

Review by Contributors: Edward Lineen and Peter Lopez

An enterocutaneous fistula (ECF) is an abnormal connection between the gastrointestinal tract and the skin or wound. Enterocutaneous fistulas can arise after abdominal trauma, inflammatory bowel disease, operations for oncologic and inflammatory processes in the abdomen, and operations for bowel obstructions. The clinical course of ECFs can range from an easily managed low-output fistula to a high-output fistula in the setting of an open abdomen requiring many months of intensive care, nutritional support, and complex reconstructive surgery (1). Immediate concerns of clinicians caring for patients with ECF include correction of fluid and electrolyte imbalance, eradication and control of peritoneal sepsis drainage of abscesses, management of fistula drainage, and skin care and nutritional support. Classic barriers to spontaneous closure of ECFs include distal obstruction, ongoing sepsis, severe malnutrition, mucocutaneous continuity (a short or epithelialized tract), malignancy, or foreign body in the tract (4). ECFs are a heavy emotional, physical, and financial burden for the patient, the patient's family, and their specialized care team. Mortality rates for patients with ECF range from 0%–33% with higher mortality rates in older patients, malnutrition, high-output fistulas, and patients with uncontrolled sepsis (2). The majority of the quality of evidence reviewed on the management of ECF is level 4 nonrandomized cohort observational trials with historical controls, or level 5 case series and expert opinion.

The management of a patient who has developed an ECF has been broken down into various phases to help simplify care (2,3,4). After discovering an ECF, the main focus of phase I is to stabilize the patient by controlling sepsis, resuscitating the patient, correcting electrolyte deficiencies, controlling fistula drainage, protecting the skin, and repleting the patient nutritionally (2,3,4). Identifying and controlling the sources of sepsis and administering appropriate and timely antibiotics is paramount, as patients with ECFs usually die from ongoing sepsis. Patients will need aggressive fluid resuscitation along with correction of electrolyte disturbances. Fistula drainage must be contained and quantified. The skin must be protected from the draining enteric contents in order to prevent a destructive cellulitis of the abdominal wall. Proper wound care that maintains the patient's skin integrity and contains fistula output is an important component in the patient's ability to manage the physical and mental stresses of living with an ECF. Vacuum-assisted wound closure devices can be used to help close wounds and control fistula output, but these devices can also cause more fistulas to develop and must be used with caution (4). The further use of irrigating vacuum-assisted devices have shown benefit in small case series (5). Control of fistula output by the use of both proton pump inhibitors and histamine

H2 blockers has been shown to decrease gastric acid output. Antidiarrheals (loperamide, diphenoxylate/atropine, codeine, and tincture of opium) have also been used to decrease fistula output. Somatostatin and octreotide can decrease both biliary and pancreatic secretions, thus decreasing fistula output. In two separate meta-analyses of the use of somatostatin and octreotide, both decreased fistula output and increased the likelihood of enterocutaneous fistula closure, with no mortality benefit (6,7).

The goal of providing nutritional support is to achieve an anabolic state with weight gain to allow for optimal healing. Parenteral nutrition should begin early to provide all of the patient's nutritional needs and prevent further protein and calorie malnutrition. If possible, the patient's gastrointestinal tract should be used to provide some or all of the calories needed by the patient in order to help prevent hepatic dysfunction and maintain some bowel immunologic and physiologic function. Enteral hypo- and iso-osmolar feeds should be provided at slow rates to give the compromised bowel time to adapt and absorb the feeds. Be aware that fistula output usually increases proportionally to the amount of tube feeds provided.

Phase II starts after the patient has been stabilized and continues until closure of the fistula. Defining the anatomy of the fistula and its organ of origin is necessary in planning the long-term care of the patient. CT scans can help give an idea of where the fistula is, and they can also be useful to help locate intraperitoneal and abdominal wall abscesses. A well-performed radiologic fistulogram defines the anatomy of the fistula tract and helps determine the patient's care. Characteristics of the fistula as defined clinically and radiologically can predict if the fistula will spontaneously close or will need a definitive operation.

During phase II, ongoing maintenance of skin care and containment of fistula output, continued nutrition support with parenteral and when possible enteral nutrition, and avoidance and early recognition of sepsis are vital in order to allow time for the patient to become optimized and be able to undergo definitive surgical closure of their ECF.

Phase III is the definitive closure of the enterocutaneous fistula. Nonoperative therapies that have been used to close ECFs include fibrin sealants, fistula plugs, and endoscopic clips. From case series, the use of fibrin sealant to help close favorable ECF, long, narrow, low output without distal obstruction or inflammatory bowel disease has been shown to increase closure rates (8). Endoscopic clips have been used to help close ECFs from small perforations from acute anastomotic leaks (9). A significant number of patients with enteric fistulas will require an operation to resect and close their fistulas. Definitive operative surgical repair is usually scheduled when the enteric fistula does not spontaneously close by 12 weeks after sepsis control. The patient must be maximized with optimal nutrition, be mentally prepared, have no evidence of ongoing sepsis, have clinical evidence of softening scars, and must be given enough time to allow their obliterative peritonitis adhesions to soften. The optimal time to operate on a patient with an ECF is a topic of ongoing debate, but can range anywhere from 3–24 months. The definitive operation should avoid any new enterotomies while performing lysis of adhesions, preserve maximal bowel length, completely resect the bowel communicating with the fistula, re-establish bowel continuity, and provide coverage of the bowel with well-vascularized soft tissue. Brenner and coauthors (10), showed that resection of the fistula with performance of a hand-sewn anastomosis had the lowest frequency of recurrent fistula.

Patients who develop enterocutaneous fistulas will require an experienced, multidisciplined, thoughtful, and long-term care team. Often this disease process quickly turns into a chronic disease state requiring complex long-term care needs. Patients find themselves isolated, frustrated, angry, hungry, and depressed, and live in fear of recurrent sepsis and appliance leaks. Patients and their families are often psychologically spent and overwhelmed from the complexity and length of time necessary to heal and be strong enough for definitive surgical repair.

The spectrum of clinical challenging problems that these patients and their caregivers encounter requires constant attention and flexibility in being able to adapt to the problems that arise in their care until definitive closure of their fistula. ECFs remain a life-altering disease process, but with time and supportive care the patient can get through and hopefully back to their previous life.

ANNOTATED REFERENCES FOR ENTEROCUTANEOUS FISTULAS: BEST EVIDENCE

1. Fisher JE, Evenson AR. Gastrointestinal-cutaneous fistulas. In: *Fischer's Mastery of Surgery*. 7th ed. Fischer JF. (Ed.). Philadelphia: Wolters Kluwer; 2019.

   The authors present an authoritative discussion on the management of enterocutaneous fistulas. This is a good start to understanding the process and complexities of managing patients with enterocutaneous fistulas.

2. Gribovskaja-Rupp I, Melton GB. Enterocutaneous fistula: Proven strategies and updates. *Clin Colon Rectal Surg.* 2016;29:130–137.

   In this article, the reader is introduced to the authors' "SNAP" protocol for the management of enterocutaneous fistulas. SNAP stands for management of skin and sepsis, nutrition, definition of the fistula anatomy, and proposing a definitive procedure to close the fistula.

3. Evenson AR, Fischer JE. Current management of enterocutaneous fistula. *J Gastrointest Surg.* 2006;10:455–464.

   A good review of the development of a process by which to manage patients with an enterocutaneous fistula.

4. Schecter WP, Asher H, Chang DS et al. Enteric fistulas: Principles of management. *J Am Coll Surg.* 2009;209(4):484.

   The multiple authors describe their helpful way to manage patients with enterocutaneous fistulas. The authors describe the three phases of enterocutaneous fistula management:

Phase 1, recognition and stabilization; Phase 2, anatomic definition and decision; and Phase 3, definitive operation.

5. Morinaga K, Rikimaru Y, Kiyokawa K. Treatment of abdominal wound dehiscence with bowel exposure and infection. Using intrawound negative pressure, irrigation, and application of artificial dermis. *Ann Plastic Surg.* 2019 Feb;82(2):213–217.

This article reviews techniques that have helped the authors manage and close difficult wounds and enterocutaneous fistulas.

6. Couglin S, Roth L, Lurati G, Faulhaber M. Somatostatin analogues for the treatment of enterocutaneous fistulas: A systemic review and meta-analysis. *World J Surg.* 2012;36(5):1016–1029.

This is a systemic review and meta-analysis of the use of somatostatin analogs in the treatment of enterocutaneous fistulas. The authors concluded that somatostatin analogs appear to decrease the duration of enterocutaneous fistulas and duration of hospital stay, but no mortality benefit was identified. The quality of evidence for outcomes in their review ranged from low to moderate.

7. Rahbour G, Siddiqui MR, Ullah MR, Gabe SM, Warusavitarne J, Vaizey CJ. A meta-analysis of outcomes following the use of somatostatin and its analogues for the management of enterocutaneous fistulas. *Ann Surg.* 2012;256(6):946–954.

A meta-analysis of outcomes following the use of somatostatin and its analogs in the management of enterocutaneous fistulas. The authors concluded that somatostatin and octreotide increase the likelihood of fistula closure. Neither drug had an effect on mortality.

8. Avalos-Gonzalez J, Portilla-deBuen E, Leal-Cortes CA et al. Reduction of the closure time of postoperative enterocutaneous fistulas with fibrin sealant. *World J Gastroenterol.* 2010;16(22):2793–2800.

This paper describes the use and success of fibrin sealant as a way to close some postoperative enterocutaneous fistulas.

9. Winder JS, Pauli EM. Comprehensive management of full-thickness luminal defects: The next frontier of gastrointestinal endoscopy. *World J Gastrointestinal Endosc.* 2015;7(8):758–768.

The authors report their experience with the endoscopic management and closure of full-thickness luminal defects that prevented or treated potential enterocutaneous fistulas.

10. Brenner M, Clayton JL, Tillou A et al. Risk factors for recurrence after repair of enterocutaneous fistula. *Arch Surg.* 2009;144(6):500–505.

These authors at a single institution reviewed their experience with the definitive surgical closure of enterocutaneous fistulas.

Additional Resources on the Management of Enterocutaneous Fistulas

11. Schecter WP. Management of enterocutaneous fistulas. *Surg Clin N Am.* 2011;91:481–491.
12. Joyce MR, Dietz DW. Management of complex gastrointestinal fistula. *Curr Probl Surg.* 2009;46:384–430.
13. Berry SM, Fisher JE. Classification and pathophysiology of enterocutaneous fistulas. *Surg Clin N Am.* 1996;76:1009–1018.

A META-ANALYSIS OF OUTCOMES FOLLOWING USE OF SOMATOSTATIN AND ITS ANALOGS FOR THE MANAGEMENT OF ENTEROCUTANEOUS FISTULAS

Rahbour G, Siddiqui MR, Ullah MR, Gabe SM, Warusavitarne J, and Vaizey CJ,
Ann Surg. 2012;256(6):946–954

ABSTRACT

Objective   Several randomized control trials (RCTs) have compared somatostatin and its analogs versus a control group in patients with enterocutaneous fistulas (ECF). This study meta-analyzes the literature and establishes whether it shows a beneficial effect on ECF closure.

Methods   We searched MEDLINE, EMBASE, CINAHL, Cochrane, and PubMed databases according to PRISMA guidelines. Seventy-nine articles were screened. Nine RCTs met the inclusion criteria. Statistical analyses were performed using Review Manager 5.1.

Results   Somatostatin analogs versus control   *Number of fistulas closed*: A significant number of ECFs closed in the somatostatin analog group compared to control group; $P = 0.002$. *Time to closure*: ECFs closed significantly faster with somatostatin analogs compared to controls; $P < 0.0001$. *Mortality*: No significant difference between somatostatin analogs and controls; $P = 0.68$.
   Somatostatin versus control   *Number of fistulas closed*: A significant number of ECFs closed with somatostatin as compared to control; $P = 0.04$. *Time to closure*: ECFs closed significantly faster with somatostatin than controls; $P < 0.00001$. *Mortality*: No significant difference between somatostatin and controls; $P = 0.63$.

Conclusions   Somatostatin and octreotide increase the likelihood of fistula closure. Both are beneficial in reducing the time to fistula closure. Neither has an effect on mortality. The risk ratio (RR) for somatostatin was higher than the RR for analogs. This may suggest that somatostatin could be better than analogs in relation to the number of fistulas closed and time to closure. Further studies are required to corroborate these apparent findings.

Editor Notes

Assessment: This was a meta-analysis of nine randomized control trials. Results suggested that somatostatin and somatostatin analogs closed a significantly higher number of enterocutaneous fistulas, and that the time to closure was significantly reduced. The mortality was not statistically impacted by the drugs.

Limitations: This was a meta-analysis of randomized control trials and has issues with scientific validity due to the variance in the studies. The study separated the randomized trials into somatostatin or its analogs. All the studies did have controls, but the studies had tremendous heterogeneous variability and spanned from 1990–2009. The study populations varied in composition (age, type [high vs. low output], location, and source of fistulas). The treatment was also heterogeneous. Varied doses and methods of dosing as well as duration of therapy were different from study to study.

Conclusions: This meta-analysis concluded that a large randomized multicenter control trial is needed. However, it does suggest that somatostatin and octreotide increase the likelihood of fistula closure. Both may be beneficial in reducing the time to fistula closure. The study supported the notion that optimal results occur after the use of somatostatin or the long-acting somatostatin analog, lanreotide. The relative risk for somatostatin was higher than for the analogs in relation to the number of fistulas closed and the time until closure, suggesting that somatostatin was more effective than its analogs.

CHAPTER 8

Acute Mesenteric Ischemia

Review by Contributor: Juan C. Duchesne

Acute mesenteric ischemia (AMI) is life-threatening and requires early multimodal medical and surgical interventions. Boley et al. (1997) identified Antonio Benivieni from Florence in the latter part of the fifteenth century as the first author in describing AMI in a classical review of the history of AMI. Although Hodgson reported another case from Guy's Hospital in 1815, it was not until further descriptions by Tiedman and Virchow in the mid-1800s that the medical profession really became interested in this condition.

In the late 1960s, the mortality rate for patients with AMI was 70%–90%. There has been little change in mortality due to the following factors: failure to make early diagnosis before intestinal infarction, progression of ischemia and infarction even after the initiating cardiac or vascular cause had been corrected, and finally, high proportion of patients with nonocclusive AMI who have an unforgiven mortality above 90%. In a systematic review and meta-analysis for effective early diagnosis of AMI, Cudnik et al. (2013) identified the sensitivity for the two isomers of lactate (L-isomer 86%; D-isomer 96%) and for computed tomography (CT) 94% with a specificity of 95%. The authors concluded that only CT angiography had adequate accuracy to early establish the etiology of AMI in lieu of laparotomy.

Knowing the etiology of AMI plays a key role in patient management and outcomes. It is important to acknowledge two important studies with differences in etiologies for AMI. In a classical analysis by Endean (2001), AMI was diagnosed in 170 patients. The most common etiology was nonthrombotic (60%), followed by thrombotic (34%), and indeterminate (6%). In the thrombotic cohort, arterial embolism accounted for 38%, arterial thrombosis for 36%, and venous thrombosis for 26%. This is in contrast to a more recent study of 107 patients with AMI by Alhan et al. (2012) where the most common etiology was documented to be mesenteric arterial thrombosis (63.6%), followed by arterial embolism (26%), and nonocclusive mesenteric ischemia (10.2%). Although differences in etiologies exist based on current literature, it is important to remember the difference in outcomes based on origin of AMI, as demonstrated by Schoots et al. (2004), who performed a quantitative analysis of data derived from 45 observational studies containing 3692 patients. They were able to identify that survival after AMI varied between the different etiological subsets. The authors concluded that the mortality rate after surgical treatment of arterial embolism and venous thrombosis has improved over the years, whereas that after surgery for arterial thrombosis and nonocclusive ischemia remained poor.

Once knowledge of the etiology has been made, timing for treatment of AMI is of the essence. The first medical intervention for AMI is intravascular fluid replacement in order to stabilize hemodynamics. To prevent exacerbation of thromboembolic occlusion, immediate anticoagulation should be performed using 5000 IU heparin IV in addition to antibiotic treatment. This is crucial since the goal here is for early intervention in order to halt progression of transmural necrosis. Emile (2018) was able to demonstrate factors that were predictive of transmural necrosis in a retrospective study of 101 patients. The independent predictors for transmural bowel necrosis besides acute peritonitis were mesenteric arterial occlusion, leukocytosis above 18,000, acidosis, free intraperitoneal fluid, and combined portal vein and SMV thrombosis on CT.

In patients with acute peritonitis or CT evidence of preexisting gangrene of the intestine, gas in the wall of the intestine or the portal venous system requires exploratory laparotomy with possible open revascularization interventions. Park et al. (2002), in his analysis of 58 exploratory laparotomies, identified open mesenteric revascularization in 43 patients. Bypass grafting was the most common with 22, followed by thromboembolectomy in 19, patch angioplasty in 11, endarterectomy in 5, and reimplantation in 2. The authors concluded that contemporary management of AMI with revascularization during open surgical techniques, resection of nonviable bowel, and liberal use of second-look procedures resulted in early survival of up to 66% of patients with embolism and thrombosis.

In patients without peritonitis, endovascular therapy (EVT) can be attempted before laparotomy as the primary revascularization method and is gaining popularity as part of a multimodal approach. Beaulieu et al. (2014) were able to demonstrate the contribution of EVT in AMI in retrospective analysis where 165 (24.3%) patients out of 679 underwent EVT. The proportion of patients undergoing endovascular repair increased from 11.9% of patients in 2005 to 30.0% in 2009. They were able to demonstrate a decrease in mortality in the EVT group when compared to open revascularization (39.3% vs. 24.9%; P < 0.01) as well as a decrease in length of stay (12.9 vs. 17.1 days; P < 0.006) and fewer bowel resections (14.4% vs. 33.4%; P < 0.001).

Because of the complexity in the management of these patients, it is important to mention the potential role of a multimodality team approach that will improve early diagnosis and intervention. This multimodality team consists of gastroenterologists, vascular and abdominal surgeons, radiologists, and intensive care specialists. Corcos et al. (2013), in a prospective Intestinal Stroke Center analysis of 18 consecutive patients, developed a similar multimodal management strategy. Patients were followed up for a mean of 497 days; 95% survived for 30 days, 89% survived for 2 years, and 28% had morbidities within 30 days. Intestinal resection was necessary for 7 cases (39%), with mean lengths of intestinal resection of 30 and 207 cm, with or without revascularization, respectively. Among patients with early- or late-stage AMI, rates of resection were 18% and 71%, respectively. Patients with early-stage disease had shorter lengths of intestinal resection than those with late-stage disease (7 vs. 94 cm) and spent less time in intensive care (2.5 vs. 49.8). Although institution of a multimodality team can improve outcomes, we must keep in mind the determinants of mortality in this group of patients when discussing outcomes with caregivers. Kougias et al. (2007), in a 12-year analysis of 72 patients, were able to demonstrate in univariate analysis renal insufficiency, age >70, metabolic acidosis, symptom duration, and bowel resection in second-look operations were all associated with an increased mortality but on logistic regression only age >70 and prolonged symptom duration were independent predictors of mortality.

ANNOTATED REFERENCES FOR ACUTE MESENTERIC ISCHEMIA

1. Boley SJ, Brandt LJ, Sammartano RJ. History of mesenteric ischemia. The evolution of a diagnosis and management. *Surg Clin North Am.* 1997;77(2)275–278.

   In this well-written history of AMI, the authors described in a great chronological fashion the diagnosis and early management. A great citation can be found at the beginning of the manuscript: "Occlusion of the mesenteric vessels is apt to be regarded as one of those conditions of which ... the diagnosis is impossible, the prognosis hopeless and the treatment almost useless. A.J. Cokkinis, 1926."

2. Cudnik MT, Darbha S, Jones J, Macedo J, Stockton SW, Hiestand BC. The diagnosis of acute mesenteric ischemia: A systematic review and meta-analysis. *Acad Emerg Med.* 2013;20(11).

   The authors performed a systematic review and meta-analysis of the available literature to determine diagnostic test characteristics of patient symptoms, objective signs, laboratory studies, and diagnostic modalities to help rule in or out the diagnosis of acute mesenteric ischemia in the ED. The quality of the overall literature base for mesenteric ischemia is varied. Signs, symptoms, and laboratory testing are insufficiently diagnostic for the condition. Only CT angiography had adequate accuracy to establish the diagnosis of acute mesenteric ischemia in lieu of laparotomy.

3. Endean ED, Barnes SL, Kwolek CJ, Minion DJ, Schwarcz TH, Mentzer RM Jr. Surgical management of thrombotic acute intestinal ischemia. *Ann Surg.* 2001;233(6):801–808.

   The authors performed a comparative retrospective analysis on patients who were diagnosed with acute intestinal ischemia between May 1993 and July 2000. The survival rate was 87% in the venous thrombosis group versus 41% and 38% for arterial embolism and thrombosis, respectively. Compared with the collated historical series, the survival rate was 52% versus 25%.

4. Alhan E, Usta A, Çekiç A, Saglam K, Türkyılmaz S, Cinel A. A study on 107 patients with acute mesenteric ischemia over 30 years. *Int J Surg.* 2012;10:510–513.

   Hospital records and clinical data of 107 patients that underwent surgical intervention for AMI in a 30-year period were reviewed, and clinical outcomes as well as factors influencing mortality analyzed. Mesenteric arterial thrombosis, arterial embolism, and nonocclusive mesenteric ischemia were the most common causes of AMI. A high index of suspicion with prompt diagnostic evaluation with CT angiography may reduce time prior to surgical intervention which may lead to improved patient survival.

5. Schoots IG, Koffeman GI, Legemate DA, Levi M, van Gulik TM. Systematic review of survival after acute mesenteric ischemia according to disease etiology. *Br J Surg.* 2004;91:17–27.

The authors performed a systematic review of the available literature from 1966 to 2002. From a total of 3692 patients with acute mesenteric ischemia, they found surgical treatment of arterial embolism has improved outcome whereas the mortality rate following surgery for arterial thrombosis and nonocclusive ischemia remains poor.

6. Emile SH. Predictive factors for intestinal transmural necrosis in patients with acute mesenteric ischemia. *World J Surg.* 2018;42:2364–2372.

The author study aimed to identify the clinical, laboratory, and radiologic parameters that can successfully predict the onset of intestinal transmural necrosis in patients with AMI. From 101 patients, the independent predictors for transmural bowel necrosis were mesenteric arterial occlusion, leukocytosis, acidosis, free intraperitoneal fluid, combined portal vein, and SMV thrombosis in CT scan.

7. Park WM, Gloviczki P, Cherry KJ Jr. et al. Contemporary management of acute mesenteric ischemia. Factors associated with survival. *J Vasc Surg.* 2002;35:445–452.

The authors concluded that the contemporary management of AMI with revascularization with open surgical techniques, resection of nonviable bowel, and liberal use of second-look procedures results in the early survival of two-thirds of the patients with embolism and thrombosis. Older patients, those who did not undergo bowel resection, and those with nonocclusive AMI have the highest mortality rates. The long-term survival rate remains dismal. Timely revascularization in patients who are symptomatic with chronic mesenteric ischemia should be considered to decrease the high mortality rate of AMI.

8. Beaulieu RJ, Arnaoutakis KD, Abularrage CJ, Efron DT, Schneider E, Black JH III. Comparison of open and endovascular treatment of acute mesenteric ischemia. *J Vasc Surg.* 2014;59:159–164.

From their review of 679 patients with AMI, the authors demonstrated that endovascular intervention for AMI had increased significantly in the modern era. Among AMI patients undergoing revascularization, endovascular treatment was associated with decreased mortality and shorter length of stay. Furthermore, endovascular intervention was associated with lower rates of bowel resection and need for TPN. Further research is warranted to determine if increased use of endovascular repair could improve overall and gastrointestinal outcomes among patients requiring vascular repair for AMI.

9. Corcos O, Castier Y, Sibert A, Gaujoux S et al. Effects of a multimodal management strategy for acute mesenteric ischemia on survival and intestinal failure. *Clin Gastroenterol Hepatol.* 2013;11:158–165.

The authors performed a prospective study to assess a multidisciplinary and multimodal management approach, focused on intestinal viability. They concluded that a multidisciplinary and multimodal management approach might increase survival of patients with AMI and prevent intestinal failure.

10. Kougias P, Lau D, El Sayed HF, Zhou W, Huynh TT, Lin PH. Determinants of mortality and treatment outcome following surgical interventions for acute mesenteric ischemia. *J Vasc Surg.* 2007;46:467–474.

The purpose of this study was to review the authors' experience with surgical management in patients with AMI and to identify variables associated with adverse outcomes following surgical interventions. Authors concluded that elderly patients and those with a prolonged duration of symptoms had worse outcomes following surgical intervention for AMI.

SURGICAL MANAGEMENT OF THROMBOTIC ACUTE INTESTINAL ISCHEMIA

Endean ED, Barnes SL, Kwolek CJ, Minion DJ, Schwarcz TH, and Mentzer RM Jr, *Ann Surg.* 2001;233(6):801–808

ABSTRACT

Objective To evaluate the University of Kentucky experience in treating acute intestinal ischemia to elucidate factors that contribute to survival.

Summary Background Data Acute intestinal ischemia is reported to have a poor prognosis, with survival rates ranging from 0% to 40%. This is based on several reports, most of which were published more than a decade ago. Remarkably, there is a paucity of recent studies that report on current outcome for acute mesenteric ischemia.

Methods A comparative retrospective analysis was performed on patients who were diagnosed with acute intestinal ischemia between May 1993 and July 2000. Patients were divided into two cohorts: nonthrombotic and thrombotic causes. The latter cohort was subdivided into three etiologic subsets: arterial embolism, arterial thrombosis, and venous thrombosis. Patient demographics, clinical characteristics, risk factors, surgical procedures, and survival were analyzed. Survival was compared with a collated historical series.

Results Acute intestinal ischemia was diagnosed in 170 patients. The etiologies were nonthrombotic (102/170, 60%), thrombotic (58/170, 34%), or indeterminate (10/170, 6%). In the thrombotic cohort, arterial embolism accounted for 38% (22/58) of the cases, arterial thrombosis for 36% (21/58), and venous thrombosis for 26% (15/58). Patients with venous thrombosis were younger. Venous thrombosis was observed more often in men; arterial thrombosis was more frequent in women. The survival rate was 87% in the venous thrombosis group versus 41% and 38% for arterial embolism and thrombosis, respectively. Compared with the collated historical series, the survival rate was 52% versus 25%.

Conclusions These results indicate that the prognosis for patients with acute intestinal ischemia is substantially better than previously reported.

Original Author Commentary: Eric D. Endean

Vascular causes for acute mesenteric ischemia (AMI) include arterial embolus, arterial thrombosis, and portal venous thrombosis. Historically, AMI is associated with a high mortality. Many factors contribute to this poor prognosis and include the relative infrequency of mesenteric ischemia as a cause for abdominal symptoms, lack of specific physical or laboratory findings, and the fact that many patients who present with AMI are elderly with comorbid conditions and limited physiologic reserve.

While we recognized the poor prognosis associated with AMI, we felt that the contemporary outcomes may be better than the reported 10%–38% survival rate. This led us to review our experience with AMI. The study was limited to patients who had AMI either due to arterial embolus or thrombosis or mesenteric venous thrombosis.

In the entire group of patients, the survival rate was 52%, seeming to confirm our hypothesis that the survival rate was better than previously reported. However, when evaluating each cohort of patients, the survival rate for patients with arterial embolus was 41%, arterial thrombosis was 38%, and mesenteric venous thrombosis was 87%. These results, while at the low end of the reported survival rates, continued to demonstrate poor prognosis. As other authors have emphasized, we also highlighted the need for early diagnosis and intervention as a strategy to improve survival. Interestingly, in our series, 13 patients (5 embolus, 8 thrombosis) had no intervention due to the extensive bowel infarction found at laparotomy. We suggest that these patients had progressed to this point in part because of delay in diagnosis and/or intervention. If these patients were excluded from the analysis, the survival rate in those who had an intervention would have been 53% for those with an embolus and 62% for those with arterial thrombosis.

Our study again emphasizes the need for early diagnosis and intervention for patients with AMI. Since our study was done prior to the era when CT was routinely utilized for patients who presented with abdominal pain, it may be that with routine CT scanning, AMI will be diagnosed earlier, leading to earlier intervention and, hopefully, improved outcomes.

CHAPTER 9

Appendicitis

Review by Contributor: Stephen M. Cohn

For about 12 centuries we were not aware that the appendix existed, as our early understanding of anatomy was based upon the teachings of Galen, who failed to identify this anatomic structure. Galen dissected monkeys, which lack an appendix (found only in humans and a few animal species such as dogs, rabbits, and some marsupials). It has been postulated that the appendix may represent a "safe house" for commensal bacteria, capable of repopulating the colon after a catastrophic event which might eradicate gut flora. (This concept is supported by the success of fecal transplantation in recurrent *Clostridia difficile* colitis.) Probably the first description of appendicitis, termed "passio iliaca," was by John of Arderne, a noted physician of the fourteenth century. This "barber surgeon" was recognized as the individual who devised methods to dramatically reduce mortality in treating fistula-in-ano, a common nearly universally fatal ailment of the Middle Ages. The "worm" (vermiformis) is visible in the drawings of Da Vinci (1492) and Vesalius (1543). Inflammation of the appendix was first described at autopsy in the eighteenth century, after perforation (Heister) and gangrene (Hunter). Appendectomies were attempted without much success in the 1700s, but in 1843 Parker reported the successful drainage of an appendiceal abscess, and Tate later described removing a gangrenous appendix from a young girl who survived in 1880. The term appendicitis was coined by Fitz in 1886 in describing the pathology of perforating appendiceal inflammation which he identified in 25 cases. By the turn of the twentieth century, appendectomy was becoming commonplace and its resultant mortality more limited (Williams, 1983).

Today, the risk of appendicitis is about 10% in the US population, with a mean age of 31. About 20% of patients present with perforation. The appendix is retrocecal in 65% of cases, and pelvic in location in 31%, a fact which certainly contributes to its confusing and often atypical clinical presentation. While abdominal pain is universal, fever and leukocytosis are variable findings. Of note, pain medications have been proven to reduce patient discomfort without obscuring physical findings or delaying intervention (Attard et al., 1992). The Alvarado score has aided in stratifying patients at risk (Alvarado, 1986). CT is the preferred diagnostic imaging technique in adults, with an accuracy rate of about 95% (Rao et al., 1998) (similar to that found with surgeon evaluation alone). There has been a reduction in the removal of normal appendices in the CT era, but the appendiceal perforation rates have actually increased over the last 20 years. In addition, many patients who may have been observed prior to CT scanning are now undergoing removal of very "early" appendicitis. MRI is valuable during pregnancy, and studies have demonstrated that the appendix does not move cephalad (i.e., remains in the same position) during gestation, contrary to previously held beliefs. Fetal mortality is much higher with perforated appendicitis, but nontherapeutic appendectomy is not as dangerous. Therefore, early open appendectomy (laparoscopy doubles the fetal loss rate) is preferred during pregnancy when appendicitis is suspected.

Appendectomy is a common procedure (over 325,000 cases yearly in the United States). The laparoscopic approach is often used in women of childbearing age, the obese (BMI > 30), and the elderly. Non-obese males are more likely to undergo open appendectomy. The laparoscopic technique is associated with a lower wound infection rate but a higher incidence of abdominal abscesses, particularly after perforated appendicitis. In addition, laparoscopic appendectomy is associated with considerably higher costs, and small, probably irrelevant, reductions in hospital stay and return to work. Surprisingly, laparoscopy is utilized in about 90% of adults with appendicitis undergoing appendectomy in the United States (Sauerland et al., 2010). Appendicitis is a polymicrobial infection that requires antibiotic coverage of both Gram-negative pathogens and anaerobes for optimal results. Antibiotic treatment is tailored to the severity of disease, with longer duration treatment reserved for the more clinically complex situations (perforation, abscess, phlegmon) (Sawyer et al., 2015). After perforation, wound infection (~40%) and intra-abdominal abscess (~10%) are common and increase the cost of care dramatically. Complicated appendicitis including abscess and phlegmon occurs in only about 4% of patients, but the course is long and complex (20% need drainage and 7% recur). Early operative intervention in complicated appendicitis should be avoided and is associated with a 300% increase in morbidity (Andersson and Petzold, 2007). Interval appendectomy is rarely indicated in the patient with no history of abscess or a major complication, as recurrence is very unusual.

The most controversial issue regarding the management of acute appendicitis in the twenty-first century, other than whether to employ the laparoscopic versus open surgical approach, is probably whether or not to treat this condition in a similar fashion to acute diverticulitis, with antibiotics alone. There is accumulating data in adults (and some in children) which suggests that uncomplicated acute appendicitis can be successfully managed with antibiotics alone in about 80% of patients, without an increased risk of perforation or complications (Salminen et al., 2015). The higher costs of surgery and the post-surgical risks of adhesive bowel obstruction and ventral hernia (trocar site hernia incidence is underappreciated) must be balanced with the danger of appendicitis recurrence. For individuals with uncomplicated appendicitis who are about to depart on travel expeditions to remote areas such as Antarctica or the Himalayas, it appears prudent to undergo an appendectomy to eliminate the likelihood of recurrent appendicitis in such austere environments. For the rest of us, while surgery is the mainstay in management of acute appendicitis, antibiotic management is looking like a favorable alternative to going under the knife.

Note: Despite 22,643 references to acute appendicitis in the world's literature according to PubMed (and 14,911 in English), there remain limited high-quality studies, and most all of the recommendations for directing management are Grade B level based on Level II or III data).

ANNOTATED REFERENCES FOR APPENDICITIS

1. Williams GR. Presidential address: History of appendicitis. *Ann Surg.* 1983;195(5): 495–506.

   The author describes the evolution of our current understanding and management of acute appendicitis. Pioneers in this field such as Fitz and Parker are nicely portrayed, along with delineation of some famous individuals who have suffered from this ailment; that is, Harvey Cushing while a surgical resident and King Edward VII prior to his coronation.

2. Attard AR, Corlett MJ, Kidner NJ, Leslie AP, Fraser IA. Safety of early pain relief for acute abdominal pain. *BMJ.* 1992;305(6853):554–556.

   In this early randomized trial, 100 patients were randomized to papaveretum versus saline, and the narcotic medication was effective in reducing abdominal pain without interfering with the ability of the clinician to accurately diagnose appendicitis.

3. Alvarado A. A practical score for the early diagnosis of acute appendicitis. *Ann Emerg Med.* May 1986;15:557–564.

   The author describes a simple scoring system for identifying patients with abdominal pain who are at increased risk for having acute appendicitis. Analysis of 305 patients revealed eight factors to be predictive of appendicitis: localized tenderness in the right lower quadrant, leukocytosis, migration of pain, increased number of immature leukocytes, fever, nausea-vomiting, anorexia, and direct rebound tenderness.

4. Rao PM, Rhea JT, Novelline RA, Mostafavi AA, McCabe CJ. Effect of computed tomography of the appendix on treatment of patients and use of hospital resources. *N Engl J Med.* 1998;338:141–6.

   The authors performed appendiceal CT scan on 100 consecutive patients with abdominal pain as a method of early identification of acute appendicitis. They changed the treatment delivered to the majority of their population and accurately diagnosed acute appendicitis in 98% of patients (53 had appendicitis). Subsequently, the CT has come to replace clinical assessment by a surgeon in the initial evaluation of the patient with suspected appendicitis.

5. Sauerland S, Jaschinski T, Neugebauer EAM. Laparoscopic versus open surgery for suspected appendicitis (Review). *Cochrane Library.* 2010. (http://onlinelibrary.wiley.com/ doi/10.1002/14651858.CD001546.pub3/full)

   This Cochrane Library compilation of the results of 56 randomized trials compared laparoscopic with open appendectomy and found that the laparoscopic technique lowered wound infection rates (OR 0.43) but increased the risk of abdominal abscess after perforation (OR 1.87). Pain on day 1 after surgery was reduced after laparoscopy by 8 mm (CI 5 to 11 mm) on a 100-mm visual analog scale. The laparoscopic technique increased hospital costs but effectively reduced both the length of hospital stay (1.1 day) and the time to return to outside activities. Diagnostic laparoscopy reduced the risk of a negative appendectomy (RR 0.37).

6. Sawyer RG, Claridge JA, Nathens AB et al. Trial of short-course antimicrobial therapy for intraabdominal infection. *N Engl J Med.* 2015;372:1996–2005.

This large randomized trial (n = 518) supported the notion that a fixed postoperative course (4 days) of antibiotics was equivalent to a longer antibiotic course which was focused upon resolution of fever and leukocytosis. It was unfortunately limited by the fact that nearly 20% of the fixed antibiotic duration group crossed over to the longer treatment group.

7. Andersson RE, Petzold MG. Nonsurgical treatment of appendiceal abscess or phlegmon a systematic review and meta-analysis. *Ann Surg.* 2007;246:741–748.

These authors reviewed the available data on the benefits of conservative management of patients with complicated appendicitis. They found that about 20% of these patients required percutaneous abscess drainage, that early surgery was associated with a higher morbidity (OR 3.3), and that there was a 7% risk of recurrence.

Landmark Article of 21st Century

ANTIBIOTIC THERAPY VS. APPENDECTOMY FOR TREATMENT OF UNCOMPLICATED ACUTE APPENDICITIS: THE APPAC RANDOMIZED CLINICAL TRIAL

Salminen P, Paajanen H, Rautio T, Nordström P, Aarnio M, Rantanen T, Tuominen R, Hurme S, Virtanen J, Mecklin JP, Sand J, Jartti A, Rinta-Kiikka I, and Grönroos JM, *JAMA.* 2015;313(23):2340–2348

ABSTRACT

Importance An increasing amount of evidence supports the use of antibiotics instead of surgery for treating patients with uncomplicated acute appendicitis.

Objective To compare antibiotic therapy with appendectomy in the treatment of uncomplicated acute appendicitis confirmed by computed tomography (CT).

Design, Setting, and Participants The Appendicitis Acuta (APPAC) multicenter, open-label, noninferiority randomized clinical trial was conducted from November 2009 until June 2012 in Finland. The trial enrolled 530 patients aged 18–60 years with uncomplicated acute appendicitis confirmed by a CT scan. Patients were randomly assigned to early appendectomy or antibiotic treatment with a 1-year follow-up period.

Interventions Patients randomized to antibiotic therapy received intravenous ertapenem (1 g/d) for 3 days followed by 7 days of oral levofloxacin (500 mg once daily) and metronidazole (500 mg 3 times per day). Patients randomized to the surgical treatment group were assigned to undergo standard open appendectomy.

Main Outcomes and Measures The primary endpoint for the surgical intervention was the successful completion of an appendectomy. The primary endpoint for antibiotic-treated patients was discharge from the hospital without the need for surgery and no recurrent appendicitis during a 1-year follow-up period.

Results   There were 273 patients in the surgical group and 257 in the antibiotic group. Of 273 patients in the surgical group, all but 1 underwent successful appendectomy, resulting in a success rate of 99.6% (95% CI, 98.0%–100.0%). In the antibiotic group, 70 patients (27.3%; 95% CI, 22.0%–33.2%) underwent appendectomy within 1 year of initial presentation for appendicitis. Of the 256 patients available for follow-up in the antibiotic group, 186 (72.7%; 95% CI, 66.8%–78.0%) did not require surgery. The intention-to-treat analysis yielded a difference in treatment efficacy between groups of −27.0% (95% CI, −31.6% to ∞) (P = 0.89). Given the prespecified noninferiority margin of 24%, we were unable to demonstrate noninferiority of antibiotic treatment relative to surgery. Of the 70 patients randomized to antibiotic treatment who subsequently underwent appendectomy, 58 (82.9%; 95% CI, 72.0%–90.8%) had uncomplicated appendicitis, 7 (10.0%; 95% CI, 4.1%–19.5%) had complicated acute appendicitis, and 5 (7.1%; 95% CI, 2.4%–15.9%) did not have appendicitis but received appendectomy for suspected recurrence. There were no intra-abdominal abscesses or other major complications associated with delayed appendectomy in patients randomized to antibiotic treatment.

Conclusions and Relevance   Among patients with CT-proven, uncomplicated appendicitis, antibiotic treatment did not meet the prespecified criterion for noninferiority compared with appendectomy. Most patients randomized to antibiotic treatment for uncomplicated appendicitis did not require appendectomy during the 1-year follow-up period, and those who required appendectomy did not experience significant complications.

Original Author Commentary: Paulina Salminen

The APPAC study group consists mainly of senior surgeon scientists. Based on our clinical experience and the available results from the previous two Swedish trials, we wanted to assess the efficacy of antibiotic therapy for uncomplicated acute appendicitis. If antibiotic treatment would work at long-term follow-up, it might have a huge impact on surgical practice and the use of surgical resources in addition to both decreased morbidity for the patients and cost savings to society by avoiding unnecessary surgeries. Even in 2009, the trial proved to be quite controversial, raising a lot of discussion in the surgical community by challenging the over century-old strong belief of the necessity of emergency appendectomy for all appendicitis patients. This line of thinking was surprisingly prominent despite the already available data on successful nonoperative treatment starting in the 1950s (Coldrey E, *Br J Med J*. 1956;2(5007):1458–1461) and the epidemiologically and clinically proven difference between uncomplicated and complicated acute appendicitis.

At the time of APPAC study initiation, there were no trials using a computed tomography (CT) diagnosis as an inclusion criterion—the French study by Vons et al. (*Lancet* 2011;377:1573–1579) was published 2 years after the APPAC study started patient enrollment. We aimed to optimize the study setting using a CT scan–diagnosed uncomplicated acute appendicitis as an inclusion criterion. We also aimed to have a clinically sound definition of the primary endpoint for two very different treatments and using surgical logic, the treatment efficacy of appendectomy was evaluated used as successful appendectomy, i.e., no appendix, no appendicitis. In the antibiotic group, treatment success was defined as resolution of appendicitis without the need for surgical intervention at 1-year follow-up. In addition to having little clinical information about antibiotic therapy for uncomplicated acute appendicitis in order to establish the estimate for the minimal clinically important difference margin for evaluating the difference between these two treatments, there was very little information about CT scan criteria for differentiating between uncomplicated and complicated acute appendicitis. However, the used CT scan diagnosis proved to have near-perfect accuracy for both the appendicitis diagnosis (two appendectomy patients did not have histologically verified acute appendicitis) and for the appendicitis severity differential diagnosis (four appendectomy patients in the appendectomy group had complicated acute appendicitis at surgery).

Based on 1-year and 5-year follow-up results, we can conclude that antibiotic treatment for uncomplicated acute appendicitis is a viable and safe alternative to appendectomy. At 5 years, 39% (n = 100) of the antibiotic group patients underwent appendectomy either during the primary hospitalization (n = 15) or for suspected recurrence (n = 85). All of these were not initial nonresponders (n = 7) or true recurrences (n = 78); the histologically proven recurrence rate was 32% (78/241). Future research needs to focus on improving the nonoperative treatment of uncomplicated acute appendicitis by using less broad-spectrum antibiotics with shorter treatment duration or only symptomatic treatment with markedly decreased or even abolished hospital stay duration. Future studies should also assess both the optimization of the CT diagnosis using low-dose CT protocols and patient treatment preference with unbiased shared decision making between appendectomy morbidity and the risk for recurrent appendicitis after nonoperative therapy. All of these topics need to be addressed in order to fully evaluate the optimal treatment paradigm for each uncomplicated acute appendicitis patient, with options potentially ranging from symptomatic treatment to antibiotic therapy and to laparoscopic appendectomy.

Reference

Salminen P, Tuominen R, Paajanen H et al. Antibiotic therapy for uncomplicated acute appendicitis and risk of recurrent appendicitis at 5 year follow-up in the APPAC Randomized Clinical Trial. *JAMA*. 2018;320(12):1259–1265.

CHAPTER 10

Lower Gastrointestinal Bleeding

Review by Contributor: Leslie Kobayashi

Lower gastrointestinal bleeding (LGIB) is a result of blood being shed into the bowel lumen from inflamed, infected, or ischemic mucosa, friable masses, arteriovenous malformations (AVMs), or exposed/engorged vessels (diverticuli, hemorrhoids). Bleeding can be slow or rapid, and associated symptoms range from asymptomatic anemia to melena/hematochezia with shock. LGIB is a common cause of hospitalization and, in contrast to upper gastrointestinal bleeding (UGIB), has been increasing in incidence (Zhao and Encinosa, 2006). Common etiologies include diverticulosis, hemorrhoids, and masses. Other less common causes include inflammation, infection, and AVMs, although the source remains unknown in up to 30% of cases (Lee et al. 2009; Navaneethan et al. 2014). Age is the biggest risk factor for LGIB, and elderly patients account for 65% of hospitalizations (Zhao and Encinosa, 2006). Reasons for this increased risk include increased incidences of diverticulosis, AVMs, and masses, as well as the frequent usage of anticoagulant and antiplatelet agents in this population.

The first step in the management of LGIB is resuscitation with crystalloid or blood products as necessary. In patients on anticoagulants, reversal of the agent should be attempted if ongoing bleeding is suspected. This may include transfusion of fresh frozen plasma, cryoprecipitate, or platelets; activated factor VIIa or prothrombin complex concentrates; and hemodialysis. For the newer oral anticoagulants, drug-specific reversal agents exist for dabigatran, rivaroxaban, and apixaban. UGIB may present similarly to LGIB particularly in cases of rapid hemorrhage and must be excluded with nasogastric lavage. If bilious non-bloody fluid returns after lavage, UGIB can be confidently excluded. The next step in treatment is colonoscopy, which can be both diagnostic and therapeutic. Although initially urgent endoscopy was performed primarily for UGIB, a study by Jensen et al. in 2000 provided evidence to support its use in patients with LGIB as well (Jensen et al. 2000). This case controlled study of patients with diverticular bleeding demonstrated that early colonoscopy (within 6–12 hours) was associated with significantly reduced rebleeding, severe bleeding, need for surgery, and complications. The patients treated with immediate colonoscopy also had a significant reduction in time to discharge. Exact timing of colonoscopy is controversial but should ideally be performed within the first 24 hours of hospitalization, as multiple studies have confirmed higher diagnostic yield, reduced transfusions, and decreased length of stay and costs with early colonoscopy (Rios et al., 2007; Lee et al., 2009; Navaneethan et al., 2014; Strate and Gralnek, 2016).

Bowel preparation for urgent colonoscopy in patients with an active LGIB is also an area of controversy. Initially, bowel preparation in the emergent/urgent setting was felt to increase risk of perforation, and the risk of significant fluid shifting and electrolyte abnormalities with older bowel preparation methods was felt to exacerbate hemodynamic instability and potentially increase risk of associated organ dysfunction. However, more recent data suggest that modern bowel preparation is safe, may reduce the risk of perforation, and is associated with significantly improved diagnostic yield (Strate and Naumann, 2010; Strate and Gralnek, 2016). Current American College of Gastroenterology recommendations are for 6 liters of polyethylene glycol solution delivered via nasogastric tube (NGT) to be given over 3–4 hours (Strate and Gralnek, 2016). NGT delivery is recommended to increase patient tolerance of the bowel preparation, particularly in the elderly and frail. Aspiration precautions should be utilized, and promotility agents may be considered to reduce symptomatic nausea and reduce risk of vomiting and aspiration (Strate and Naumann, 2010; Strate and Gralnek, 2016).

If colonoscopy is not available or impossible due to patient intolerance or instability, angiography, computed tomography (CT), and tagged red blood cell (RBC) scans can be used to localize bleeding. Bleeding must be fairly brisk (at least 0.5–1 mL/min) to be detectable by angiography, but similar to colonoscopy it has the benefit of being potentially therapeutic as well as diagnostic (Lee et al., 2009). Diagnostic yield for angiography in LGIB ranges widely (25%–70%) but is generally higher in patients with shock and symptoms of ongoing hemorrhage (Lee et al., 2009; Strate and Naumann, 2010). Direct comparisons between diagnostic modalities are few, but suggest a higher diagnostic yield for colonoscopy (Strate and Gralnek, 2016).

Once LGIB has been localized and a specific etiology has been identified, treatment can be performed via endoscopic, angiographic, and surgical routes. Endoscopic therapies include injection of epinephrine or sclerosants, thermal contact, argon plasma coagulation, and application of clips. Optimal choice of endoscopic therapy is determined by the location, type, and characteristics of the lesion. Clips are recommended for diverticular sources, coagulation for angioectasias, and polypectomy for bleeding polyps. Injection therapy is generally recommended only to temporarily address bleeding and should be used as an adjunct to clips or coagulation/thermal hemostasis (Strate and Gralnek, 2016). Endoscopic treatments are highly effective and safe, with hemostasis rates of 80%–96%, rebleeding rates of 23%–30% (Strate and Syngal, 2005; Strate and Naumann, 2010), and complications in only 0%–2% (Strate and Naumann, 2010; Strate and Gralnek, 2016) of patients.

Angiographic therapies include angioembolization and vasopressin infusion. Angioembolization is successful in 80%–100% of patients. Rebleeding rates are variable (1%–57%), with most rates in the 10%–20% range. Vasopressin infusion is similarly successful in 62%–100% of patients, but rebleeding rates are generally higher compared to angioembolization at 40%–50% (Zuckerman and Prakash, 1999; Strate and Naumann, 2010; Kaltenbach et al., 2012). The most significant complication following angiographic intervention is bowel ischemia; however, this is rare in modern studies, occurring in 1%–4% of cases (Strate and Gralnek, 2016).

Given the efficacy and safety of endoscopic and angiographic intervention, the need for surgical intervention is low. Indications for surgery include hemodynamic instability despite adequate resuscitation, excessive transfusion requirements, and failure of endoscopic or angiographic therapies (Lee et al., 2009). For the first episode of rebleeding, repeat colonoscopy or angiography should be attempted before surgical resection is considered. Once the decision to proceed to surgery is made, it is essential that bleeding is localized prior to surgical exploration. Accurate preoperative localization reduces the amount of bowel lost, improves rates of hemostasis, and is associated with decreased morbidity and mortality (Zuckerman and Prakash, 1999; Lee et al., 2009). Morbidity and mortality in patients with LGIB treated with surgery is high and is significantly increased following blind resection compared to directed segmental colectomy (Zuckerman and Prakash, 1999; Lee et al., 2009).

LGIB is associated with a low overall mortality, with rates ranging from 0.3%–5%. Patients with shock, the elderly, those developing LGIB after hospital admission, and those requiring surgery have the highest mortality (Zuckerman and Prakash, 1999; Rios et al., 2007; Lee et al., 2009; Navaneethan et al., 2014).

ANNOTATED REFERENCES FOR LOWER GASTROINTESTINAL BLEEDING

1. Zhao Y, Encinosa W. *Hospitalizations for Gastrointestinal Bleeding in 1998 and 2006: Statistical Brief #65. Health care Cost and Utilization Project (HCUP) Statistical Briefs.* Rockville (MD): Agency for Health care Research and Quality (US); 2006.

   In this population-based study, the authors summarize the Health care Cost and Utilization Project findings for hospitalizations due to gastrointestinal bleeding from 1998–2006. Overall hospitalizations due to UGIB decreased nationwide despite increases in the diagnosis of gastroesophageal reflux. In contrast, hospitalizations due to LGIB increased 8%. In addition, while overall hospitalizations for GIB among the elderly decreased over time, patients ≥65 years accounted for 65% of all hospitalizations. The overall mortality declined 23%, from 3.9% to 3%.

2. Lee J, Costantini TW, Coimbra R. Acute lower GI bleeding for the acute care surgeon: Current diagnosis and management. *Scand J Surg.* 2009;98(3):135–142.

   This review summarizes the major studies of LGIB up to 2009 with an emphasis on the diagnostic modalities that should be familiar to the acute care surgeon who may be consulted for patients with significant acute LGIB.

3. Navaneethan U, Njei B, Venkatesh PG, et al. Timing of colonoscopy and outcomes in patients with lower GI bleeding: A nationwide population-based study. *Gastrointest Endosc.* 2014;79(2):297–306.e12.

   This study of the Nationwide Inpatient Sample from the year 2010 describes the national utilization of colonoscopy for the treatment of LGIB. Over 58,000 patients were analyzed, of which 22,720 underwent colonoscopy. Patients undergoing early colonoscopy (<24 hours of admission) were compared to those who underwent the procedure late (>24 hours). Patients in the early colonoscopy group had a shorter length of stay, decreased need for blood transfusion, and lower costs.

4. Strate LL, Gralnek IM. ACG Clinical Guideline: Management of patients with acute lower gastrointestinal bleeding. *Am J Gastroenterol.* 2016;111(5):755.

   The American College of Gastroenterology 2016 Clinical Management Guidelines for Acute LGIB provide a summary of the key studies to date on LGIB and grade the quality of the data available. Recommendations on initial evaluation, resuscitation, workup, and treatment are provided along with the strength of each recommendation based on the quality of available data evaluated by the GRADE system.

5. Rios A, Montoya MJ, Rodriguez JM, et al. Severe acute lower gastrointestinal bleeding: Risk factors for morbidity and mortality. *Langenbecks Arch Surg.* 2007;392(2):165–171.

   The authors retrospectively examined a cohort of patients with LGIB at a single center. Risk factors for emergency surgery, morbidity, mortality, and rebleeding were analyzed. The authors found urgent colonoscopy was associated with higher diagnostic yield. Urgent surgery was required in 14% of patients; shock and location of bleeding were significant predictors for the need for surgery. Presence of comorbid conditions and surgery were both associated with higher mortality.

6. Strate LL, Naumann CR. The role of colonoscopy and radiological procedures in the management of acute lower intestinal bleeding. *Clin Gastroenterol Hepatol.* 2010;8(4):333–343. quiz e44.

   The authors of this meta-analysis describe the role of colonoscopy in acute LGIB. The results favor colonoscopy as the diagnostic and therapeutic technique of choice due to increased diagnostic yield compared to CT angiography and tagged RBC scans, and lower rates of rebleeding and complications when compared to angiography. They also advocate for early colonoscopy (within 24 hours) and use of bowel preparation, as both are associated with better outcomes.

7. Strate LL, Syngal S. Predictors of utilization of early colonoscopy vs. radiography for severe lower intestinal bleeding. *Gastrointest Endosc.* 2005;61(1):46–52.

   This cohort study of 252 patients with severe acute LGIB at a single center compared early colonoscopy to angiography and radionuclide scans. The authors found that early colonoscopy was associated with higher diagnostic yield (85% vs. 45%), lower transfusion requirements (3 units vs. 5.5 units), and hospital length of stay (2.6 days vs. 4.5 days).

8. Zuckerman GR, Prakash C. Acute lower intestinal bleeding. Part II: Etiology, therapy, and outcomes. *Gastrointest Endosc.* 1999;49(2):228–238.

   The authors provide a brief but comprehensive review of the etiologies of LGIB, the risk factors associated with bleeding episodes (in particular the role of nonsteroidal anti-inflammatory agents in increasing risk of LGIB as well as rebleeding), and the endoscopic, angiographic, and surgical therapies available.

9. Kaltenbach T, Watson R, Shah J et al. Colonoscopy with clipping is useful in the diagnosis and treatment of diverticular bleeding. *Clin Gastroenterol Hepatol.* 2012;10(2):131–137.

   This retrospective review of patients with LGIB at two VA hospitals describes the utilization of colonoscopy and efficacy of endovascularly placed clips for control of diverticular LGIB. The authors found that 88% of diverticular sources of hemorrhage were successfully controlled with clips. No early rebleeding or complications were found in this study. Median follow-up of 35 months found a late rebleeding rate of 22%, of which 29% required repeat colonoscopy.

Landmark Article of 21st Century

URGENT COLONOSCOPY FOR THE DIAGNOSIS AND TREATMENT OF SEVERE DIVERTICULAR HEMORRHAGE

Jensen DM, Machicado GA, Jutabha R, and Kovacs TO, *N Engl J Med*. 2000;342(2):78–82

ABSTRACT

Background Although endoscopy is often used to diagnose and treat acute upper gastrointestinal bleeding, its role in the management of diverticulosis and lower gastrointestinal bleeding is uncertain.

Methods We studied the role of urgent colonoscopy in the diagnosis and treatment of 121 patients with severe hematochezia and diverticulosis. All patients were hospitalized, received blood transfusions as needed, and received a purge to rid the colon of clots, stool, and blood. Colonoscopy was performed within 6–12 hours after hospitalization or the diagnosis of hematochezia. Among the first 73 patients, those with continued diverticular bleeding underwent hemicolectomy. For the subsequent 48 patients, those requiring treatment received therapy, such as epinephrine injections or bipolar coagulation, through the colonoscope.

Results Of the first 73 patients, 17 (23%) had definite signs of diverticular hemorrhage (active bleeding in 6, nonbleeding visible vessels in 4, and adherent clots in 7). Nine of the 17 had additional bleeding after colonoscopy, and 6 of these required hemicolectomy. Of the subsequent 48 patients, 10 (21%) had definite signs of diverticular hemorrhage (active bleeding in 5, nonbleeding visible vessels in 2, and adherent clots in 3). An additional 14 patients in this group (29%) were presumed to have diverticular bleeding because although they had no stigmata of diverticular hemorrhage, no other source of bleeding was identified. The other 24 patients (50%) had other identified sources of bleeding. All 10 patients with definite diverticular hemorrhage were treated endoscopically; none had recurrent bleeding or required surgery.

Conclusions Among patients with severe hematochezia and diverticulosis, at least one-fifth have definite diverticular hemorrhage. Colonoscopic treatment of such patients with epinephrine injections, bipolar coagulation, or both may prevent recurrent bleeding and decrease the need for surgery.

Editor Notes

Assessment: This small study compared outcomes following urgent colonoscopy for hematochezia (within 12 hours of admission) during two different time periods. The authors found that therapeutic endoscopy decreased the likelihood of both recurrence of bleeding and the need for surgical intervention. During the first time period (1986–1992), 17 of 73 (23%) patients had diverticular hemorrhage, and 6 underwent colectomy. In the second time period (1994–1998), 10 of 48 patients had diverticular hemorrhage and were treated with therapeutic endoscopy (none required surgery). The principle innovation of this study was aggressive employment of the hemorrhage control via endoscopy. This led to the current era where therapeutic endoscopy is nearly always successful, and surgery is rarely necessary.

Limitations: This was a prospective data collection compared to a historical control. These were two different time periods with two alternate approaches applied to patients with lower gastrointestinal bleeding. The definition of active diverticular bleeding included adherent clot and visible vessel, so many of the patients operated upon in the first group may in fact not have needed any intervention, but rather observation may have been successful. Essentially, the authors reported the outcomes when they changed their approach to bleeding (to avoid surgery).

Conclusions: This paper describes the experience of one institution during two time periods and was one of the first publications to suggest that therapeutic endoscopy could eliminate the majority of surgical interventions in the setting of lower gastrointestinal bleeding.

CHAPTER 11

Acute Diverticulitis

Review by Contributor: Akpofure Peter Ekeh

The incidence of diverticulosis has increased in Western societies over the last century and has paralleled industrialization as well as increased consumption of refined products with reduced dietary fiber. Acute diverticulitis occurs in a small subset of individuals with diverticulosis, and the majority of attacks (95%) occur in the sigmoid colon. It remains a common clinical condition that general surgeons have to manage in both the acute and long-term settings.

There has, over the last few decades, been a paucity of randomized prospective studies and high-quality studies relating to the management of acute diverticulitis. While several studies have been published, they have been mostly case series retrospective reviews, which have sometimes produced conflicting results supporting or denouncing specific management styles and interventions. Groups such as the American Society of Colon and Rectal Surgery (ASCRS) and the World Society of Emergency Surgery (WSES) have published comprehensive evidence-based guidelines on the management of colonic diverticular disease derived from the best available data to guide contemporary management. In addition, a few high-quality randomized clinical trials, some of which are referenced in this chapter, have emerged in the last decade that have added solid information to the body of literature that exists for this common malady.

The Hinchey classification, which was first described in a 1978 publication, has remained the primary method of characterizing the severity of acute diverticulitis, despite multiple alternate classification schemes that have been developed over the years. The simplicity of this classification system has led to its enduring legacy (Hinchey et al., 1978).

Acute diverticulitis can present in both uncomplicated and complicated fashions. Uncomplicated presentations can often be treated with simple antimicrobial therapy. Traditionally, this has involved initial intravenous administration with hospital admission. Increasingly, mild episodes of diverticulitis are being treated in an outpatient fashion when appropriate. Some studies have questioned the treatment of early uncomplicated diverticulitis with antimicrobial agents and have demonstrated no difference in recovery and subsequent complications in patients who received no antibiotics (Daniels et al., 2017). This is an interesting finding that will certainly be explored further in the future.

Complicated presentations involve the development of abscesses, perforations, strictures, or fistulas. These presentations occur about a quarter of the time and often require intervention (surgical or interventional radiology) beyond just antibiotic therapy.

A major change in surgical practice over the last decade has been with regard to the indications for elective sigmoid resection after repeated episodes of acute uncomplicated diverticulitis. The traditional teaching from the past had been to proceed with elective sigmoid colectomy after two attacks of acute uncomplicated diverticulitis, or after one attack in patients under 50 years of age. This was partly based on studies by Parks and others that had studied a large population of patients with acute diverticulitis and determined the risks of subsequent attacks necessitated preemptive resection. The current recommendation based on contemporary data is to individualize the decision for elective surgery on a case-by-case basis, and not based on the number of attacks or patient age (Chapman et al., 2006).

Most of the controversies and proposals for new therapeutic approaches in diverticular disease of the colon have centered on the management of complicated diverticulitis that requires emergent operative intervention. The long-standing treatment approach in complicated diverticulitis with perforation has been the Hartmann procedure (HP)—resection of the sigmoid colon, leaving a rectal stump and a sigmoid colostomy. It is, however, recognized that up to half of these patients who have undergone HP may end up never having their ostomies reversed. In addition, the ostomy reversal operation could be fraught with significant surgical complications. Consequently, other operative approaches have been considered as alternatives to the traditional HP. These include sigmoid resection with primary anastomosis (PA), sigmoid resection with primary anastomosis plus diverting ileostomy, laparoscopic sigmoid resection with/without primary anastomosis, and laparoscopic lavage.

Two randomized studies have compared HP to PA in Hinchey III and IV patients. (Oberkofler et al., 2012; Bridoux et al., 2017) They both demonstrate a similar mortality and complication profile in both groups but a consistently significantly higher ostomy reversal rate in the PA groups. These two studies were performed with the use of proximal diverting loop ileostomies. Other papers have described the use of primary anastomoses without any diverting ileostomy in acute diverticulitis with good results.

In the acute setting, laparoscopic sigmoid resection with or without PA has been described and can be considered in the emergency setting in situations where the surgeon has adequate requisite laparoscopic experience. Furthermore, the use of "damage control surgery" strategies involving sigmoid colon excision and temporary abdominal closure in clinically unstable patients has been described with the patients returning to the operating room following adequate resuscitation and restoration physiologic parameters.

Laparoscopic lavage in acute complicated diverticulitis with purulent perfo-rated diverticulitis is a method that had been increasingly described in recent publications. Two Scandinavian randomized prospective trials examined closely the use of this modality. The larger of these two studies (SCANDIV, referenced below), which had a longer follow-up period, demonstrated laparoscopy did not necessarily lead to fewer complications but noted more reoperations due to failure of the modality as well as worse secondary outcomes. Laparoscopic lavage has therefore not been largely recommended as the "replacement" for surgical resec-tion. The danger of misdiagnosing a colonic malignancy due to the lack of patho-logic assessment of the specimen is also a risk, as demonstrated in this SCANDIV study.

The management of acute diverticulitis continues to evolve. Practice patterns will cor-respondingly continue to change as more clinical trials and high-quality data on the subject is published.

ANNOTATED REFERENCES FOR ACUTE DIVERTICULITIS

1. Parks TG. Natural history of diverticular disease of the colon. A review of 521 cases. *Br Med J*. 1969;4:639–645.

   This was a case series from Northern Ireland in which the clinical course of 521 patients with diverticular disease of the colon was followed. This publication expounded on the natural history of diverticulitis as it was comprehended at the time and contributed to the understanding the course of the disease in the pre-CT era.

2. Hinchey EF, Schaal PG, Richards GK. Treatment of perforated diverticular disease. *Adv Surg*. 1978;12:85–109.

   Hinchey et al. first proposed a simple classification scheme in this paper that remains the gold standard today.

3. Aldoori WH, Giovannucci EL, Rimm EB, Wing AL, Trichopoulos DV, Willet WC. A prospective study of diet and the risk of symptomatic diverticular disease in men. *Am J Clin Nutr*. 1994;60:757–764.

   In this study, the dietary patterns of 47,888 men in the United States were followed prospectively for a 4-year period and observed for the development of new onset of acute diverticulitis. This was noted to occur in 385 of the subjects. There was an increased risk of developing symptomatic diverticular disease in men with low dietary fiber consump-tion. The consumption of a high intake of total fat and large red meat consumption also was noted to augment the risk.

4. Chapman JR, Dozois EJ, Wolff BG, Gullerud RE, Larson DR. Diverticulitis: A pro-gressive disease? Do multiple recurrences predict less favorable outcomes? *Ann Surg*. 2006;243:876–830.

   An important study that demonstrated the severity and risks of an attack of diverticulitis did not necessarily correlate with the number of prior attacks. This was one of the pub-lications that challenged the long-standing dogma of the need for elective sigmoid colon resection following two attacks of acute diverticulitis.

5. Oberkofler CE, Rickenbacher A, Raptis DA et al. A multicenter randomized clinical trial of primary anastomosis or Hartmann's procedure for perforated left colonic diverticulitis with purulent or fecal peritonitis. *Ann Surg.* 2012;256:819–827.

Landmark Papers

6. Feingold D, Steele SR, Lee S et al. Practice parameters for the treatment of sigmoid diverticulitis. *Dis Colon Rectum.* 2014;57:284–294.

A useful resource for addressing typical questions relating to the management of diverticular disease with multiple references on different aspects of care.

7. Schultz JK, Yaqub S, Wallon C et al.; SCANDIV Study Group. Laparoscopic lavage vs. primary resection for acute perforated diverticulitis: The SCANDIV randomized clinical trial. *JAMA.* 2015;314:1364–1375.

This important study performed at 21 sites in Sweden and Norway randomized 199 patients with perforated diverticulitis requiring surgery into either a laparoscopic lavage or perforated diverticulitis group. Postoperative complications in both groups were equivalent, as were colon resection rates, postop quality of life, and 90-day mortality rate. The reoperation rate was, however, significantly higher in the laparoscopic lavage group, which however had shorter operating times. Importantly, four carcinomas (about 4%) were missed in the laparoscopic lavage group. The authors' conclusion was that their data did not support the use of laparoscopic lavage in perforated diverticulitis.

8. Sartelli M, Catena F, Ansaloni L et al. WSES Guidelines for the management of acute left sided colonic diverticulitis in the emergency setting. *World J Emerg Surg.* 2016;11:37.

This paper was a comprehensive review of several issues surrounding treatment controversies in acute diverticulitis and proffering a number of evidence-based guidelines based on the available data at the time of publication. It is a good source for reference.

9. Bridoux V, Regimbeau JM, Ouaissi M et al. Hartmann's procedure or primary anastomosis for generalized peritonitis due to perforated diverticulitis: A prospective multicenter randomized trial (DIVERTI). *J Am Coll Surg.* 2017;225:798–805.

This multi-institutional study from France randomized 102 patients with acute diverticulitis requiring emergency surgical intervention to either HP or PA (with ileostomy) over a 4-year period with a subsequent 18-month follow up. Mortality, which was the primary outcome, was similar in both groups, as were other secondary outcomes such as morbidity and length of stay. The reversal rate, however, was markedly significant: 96% versus 65% in the PA versus HP groups. They concluded based on their data that PA (with diversion) was a more favorable option than HP.

10. Daniels L, Ünlü Ç, de Korte N et al.; Dutch Diverticular Disease (3D) Collaborative Study Group. Randomized clinical trial of observational versus antibiotic treatment for a first episode of CT-proven uncomplicated acute diverticulitis. *Br J Surg.* 2017;104:52–61.

In this multi-site study from the Netherlands, 528 patients with a first episode of CT-proven uncomplicated diverticulitis were randomized into two groups—antibiotic treatment versus observation. There was no difference in the endpoints, which were median time to recovery, complicated diverticulitis, ongoing diverticulitis, sigmoid resection, readmission, adverse events, and mortality. Hospital stay was shorter in the observation group.

A MULTICENTER RANDOMIZED CLINICAL TRIAL OF PRIMARY ANASTOMOSIS OR HARTMANN'S PROCEDURE FOR PERFORATED LEFT COLONIC DIVERTICULITIS WITH PURULENT OR FECAL PERITONITIS

Oberkofler CE, Rickenbacher A, Raptis DA, Lehmann K, Villiger P, Buchli C, Grieder F, Gelpke H, Decurtins M, Tempia-Caliera AA, Demartines N, Hahnloser D, Clavien PA, and Breitenstein S, *Ann Surg.* 2012;256(5):819–827

ABSTRACT

Objectives   To evaluate the outcome after Hartmann's procedure (HP) versus primary anastomosis (PA) with diverting ileostomy for perforated left-sided diverticulitis.

Background   The surgical management of left-sided colonic perforation with purulent or fecal peritonitis remains controversial. PA with ileostomy seems to be superior to HP; however, results in the literature are affected by a significant selection bias. No randomized clinical trial has yet compared the two procedures.

Methods   Sixty-two patients with acute left-sided colonic perforation (Hinchey III and IV) from four centers were randomized to HP (n = 30) and to PA (with diverting ileostomy, n = 32), with a planned stoma reversal operation after 3 months in both groups. Data were analyzed on an intention-to-treat basis. The primary endpoint was the overall complication rate. The study was discontinued following an interim analysis that found significant differences of relevant secondary endpoints as well as a decreasing accrual rate.

Results   Patient demographics were equally distributed in both groups (Hinchey III: 76% vs. 75% and Hinchey IV: 24% vs. 25%, for HP vs. PA, respectively). The overall complication rate for both resection and stoma reversal operations was comparable (80% vs. 84%, P = 0.813). Although the outcome after the initial colon resection did not show any significant differences (mortality 13% vs. 9% and morbidity 67% vs. 75% in HP vs. PA), the stoma reversal rate after PA with diverting ileostomy was higher (90% vs. 57%, P = 0.005) and serious complications (Grades IIIb-IV: 0% vs. 20%, P = 0.046), operating time (73 minutes vs. 183 minutes, P < 0.001), hospital stay (6 days vs. 9 days, P = 0.016), and lower in-hospital costs (US $16,717 vs. US $24,014) were significantly reduced in the PA group.

Conclusions   This is the first randomized clinical trial favoring PA with diverting ileostomy over HP in patients with perforated diverticulitis.

Editor Notes

Assessment: This was a small study in patients with perforated left-sided diverticulitis performed at four centers in Switzerland. Patients were randomized to Hartmann's procedure (HP) versus primary anastomosis (PA) with diverting ileostomy. The mortality and morbidity appeared similar between the two groups. The overall complication rate for both resection and stoma reversal was high (80% vs. 84%, P = 0.813). Stoma reversal rate was higher for PA with diverting ileostomy compared to HP (90% vs. 57%, P = 0.05). PA also was shown to have significantly reduction in secondary outcomes (lower complications, operating time, hospital stay, and lower in-hospital costs). After the inclusion of 62 patients, the data-monitoring committee recommended to stop the trial, not only because of the lowered accrual rate but also for reasons of safety.

Limitations: This was complex study to complete, with four centers comparing two substantially different surgical procedures. Several patients could have been assessed for eligibility, but some surgeons declined trial participation, making the recruitment process difficult. Although this trial had a relatively small population (n = 62), the secondary outcome differences benefits in the PA group were notable.

Conclusions: While overall complication rate did not differ between the Hartmann procedure and primary anastomosis with diverting ostomy in the treatment of acute left-sided colonic perforation, secondary outcomes strongly favored PA.

CHAPTER 12

Large Bowel Obstruction Management

Review by Contributors: Pamela Daher-Tobia and Carlos V.R. Brown

The management of large bowel obstructions (LBO), a relatively uncommon acute care surgery problem, is a complicated and controversial topic. Traditionally treated operatively, the addition of nonoperative approaches has further expanded the treatment algorithm.

The most common etiology of LBOs is colorectal malignancy (50%), followed by complications of diverticular disease and strictures (10%–20%), volvulus of the sigmoid and cecum (10%–17%), and less commonly, inflammatory bowel strictures, extrinsic compression by carcinomatosis or extracolonic malignancies, and finally, adhesions (Yeo et al., 2013). Evidence to date conclusively supports CT scanning as the gold standard for the initial diagnosis and possible staging if applicable, with a sensitivity and specificity of over 90%, which increases with addition of combined IV, PO, and rectal contrast routes. Barium enema can be a useful adjunct at time of diagnosis in stable patients, as it can provide additional information regarding the size and tortuosity of obstructing lesions.

Much of the recent literature surrounding the treatment approaches for LBOs not only seeks to identify the ideal operative approach, but also the ideal timing of surgery and whether nonoperative bridging methods can help avoid emergent operations and improve outcomes. Most agree that surgery for acutely presenting LBO should be performed in an oncologic fashion even if no formal diagnosis of a malignancy is available.

Ascending colon obstructions are less common given the larger diameter of the colon, but often present with higher tumor burden and more advanced disease in setting of colorectal malignancies (Baer et al., 2017). Earlier studies have found significant differences in anastomotic leaks when comparing right hemicolectomies performed under emergent versus non-emergent conditions (4.3% vs. 0.5%) (Bokey et al., 1995). Others have quoted anastomotic leak rates in emergent right colectomies with primary anastomosis of up to 16% and thus advocate for terminal stoma in high-risk patients (Frago et al., 2011). Specific criteria do not exist to define this high-risk population subset, with the exception of patients that present hemodynamically unstable or with generalized peritonitis, in which resection and end ileostomy with possible distal mucous fistula is the agreed-upon treatment. Despite these issues, the majority of the literature heavily supports a right colectomy with primary ileocolic anastomosis in these cases.

The literature regarding the treatment of acute descending colon obstructions, most commonly found in the sigmoid given its smaller diameter and thicker stool burden, is more varied and controversial. In the absence of hemodynamic instability or diffuse peritonitis, a transverse loop colostomy diversion has been shown to successfully alleviate pathology, while allowing time for staging and eventually definitive oncologic treatment when needed, as well as minimizing operation times. Stomas, however, are known to have complications, such as prolapse and hernias, and efforts have centered around identifying patients where these can be avoided while preserving good outcomes. In fact, the World Society of Emergency Surgery (WSES) concluded that primary resection with primary anastomosis is a safe option in stable patients with low operative risk factors (Ansaloni et al., 2010), such as ASA <3, age <70, absence of renal failure pathology, no advanced cancer, and no severe dilation proximal colon (Biondo et al., 2004).

Despite this evidence, a Hartmann's resection is still the most common operation currently performed in setting of acute LBO requiring emergent surgery. Kronborg et al.'s randomized controlled study compared outcomes between loop colostomy diversion and Hartmann's resection and concluded no significant differences exist regarding mortality, recurrence rates, or cancer-specific survival between groups. These findings were further confirmed by a large Cochrane review in 2004 as well as a more recent randomized controlled trial by Krstic et al. (2014), which showed no difference in complication rates, transfusion rates, hospital length of stay, or mortality between these patient cohorts. Thus, loop diversion has been reserved for damage control surgery or in the setting of unresectable tumors requiring a staged approach.

Current literature identifies different treatment modalities for LBOs based on the acuity of presentation and the location of the obstruction, as the etiology and pathology behind these differ slightly. For colorectal malignancies, 15%–20% are diagnosed on presentation as an acute obstruction requiring emergent intervention. In this setting, patients often present with high tumor burden, severe malnutrition, and electrolyte imbalances, all factors contributing to high rates of stoma creations, and high morbidity and mortality when compared to colectomies in non-emergent settings. Considering this, temporizing therapies to bridge between emergent and non-emergent surgery in stable patients, such as the placement of self-expanding metallic stents (SEMs), have received considerable attention and support. SEM decompression allows for bowel prep, histologic diagnosis, evaluation for synchronous lesions, and planning for possible minimally invasive resections with primary anastomosis in an elective, controlled fashion. Many studies to date suggest a reduction in the risk of stoma creation, morbidity and mortality, improved quality of life, and lower rates of total colectomies. The largest prospective multicenter trial to date assessing safety and effectiveness of SEMs in the bridging treatment of malignant LBOs found high rates of successful stent deployment and effective decompression, resulting in 98% of their subjects receiving eventual elective surgery with minimal intervention-associated morbidity (3.3%) (Jimenez et al., 2011). Jimenez et al. further concluded that the use of SEMs avoided emergent surgery and successfully bridged toward single-stage elective resections with primary anastomosis rates twice as high as those in emergent resections, and a significant decrease in colostomy rates. Some studies have also found improved oncologic resection and prognosis after non-emergent resections allowed by use of SEMs, thus further supporting the use of these temporizing measures (Cheung et al., 2009). Others, such as Arezzo et al.'s (2017) multicenter RCT, showed similar morbidity, mortality, and oncologic outcomes between patients bridged with SEMs and those undergoing emergent colectomies. Despite conflicting data surrounding SEMs and overall underpowered RCTs, guidelines from the American Society of Colorectal Surgeons support the use of SEMs in the setting of more complicated malignant obstructive disease and high-risk patients in order to decrease the need for emergent resections, reduce rates of stoma creations, and allow for full preoperative planning and optimization to increase the rates of single-stage curative resections (Vogel et al., 2017).

ANNOTATED REFERENCES FOR LARGE BOWEL OBSTRUCTION MANAGEMENT

1. Yeo HL, Lee SW. Colorectal emergencies: Review and controversies in the management of large bowel obstruction. *J Gastrointest Surg*. 2013;17(11):2007–2012.

   Evidence-based management guidelines for the treatment for LBOs. Discusses controversies surrounding key RCTs looking at colonic stenting as bridge to elective surgery.

2. Baer C, Menon R, Bastawrous S, Bastawrous A. Emergency presentations of colorectal cancer. *Surg Clin N Am*. 2017;97:529–545.

   Review of the current literature identifying the complexities and variations surrounding the treatment of a distal large bowel and rectal obstructions versus a more standardized approach for proximal large bowel obstructions.

3. Bokey EL, Chapuis PH, Fung C et al. Postoperative morbidity and mortality following resection of the colon and rectum for cancer. *Dis Colon Rect*. 1995;5:480–486.

   Prospectively collected clinical and operative data on 1846 patients during a 20-year period was analyzed to determine the prevalence of postoperative complications after conventional surgical treatment of left and right colonic malignancies. This study evaluates the rates of anastomotic leaks after emergent versus non-emergent hemicolectomies.

4. Frago R, Biondo S, Millan M et al. Differences between proximal and distal obstructing colonic cancer after curative surgery. *Colorectal Dis*. 2011;13:e116–e122.

   Retrospective observational study of 377 patients between 1994 and 2006 evaluating morbidity, mortality, and survival rates in patients undergoing surgery for obstructive colorectal malignancies stratified based on tumor location. This study found higher anastomotic leak rates in proximal colonic tumors undergoing primary anastomosis after resection.

5. Ansaloni L, Andersson RE, Bazzoli F et al. Guidelines in the management of obstructing cancer of the left colon: Consensus Conference of the World Society of Emergency Surgery (WSES) and Peritoneum and Surgery (PnS) Society. *World J Emerg Surg*. 2010;5:29.

   Expert recommendations from WSES and PnS societies from 2010 based on one of the most extensive and comprehensive PubMed and Cochrane database literature reviews. These recommendations support use of loop colostomy diversion in complicated cases or those requiring neoadjuvant treatment and the use of Hartmann's procedure in patients at high risk for anastomotic dehiscence. Experts agree stenting as a bridge to elective surgery should be undertaken when appropriate expertise is available.

6. Biondo S, Pares D, Frago R et al. Large bowel obstruction: Predictive factors for postoperative mortality. *Dis Colon Rectum*. 2004;47:1889–1897.

Retrospective comparison of outcomes and mortality collected between 1994 and 2001 in 234 patients undergoing emergent resection for LBO. Primary anastomosis outcomes were compared to Hartmann's resection, subtotal colectomy, and diverting colostomy outcomes. This study did not find significant differences in mortality between proximal and distal colonic obstructions requiring emergent surgical intervention. Risk factors for postoperative mortality were identified across groups.

7. Kronborg O. Acute obstruction from tumor in the left colon without spread. A randomized trial of emergency colostomy versus resection. *Int J Colorectal Dis*. 1995;10:1–5.

First randomized controlled study of 121 patients undergoing emergent surgery secondary to left-sided colon obstructions between 1978 and 1993. Outcomes were compared between diverting transverse colostomies and Hartmann's resection subgroups. The colostomy subset of patients underwent shorter surgery times, fewer blood transfusions, fewer wound infections, and smaller rates of ostomy creation at the time of second stage definitive resection. Mortality and recurrence rates were not found to be significantly different.

8. De Salvo GL, Gava C, Lise M. Curative surgery for obstruction from primary left colorectal carcinoma: Primary or staged resection? *Cochrane Database Syst Rev*. 2004;(2):CD002101.

Reviews of randomized controlled trials have been limited by conflicting data and low associated statistical power.

9. Krstic S, Resanovic V, Alempijevic T et al. Hartmann's procedure vs. loop colostomy in the treatment of obstructive rectosigmoid cancer. *World J Emerg Surg*. 2014;9:52.

Randomized controlled trial aimed to identify significant differences in hospital length of stay, complication rates, and mortality in 75 patients with malignant LBOs treated with either loop colostomies or Hartmann's resection and found no significant differences between surgical approaches, thus concluding neither provided a significant advantage in this patient subset.

10. Jiménez-Pérez J, Casellas J, García-Cano J et al. Colonic stenting as a bridge to surgery in malignant large-bowel obstruction: A report from two large multinational registries. *Am J Gastroenterol*. 2011;106(12):2174–2180.

Largest prospective multicenter trial to date assessing the safety and effectiveness of SEMs (WallFlex) in malignant colorectal obstructions as a bridge between emergent and elective colectomy in a subset of 182 patients. The authors concluded SEMs were effective and carried an acceptable complication rate as a bridging method to elective surgical intervention, allowing for primary anastomosis with decreased rates of stoma creations in most patients.

11. Cheung HY, Chung CC, Tsang WW, Wong JC, Yau KK, Li MK. Endolaparoscopic approach vs. conventional open surgery in the treatment of obstructing left-sided colon cancer: A randomized controlled trial. *Arch Surg*. 2009;144(12):1127–1132.

Randomized controlled trial comparing laparoscopic colectomy after bridging with SEM placement versus immediate emergent colectomy. This study found SEM placement reduced blood loss, wound infection, anastomotic fistulas, and postoperative complications. They also found a significant increase in rates of one-stage resections and a significant decrease in rates of permanent colostomy formations.

12. Arezzo A, Balague C, Targarona E et al. Colonic stenting as a bridge to surgery versus emergency surgery for malignant colonic obstruction: Results of a multicentre randomised controlled trial (ESCO trial). *Surg Endosc.* 2017;31:3297–3305.

    This multicenter randomized controlled trial assessed the 60-day morbidity in acute left-sided large bowel obstructions secondary to malignancy bridged to elective surgery with SEMs versus those patients treated with emergent surgery. At the median follow-up of 36 months, the authors found similar morbidity and mortality rates in both groups, similar stoma formation rates, and similar oncological outcomes.

13. Vogel JD, Eskicioglu C, Weiser M, Feingold D, Steele S. The American Society of Colon and Rectal Surgeons Clinical Practice Guidelines for the Treatment of Colon Cancer. *Dis Colon Rectum.* 2017;60(10):999–1017.

    Clinical practice guidelines based on best available up-to-date evidence for management of obstructing colorectal pathology. Guidelines recommend bridging to non-emergent surgery with use of SEMs in left- and right-sided colonic obstructions in order to ensure preoperative optimization and allow for curative resections.

Landmark Study

Jiménez-Pérez J, Casellas J, García-Cano J et al. Colonic stenting as a bridge to surgery in malignant large-bowel obstruction: A report from two large multinational registries. *Am J Gastroenterol.* 2011;106(12):2174–2180.

COLONIC STENTING AS A BRIDGE TO SURGERY VERSUS EMERGENCY SURGERY FOR MALIGNANT COLONIC OBSTRUCTION: RESULTS OF A MULTICENTRE RANDOMISED CONTROLLED TRIAL (ESCO TRIAL)

Arezzo A, Balague C, Targarona E, Borghi F, Giraudo G, Ghezzo L, Arroyo A, Sola-Vera J, De Paolis P, Bossotti M, Bannone E, Forcignanò E, Bonino MA, Passera R, and Morino M, *Surg Endosc.* 2017;31:3297–3305

ABSTRACT

Background   The aim of colonic stenting with self-expandable metallic stents in neoplastic colon obstruction is to avoid emergency surgery and thus potentially reduce morbidity, mortality, and need for a stoma. Concern has been raised, however, about the effect of colonic stenting on short-term complications and long-term survival. We compared morbidity rates after colonic stenting as a bridge to surgery (SBTS) versus emergency surgery (ES) in the management of left-sided malignant large-bowel obstruction.

Methods   This multicenter randomized controlled trial was designed with the endorsement of the European Association for Endoscopic Surgery. The study population was consecutive patients with acute, symptomatic malignant left-sided large-bowel obstruction localized between the splenic flexure and 15 cm from the anal margin. The primary outcome was overall morbidity within 60 days after surgery.

Results Between March 2008 and November 2015, 144 patients were randomly assigned to undergo either SBTS or ES; 29/144 (13.9%) were excluded post-randomization mainly because of wrong diagnosis at computed tomography examination. The remaining 115 patients (SBTS n = 56, ES n = 59) were deemed eligible for analysis. The complications rate within 60 days was 51.8% in the SBTS group and 57.6% in the ES group (p = 0.529). Although long-term follow-up is still ongoing, no statistically significant difference in 3-year overall survival (p = 0.998) and progression-free survival rates between the groups has been observed (p = 0.893). Eleven patients in the SBTS group and 23 in the ES group received a stoma (p = 0.031), with a reversal rate of 30% so far.

Conclusions Our findings indicate that the two treatment strategies are equivalent. No difference in oncologic outcome was found at a median follow-up of 36 months. The significantly lower stoma rate noted in the SBTS group argues in favor of the SBTS procedure when performed in expert hands.

Editor Notes

Assessment: Patients presenting with left-sided colon obstruction from malignancy were enrolled in a prospective multicenter randomized controlled trial from three hospitals in Italy and two in Spain. The primary outcome was overall morbidity within 60 days after surgery. The study compared patients who underwent colonic stenting as a bridge to surgery (SBTS) versus emergency surgery (ES). The median time from stent placement to elective surgery was 5 days. The complication rates were not statistically different between groups (52% in the SBTS versus 57% in the ES group (p = 0.6)). The stoma rate was significantly lower in the SBTS group compared to the ES group (20% vs. 39%, p = 0.03) and only 30% of these temporary stomas were reversed. There was no survival difference over 3 years and progression-free survival rate was similar.

Limitations: The study duration was 7 years, and five centers were involved in the study. Technical success was reported in 88% (49/56) of the stented patients. Eight stent-related complications occurred, with five perforations, one bleeding, one relevant pain, and one aspiration resulting in pulmonary infection.

Conclusions: The two options of treating left-sided large bowel obstruction from malignancy appear equivalent in terms of morbidity. However, emergency surgery required stoma creation twice as often as those receiving stent placement and the authors recommended stenting as a bridge to surgery over emergency surgery when expertise is available.

CHAPTER 13

Ogilvie Syndrome or Acute Colonic Pseudo-Obstruction

Review by Contributors: Matthew J. Forestiere and Kenji Inaba

Prior to 1948, there had not been any accounts or descriptions of acute colonic pseudo-obstruction in the medical literature. Sir William Heneage Ogilvie, a dedicated British surgeon who served during both World Wars, wrote about two cases he attributed to a new clinical syndrome while working at Guy's Hospital in London. This syndrome that would soon eponymously bear his name was elegantly described as "large intestine colic due to sympathetic deprivation." Sir Ogilvie's initial description of the disease process proposed three different possibilities as to the cause of the signs and symptoms of colonic obstruction without any obstruction or colonic abnormality at surgery. The theories were that the "tumor" stimulated the parasympathetic supply to the colon, or stimulated peristalsis, or that malignant invasion interrupted the sympathetic supply to the large intestine (Ogilvie, 1948). Although to this day the exact cause is still not known, Sir Ogilvie was not far off on his postulations involving neural pathways. Today, the cause is thought to be a consequence of decreased parasympathetic activity from the sacral plexus (S2, S3, S4). The majority of the cases (~40%) in a large review of more than 400 patients involved patients who had orthopedic or pelvic surgery, recent childbirth, or spinal cord trauma, all of which could contribute to decreased parasympathetic activity (Vanek and Al-Salti, 1986).

The diagnosis of Ogilvie syndrome classically starts with a clinical picture of obstipation and increasing gaseous abdominal distention. All patients with suspected Ogilvie syndrome should have an acute low colorectal mechanical obstruction ruled out. Historically this was done with a contrast enema, but IV contrast-enhanced CT scan of the abdomen and pelvis is now routinely used in the emergent evaluation of patients with large bowel obstruction or suspected Ogilvie syndrome. Compared to contrast enemas, contemporary CT imaging is of such high quality that it is highly sensitive and specific for delineating obstruction (96% and 93% vs. 80% and 100%). They can also readily show evidence of ischemia or perforation, as well as reliably exclude intrinsic or extrinsic compression (Frager et al. 1998; Choi et al. 2008). Another important element to consider in the evaluation is the size of the dilated colon and the risk of colonic perforation. Dilation of the cecum of 12 cm warrants intervention, as the risk of perforation increases significantly when greater than 12 cm, and the associated mortality can exceed 40% (Vanek and Al-Salti, 1986; Tsirline et al., 2012).

Treatment begins by allowing nothing by mouth, nasogastric decompression, correction of electrolyte abnormalities, and removal of offending agents. While there is no standard for the duration of a trial of non-interventional management, the risk of perforation increases after failure of conservative treatment for greater than 3 days or when the colon diameter exceeds 12 cm (Vanek and Al-Salti, 1986; Tsirline et al., 2012). For patients who persist with colonic obstruction, the next step in their treatment remains neostigmine. This is a cholinesterase inhibitor that allows more acetylcholine to be present at the synapses for parasympathetic stimulation and increased contractility. When compared to placebo, neostigmine was effective in decompressing the colon in greater than 80% of patients in two randomized trials (Ponec et al., 1999; Van der Spoel et al., 2001). The side effects of neostigmine are not inconsequential and require close monitoring for severe colicky abdominal pain and bradycardia. Polyethylene glycol has also been used and shown to prevent relapse of symptoms after successful colonic decompression with either neostigmine or colonoscopy (Sgouros et al., 2006). Other medical modalities, including tegaserod, erythromycin, metoclopramide, Narcan, and methylnaltrexone, have been reported in individual case reports but have not been confirmed with larger studies.

Colonoscopic decompression as a treatment modality surfaced in the late 1970s when surgical therapy was consistently showing a high mortality rate of greater than 50%. However, colonoscopy never took over as a primary treatment option. Over the next two decades, colonoscopy with or without a long colonoscopic decompression tube increased in popularity and was shown to have success rates comparable to neostigmine, with a low risk of complications (Geller et al., 1996). The risk of recurrence after colonoscopic decompression is reported to be anywhere from 18%–40% (Geller et al., 1996; Tsirline et al., 2012). In the last few years, two larger studies have shown that colonoscopy can have similar success rates to neostigmine administration when used both as first-line therapy and as rescue therapy (Tsirline et al., 2012; Peker et al., 2017). These studies were retrospective and nonrandomized, so there is still a need for randomized, prospective, larger volume data to definitively compare colonoscopy to neostigmine.

Surgery for Ogilvie syndrome, although once considered the standard of care, is now used as a last resort and reserved for patients with ischemia or perforation. Historically, cecostomy or tube cecostomy were the most common surgical procedures of choice in this usually frail, debilitated patient population before neostigmine or endoscopy became more prominent. These procedures had higher success rates with lower morbidity and mortality when compared to more invasive surgical procedures (Vanek and Al-Salti, 1986).

Ogilvie syndrome, or acute colonic pseudo-obstruction, is a syndrome marked by massive colonic dilation without mechanical obstruction. The clinical history is important to consider as it usually occurs in patients who tend to be debilitated, with prolonged hospitalizations or a variety of contributing medical conditions and pelvic or spinal pathology. Despite this, with conservative treatment alone, it is reported that up to

30%–50% of patients will resolve within 3 days (Vanek and Al-Salti, 1986, Tsirline et al., 2012; Peker et al., 2017). Patients with persistent obstruction after conservative management should progress to the next treatment modality, as the risk of perforation increases after 3 days. The only randomized, double-blinded data available for a treatment modality is the use of neostigmine, which to this day remains a very safe, practical, and cost-effective treatment. The administration of neostigmine is not without side effects, and administration should be in a monitored setting. There is a role for colonoscopic decompression in patients who do not respond to conservative management or neostigmine therapy. Surgery should be reserved as the last treatment option for those with evidence of peritonitis, ischemia, or perforation.

ANNOTATED REFERENCES FOR OGILVIE SYNDROME OR ACUTE COLONIC PSEUDO-OBSTRUCTION

1. Ogilvie H. Large-intestine colic due to sympathetic deprivation: A new clinical syndrome. *Br Med J.* 1948;2(4579):671–673.

   The author describes the first two cases of diffuse large bowel dilation concerning for obstruction that would ultimately be labeled colonic pseudo-obstruction, or Ogilvie syndrome. Both of these cases were patients with progressive large bowel dilation and non-obstructive pattern on barium enema. At laparotomy, both patients were found to have no obvious mechanical obstruction and only metastatic disease with carcinomatosis and the majority of the disease surrounding the celiac axis or foregut. Being the first to describe this pseudo-obstruction phenomenon, the disease now bears his name.

2. Addison NV. Pseudo-obstruction of the large bowel. *JRSMV.* 1983;76:252–255.

   In this early case series of 30 patients, the author reports his findings over 25 years on pseudo-obstruction of the large bowel. Seventeen of the patients went emergently to the operating room and no mechanical obstruction was found. Of the remaining thirteen patients, five were managed with cecostomy tube and the remaining eight were treated conservatively. This author recognized that the patients without any apparent mechanical obstruction could be managed conservatively with correction of electrolytes and treatment of the primary pathology. This author also recognized that segmental colectomy is not always effective in relief of the pseudo-obstruction and that decompression is the best treatment. However, the author recommends cecostomy as primary surgical treatment.

3. Vanek VW, Al-Salti M. Acute pseudo-obstruction of the colon (Ogilvie's syndrome). An analysis of 400 cases. *Dis Colon Rectum.* 1986;29:203–210.

   The authors performed a review of the literature to that time and reviewed 400 cases of acute colonic pseudo-obstruction. This was the biggest publication of cases to date looking at surgical management of this disease. In total, 179 patients underwent a surgical procedure, with tube cecostomy and cecostomy being the most common, with morbidity (9% and 3%) and mortality (15% and 21%) being much lower than exploratory laparotomy, which had a mortality >40%. They recommended tube cecostomy or cecostomy as the surgical procedure of choice in cases without ischemia or perforation.

4. Geller A, Peterson BT, Gostout CJ. Endoscopic decompression for acute colonic pseudo-obstruction. *Gastrointest Endosc.* 1996;2:144–150.

   The authors conducted the largest to date, retrospective, single-center analysis of all colonoscopic decompression for 50 patients with acute colonic pseudo-obstruction over a 6-year period. The authors reported clinical success of 88% (44/50) of patients with colonoscopic decompression, with some of the patients also having a colonoscopically placed rectal tube. Prior studies have examined colonoscopic decompression, but this study showed you just need decompression to the splenic flexure. The report was not large enough to identify clinical predictors of success or recurrence, which had a rate of almost 20% after decompression.

5. Frager D, Rovno HDS, Baer JW, Bashist B, Friedman M. Prospective evaluation of colonic obstruction with computed tomography. *Abdom Imaging.* 1998;23:141–146.

The authors conducted the first prospective, single-center analysis of patients with suspected large bowel obstruction evaluating the diagnostic capabilities of CT compared to contrast enema (CE). The authors reported that CT correctly diagnosed obstruction in 45/47 patients (96% sensitive) and non-obstruction in 26/28 patients (93% specific). CT scan was also extremely accurate at localizing the obstruction point in 44/47 patients (94%). Comparing this to CEs, which were done in 25 patients in addition to the CT scans, the sensitivity of CE was 80%. This study was the first major study to show that CT is a viable option over CE in diagnosing and localizing large bowel obstruction.

6. Van der Spoel JL, Oudemans-van Straaten HM, Stoutenbeek CP, Bosman RJ, Zandstra DF. Neostigmine resolves critical illness-related colonic ileus in intensive care patients with multiple organ failure – A prospective, double-blind, placebo-controlled trial. *Int Care Med.* 2001;27:822–827.

The authors performed a double-blinded, placebo-controlled prospective study on 30 patients in the ICU with colonic ileus. This randomized trial confirmed the landmark paper's new and standardized treatment for colonic ileus (i.e., Ogilvie syndrome) with neostigmine. All patients in the placebo arm failed to pass stools, whereas the neostigmine arm proved successful >80%. The placebo and failed neostigmine patients were then randomly crossed over into the neostigmine arm successfully, giving the neostigmine arm 19/24 patients receiving neostigmine passing bowel movements. This study was the first major study to reaffirm the landmark paper's findings of neostigmine and acetylcholine deprivation as a potential source for colonic pseudo-obstruction, laying out a treatment standard for this rare syndrome.

7. Sgouros SN, Vlachogiannakos J, Vassiliadis K et al. Effect of polyethylene glycol electrolyte balances solution on patients with acute colonic pseudo-obstruction after resolution of colonic dilation: A prospective, randomised, placebo controlled trial. *Gut.* 2006;55:638–642.

The authors performed a prospective, randomized, placebo-controlled study on 30 patients in a single center with colonic ileus who had failed conservative management. All patients then underwent either neostigmine administration or endoscopic decompression. Here patients were randomized to receive either 29.5 g of PEG balanced solution or placebo, and patients were monitored for stool, flatus, abdominal distention, and colonic dilation on plain radiograph for 7 days. Patients who were given PEG after treatment for Ogilvie syndrome showed marked improvement in colonic dilation, abdominal circumference, number of stools, and flatus, and had no relapses. This study was the first to show promise of osmotic laxatives in preventing relapse of colonic pseudo-obstruction symptoms, although further and larger-powered studies are needed.

8. Choi JS, Lim JS, Kim H et al. Colonic pseudo-obstruction: CT findings. *AJR.* 2008;190:1521–1526.

The authors present a radiographic review of all patients with colonic pseudo-obstruction at their institution over a 5-year period. CT radiograph in all patients showed dilated proximal and transverse colon without discrete mechanical obstruction or complete transition zone. In nearly all cases, there was an intermediate transition zone which was located at or near the splenic flexure. The authors suggest that this is likely the transition of the colonic innervation from vagal to sacral nerve fibers, and the presence of this finding differentiates the disease from paralytic ileus. In this study, 75% of patients underwent surgical resection, and final histopathology showed abnormal or degenerative ganglion cells in 66%.

9. Tsirline VB, Zemlyak AY, Avery MJ et al. Colonoscopy is superior to neostigmine in the treatment of Ogilvie's syndrome. *Am J Surg.* 2012;204:849–855.

   The authors reviewed a large retrospective series of 100 patients with Ogilvie syndrome at a single institution. This paper showed that the success rate of colonic decompression with colonoscopy was 85% with 1–2 interventions compared to 55% with the same number of treatments with neostigmine, $p = 0.031$. This early success was also confirmed with radiographic evidence of improved colonic decompression with colonoscopy versus neostigmine (improvement in cecal diameters of 10.2 cm−7.1 cm with colonoscopy vs. 10.5 cm−8.8 cm with neostigmine, $p = 0.026$).

10. Peker KD, Cikot M, Bozkurt MA et al. Colonoscopic decompression should be used before neostigmine in the treatment of Ogilvie's syndrome. *Eur J Trauma Emerg Surg.* 2017;43:557–566.

    The authors reported a large retrospective, nonrandomized clinical study of sequential patients from 2008−2015 separated into two groups of patients. Group 1 (31 patients) received neostigmine as first-line treatment and subsequently had colonoscopy; Group 2 (37 patients) received colonoscopy first, followed by neostigmine. They found that patients receiving colonoscopy first had a significantly better first-line treatment response than patients receiving neostigmine first (83.8% vs. 48.4%, $p = 0.002$). The authors recommend colonoscopic decompression as first-line therapy by an experienced endoscopist after failed conservative management.

Landmark Article

NEOSTIGMINE FOR THE TREATMENT OF ACUTE COLONIC PSEUDO-OBSTRUCTION

Ponec RJ, Saunders MD, and Kimmey MB, *N Engl J Med.* 1999;341(3):137–141

ABSTRACT

Background   Acute colonic pseudo-obstruction—that is, massive dilation of the colon without mechanical obstruction—may develop after surgery or severe illness. Although it may resolve with conservative therapy, colonoscopic decompression is sometimes needed to prevent ischemia and perforation of the bowel. Uncontrolled studies have suggested that neostigmine may be an effective treatment.

Methods   We studied 21 patients with acute colonic pseudo-obstruction. All had abdominal distention and radiographic evidence of colonic dilation, with a cecal diameter of at least 10 cm, and had had no response to at least 24 hours of conservative treatment. We randomly assigned 11 to receive 2.0 mg of neostigmine intravenously and 10 to receive intravenous saline. A physician who was unaware of the patients' treatment assignments recorded clinical response (defined as prompt evacuation of flatus or stool and a reduction in abdominal distention), abdominal circumference, and measurements of the colon on radiographs. Patients who had no response to the initial injection were eligible to receive open-label neostigmine 3 hours later.

Results   Ten of the eleven patients who received neostigmine had prompt colonic decompression, as compared with none of the ten patients who received placebo ($P < 0.001$). The median time to response was 4 minutes (range, 3–30). Seven patients in the placebo group and the one patient in the neostigmine group without an initial response received open-label neostigmine; all had colonic decompression. Two patients who had an initial response to neostigmine required colonoscopic decompression for recurrence of colonic distention; one eventually underwent subtotal colectomy. Side effects of neostigmine included abdominal pain, excess salivation, and vomiting. Symptomatic bradycardia developed in two patients and was treated with atropine.

Conclusions   In patients with acute colonic pseudo-obstruction who have not had a response to conservative therapy, treatment with neostigmine rapidly decompresses the colon.

Editor Notes

Assessment: In this small randomized trial, 21 patients with acute colonic pseudo-obstruction who had failed 24 hours of conservative management were randomized to neostigmine or placebo. While 90% of patients experienced colonic decompression after 2.0 mg of neostigmine within a median of 4 minutes, none of the placebo patients resolved initially. Nonresponders had a high response rate (70%) after crossing over to receive neostigmine.

Limitations: The power analysis in this study assumed a huge effect of the neostigmine (which was borne out in the trial). This study ideally would have included a control group undergoing colonoscopy as primary treatment, in addition to the "conservative management" arm. Patients were included with a 10-cm cecal diameter, which is the upper limit of normal size. Therefore, a higher number of patients may have responded to colonoscopy. Approximately 10% of patients had recurrence of colonic distention after neostigmine and about 20% of patients developed symptomatic bradycardia.

Conclusions: This trial changed our approach to colonic pseudo-obstruction, supporting the value of initial medical management with neostigmine.

CHAPTER 14

Colonic Volvulus

Review by Contributor: Joseph Love

The twisting or torsion of the alimentary track was first described in the Ebers Papyrus, an Egyptian medical document from around 1550 BC in which the natural course was documented as leading to intestinal "rotting." Volvulus was managed by an injection of a large quantity of air through the anus along with placement of a suppository to assist with detorsion of the bowel. It was not until 1841 when the first description of volvulus was documented in Western medical literature. By the end of the twentieth century, surgical management of intestinal volvulus was the standard of care. In 1883, Atherton described laparotomy with lysis of adhesions for the treatment of volvulus (Gingold and Murrell, 2012). Over time, three separate approaches were developed, including decompression and plication of the mesentery, resection with anastomosis, and Hartmann's procedure. In 1947, Bruusgaard introduced the idea of decompression with sigmoidoscopy for distal colonic volvulus with a rigid proctoscope. They reported on 91 patients with a 14% mortality. With this approach there was a recurrence rate of 90% and a mortality rate upwards of 40% (Bruusgaard, 1947). However, this approach led to the idea of transanal decompression of sigmoid volvulus, which is a standard practice today. With the creation of flexible endoscopy, many have advocated for its use as an adjunctive procedure in those who would not tolerate laparotomy. This modality allows for a rectal tube to be placed as a means of temporizing in preparation for surgical intervention.

Colonic volvulus is the third leading cause of bowel obstruction worldwide. Populations most affected live in Africa, the Middle East, India, and Russia, which together are known as the "volvulus belt." The population in this region tend to be affected at a younger age (40–50) compared to Western countries, and as such tend to be healthier (Heis et al., 2008). In the United States, volvulus accounts for 10%–15% of colonic obstruction behind diverticulitis and colon cancer, and is responsible for 1%–20% of intestinal obstructions. The cause is thought to be related to a mobile portion of bowel that twists around a fixed base or mesentery, creating a closed-loop obstruction. The most common site of colonic volvulus involves the sigmoid (60.9%), followed by the cecum (34.5%), transverse (3.6%), and splenic flexure (1%) (Ballantine et al., 1985). In the United States, it is more common in the elderly population, with risk factors including previous volvulus, abdominal surgery, institutionalization, megacolon, and chronic constipation (Gingold and Murrell, 2012). These differences in demographics necessitate caution when interpreting management described from outside one's geographic region. There are no randomized control trials to guide decision management in the setting of acute colonic volvulus. However, several patterns of practice have developed as a result of describing the care of this patient population.

For complicated forms of volvulus, the management is straightforward, based on severity, consisting of laparotomy and resection of the necrotic segment. Whether or not to restore intestinal continuity depends on physiologic status and location. One Turkish series of 271 patients demonstrated 61% of their patients presented with colonic necrosis. The presence of shock, prolonged duration of symptoms, and combined colonic ileal volvulus along with severe comorbid conditions (COPD, hypertension, ischemic heart disease, heart failure, diabetes, renal failure, Parkinson disease) were associated with necrosis (Atamanalp et al., 2013). The decision to establish continuity can be immediate with an ileocolic anastomosis in the absence of peritoneal contamination for cecal volvulus. The decision differs in relation to the sigmoid colon, where a proximally dilated stool-filled segment of colon may carry a higher risk of anastomotic leak. Oren et al. evaluated the use of Hartmann's and resection with anastomosis in patients with sigmoid volvulus and found no differences in mortality (22% vs. 19%, respectively), in patients without peritoneal contamination (Oren et al., 2007). For uncomplicated cases of colonic volvulus, colonoscopy is often the initial modality for diagnosis of ischemia and treatment. In the absence of necrosis, endoscopy can convert an urgent into a "semi-elective" situation. The use of flexible endoscopy as an initial means of treatment has demonstrated variable success rates depending on the anatomy of the segment involved. While it is a relatively simple procedure, it carries a success rate of 20%–95% and a 4% mortality (Turns et al., 2004; Oren et al., 2007). It is recommended that detorsion be followed by definitive resection because of the reported recurrence rate of greater than 60% and its associated increase in mortality among patients who could otherwise tolerate surgery (Tan et al., 2010). In the absence of a randomized trial, the consensus is to perform resection within 2–5 days at the first episode. For cecal volvulus, colonoscopy is not recommended, as the efficacy for detorsion is low at around 30%. Cecal volvulus should be considered a surgical emergency (Bauman and Evans, 2018).

One of the only recent publications to address the care of colonic volvulus in the United States evaluated a nationwide inpatient sample from 2002–2010 retrospectively for admitted colonic volvulus cases. Of the estimated 3,351,152 cases admitted for bowel obstruction, only 63,749 cases (1.9%) were attributed to colonic volvulus. During this period, the incidence of cecal volvulus increased 5.53% per year and was more prevalent in young females (mid-50s). The incidence of sigmoid volvulus remained unchanged with an older population (70s) and more frequent in African Americans. With the aging population one would expect this number to increase; however, it has remained steady. The epidemiological trends may be explained by anatomic changes associated with the use of screening colonoscopy, increased use of laparoscopy, and link between pregnancy and displacement of the cecum. Colonoscopic decompression was the most common modality, with a success rate of 70%–90% mainly in sigmoid volvulus, as the cecal volvulus was mostly unsuccessful. It was rare for colonic decompression to be the sole treatment with its associated recurrence rate of 20%–70%. Moreover, the mortality rate for recurrent sigmoid volvulus presenting emergently can be as high as 33% (Halabi et al., 2014).

Surgical resection can be described broadly as resective or non-resective. Resective surgery with or without ostomy was found to be the most commonly performed surgical procedure (89.3%). Additional procedures included decompression with or without fixation or enterostomy, and laparoscopy, which was performed rarely (3.7%) for both resection and pexy of the colon. Anastomotic complications were similar between sigmoid and cecal volvulus (15.8% vs. 15.2%), indicating that the anatomic location may not play as significant a role as previously thought. Primary anastomosis may be safe in this setting and consistent with other studies with uncomplicated cases (Chauhan et al., 2015). The presence of peritonitis, bowel gangrene, and coagulopathy (includes DIC) were strongly associated with mortality (Halabi et al., 2014). This suggests that prompt management of colonic volvulus patients is essential to the optimal outcomes for this patient population.

ANNOTATED REFERENCES FOR COLONIC VOLVULUS

1. Gingold D, Murrell Z. Management of colonic volvulus. *Clin Colon Rectal Surg.* 2012;25:236–244.

   The authors present the history of colonic volvulus along with the predisposing features thought to cause its development. The early historical management along with current thoughts with references to more recent investigations are presented based on the anatomic location of the volvulized segment.

2. Bruusgaard C. Volvulus of the sigmoid colon and its treatment. *Surgery.* 1947;22(3):466–478.

   A historical study examining the presentation and management of 91 patients admitted 168 times with sigmoid volvulus. This publication presented the idea of colonic decompression with rigid proctoscopy along with its dismal recurrence rate and associate mortality.

3. Heis HA, Bani-Hani KE, Rabadi DK et al. Sigmoid volvulus in the Middle East. *World J Surg.* 2008;32(3):459–464.

   This study was a retrospective review of patients admitted over a 6-year period with diagnosis of large bowel obstruction in a region of the world reported to have higher prevalence of colonic volvulus. While they reported rates similar to Western countries (9.2%), they did comment on the younger ages seen at presentation compared to Western countries.

4. Ballantine GH, Brandner MD, Beart RW, Listrup DM. Volvulus of the colon. Incidence and mortality. *Ann Surg.* 1985;202(1):83–92.

   Patients admitted to a prominent US medical center over a 20-year period were reviewed. The modality of therapy, outcomes, and anatomic relationship were described. In addition, the authors noted the relatively low mortality rate (7%) and attributed this to the low number of patients presenting with necrotic colon. They noted other American studies reporting mortality rates of 80% for patients with gangrenous colons.

5. Ballantyne GH. Review of sigmoid volvulus: History and results of treatment. *Dis Colon Rect.* 1982;25(5):494–501.

   The author presents a history of diagnosing and managing patients with colonic volvulus. Included is a review of treatment modalities described in US literature in comparison to other regions of the world to include incidence, management, and mortality.

6. Atamanalp SS, Kisaoglu A, Ozogul B. Factors affecting bowel gangrene development in patients with sigmoid volvulus. *Ann Saudi Med.* 2013;33(2):144–148.

The authors retrospectively reviewed patients with sigmoid volvuli in a region in which sigmoid volvulus is endemic. The authors found a correlation between hypovolemic shock, prolonged duration of symptoms, over-rotation of the volvulized segment, combined ileocolonic volvulus, and significant comorbid diseases with the development of sigmoid gangrene.

7. Oren D, Atamanalp SS, Aydinli B et al. An algorithm for the management of sigmoid colon volvulus and safety of primary resection: Experience with 827 cases. *Dis Colon Rectum.* 2007;50:489–497.

The authors reviewed records of patients who underwent emergent nonoperative or operative treatment for sigmoid colon volvulus in a university setting. The authors recommend the initial management of flexible endoscopy with rectal tube placement followed by "semi-elective" resection with anastomosis of the involved segment. In the emergent setting (gangrene, peritonitis, failure to decompress) little if any delay to surgical intervention should occur to decrease morbidity and mortality.

8. Turns M, Sen M, Karadayi A, Topcu O, Yildirir C, Duman M. Our sigmoid colon volvulus experience and benefits of colonoscope in the detorsion process. *Rev ESP Enferm Dig.* 2004;96:32–35.

The authors present two distinct time frames using either rigid or flexible sigmoidoscopy for the initial management of sigmoid volvulus. They reported a higher detortion rate with the use of flexible endoscopy (60% vs. 42%) without any complications, allowing for preparation of patients for surgical resection.

9. Tan K, Chong C, Sim R. Management of acute sigmoid volvulus: An institution's experience over 9 years. *World J Surg.* 2010;83:74–78.

Authors retrospectively reviewed all patients admitted over an 8-year period and reported a high recurrence rate (>60%) for those treated conservatively with decompression and no resection. However, they did report a high successful decompression rate nonoperatively (75%). In their series, those patients needing emergent surgery had a high associated mortality rate compared to "elective" surgery (17.6% vs. 0%). They concluded patients are better served with elective resection in view of the high recurrence rate and considerable risk of emergent surgery.

10. Bauman Z, Evans C. Volvulus. *Surg Clin North Am.* 2018;98:973–993.

Authors provide a detailed review article covering intestinal volvulus. In review of cecal volvulus, they recommend all patients be considered a surgical emergency as endoscopic decompression is rarely successful (30%) and most patients will tolerate a non-oncologic resection with immediate anastomosis.

11. Halabi W, Jabari M, Kang C et al. Colonic volvulus in the United States: Trends, outcomes and predictors of mortality. *Ann Surg.* 2014;259:293–301.

12. Chauhan A, Gangji A, Menon A. Comparison of primary resection and anastomosis with defunctioning stoma in cases of uncomplicated sigmoid volvulus patients: A retrospective study. *Sch J App Med Sci.* 2015;3(2G):991–994.

Authors describe patients admitted and operated on for sigmoid volvulus over an 8-year period. Patients found to have gangrene at time of surgery were excluded. In patients with uncomplicated sigmoid volvulus, resection with primary anastomosis did not increase morbidity or mortality, decreased length of stay, and avoided the need for a second operation to reverse the patient's stoma.

COLONIC VOLVULUS IN THE UNITED STATES: TRENDS, OUTCOMES, AND PREDICTORS OF MORTALITY

Halabi WJ, Jafari MD, Kang CY, Nguyen VQ, Carmichael JC, Mills S, Pigazzi A, and Stamos MJ, *Ann Surg.* 2014;259:293–301

ABSTRACT

Introduction Colonic volvulus is a rare entity associated with high mortality rates. Most studies come from areas of high endemicity and are limited by small numbers. No studies have investigated trends, outcomes, and predictors of mortality at the national level.

Methods The Nationwide Inpatient Sample 2002–2010 was retrospectively reviewed for colonic volvulus cases admitted emergently. Patient demographics, hospital factors, and outcomes of the different procedures were analyzed. The LASSO algorithm for logistic regression was used to build a predictive model for mortality in cases of sigmoid volvulus (SV) and cecal volvulus (CV) taking into account preoperative and operative variables.

Results An estimated 3,351,152 cases of bowel obstruction were admitted in the United States over the study period. Colonic volvulus was found to be the cause in 63,749 cases (1.90%). The incidence of CV increased by 5.53% per year, whereas the incidence of SV remained stable. SV was more common in elderly males (aged 70 years), African Americans, and patients with diabetes and neuropsychiatric disorders. In contrast, CV was more common in younger females. Nonsurgical decompression alone was used in 17% of cases. Among cases managed surgically, resective procedures were performed in 89% of cases, whereas operative detorsion with or without fixation procedures remained uncommon. Mortality rates were 9.44% for SV, 6.64% for CV, 17% for synchronous CV and SV, and 18% for transverse colon volvulus. The LASSO algorithm identified bowel gangrene and peritonitis, coagulopathy, age, the use of stoma, and chronic kidney disease as strong predictors of mortality.

Conclusions Colonic volvulus is a rare cause of bowel obstruction in the United States and is associated with high mortality rates. CV and SV affect different populations, and the incidence of CV is on the rise. The presence of bowel gangrene and coagulopathy strongly predicts mortality, suggesting that prompt diagnosis and management are essential.

Editor Notes

Assessment: This study investigated the outcomes of colonic volvulus using a large national database spanning an 8-year time period. The authors reviewed 63,749 cases of colonic volvulus admitted as a cause of bowel obstruction. This population makes up just 1.9% of all cases admitted during this time for bowel obstruction. While initial endoscopy is typically attempted in stable patients, nearly half of the patients with sigmoid volvulus received a stoma at the initial operation. In the setting where there is no evidence of peritonitis or gangrene, a primary anastomosis may be safely performed; however, the rates of anastomotic complications remain quite high (over 15%). The presence of intestinal gangrene and/or peritonitis were strong predictors of mortality in the setting of colonic volvulus (9.4% sigmoid vs. 6.7% cecal).

Limitations: The accuracy of a large administrative database is always dependent on the accuracy of the data entry. In addition, there was no ICD code that differentiated cecal from sigmoid volvulus. This retrospective review of national data represents the predominant paper in recent years. No single institution has sufficient volume and experience with volvulus to warrant prospective trials.

Conclusions: This paper established the paucity of data on volvulus in the literature and the high associated morbidity and mortality associated with this condition.

CHAPTER 15

Clostridium difficile *Infection*

Review by Contributors: Sarah Mathew, Jessica Barton, and Adrian W. Ong

Postoperative colitis as a disease entity was first described in 1893 by Finney, a Johns Hopkins surgeon who found "pseudodiptheritic enteritis" on the autopsy of a postoperative patient who developed severe diarrhea. Over the next several decades, it remained a rarely reported condition. This changed in the 1950s with reports of postoperative diarrhea and pseudomembranous colitis linked to antibiotics. The culprit was thought to be a *Staphylococcus* species, but it was not until 1977 that *Clostridium difficile* was correctly identified as the cause with the demonstration of neutralization of stool filtrate-induced cytotoxicity by *Clostridial* anti-toxin (Bartlett et al., 1978). With the identification of *C. difficile* as the pathogen, the modern era of diagnosis and treatment had begun.

The production of cytotoxins A and B has been considered as the sine qua non of *C. difficile* infection (CDI). The cytotoxicity assay used in initial studies developed into the gold standard for diagnosing patients in the 1980s and 1990s. It was a sensitive test but required 24 to 48 hours to complete and was impractical for clinical use. Enzyme-linked immunoassays (EIA) to detect toxin were faster but not as sensitive. In 1997, polymerase chain reaction (PCR) amplification of *C. difficile* toxin B in stool was reported as a fast and accurate way of diagnosing CDI with sensitivity and specificity of >95% (Alonso et al., 1997). Detection of glutamate dehydrogenase (GDH) in stool also emerged as a quick way to detect cytotoxin. When PCR was subsequently compared with all available tests it was found to be the most accurate way to rapidly diagnose CDI (Eastwood et al., 2009). For cost effectiveness, current clinical practice guidelines recommend a two-step diagnostic algorithm with PCR often used as one of the confirmatory tests after EIA or GDH detection. When there are clinical symptoms to suggest CDI, PCR can be used alone (McDonald et al., 2018).

With the recognition of *C. difficile* as the pathogen responsible for pseudomembranous colitis, metronidazole and vancomycin were recognized as effective antimicrobial agents. Risk factors for CDI were also identified, and included antibiotic exposure (the most important), age, prior hospitalization, prior stay at a long-term care facility, abdominal surgery, immunosuppression, and chronic kidney disease. Prior to 2000, failure rates for antibiotic therapy were less than 5% for both metronidazole and vancomycin. After 2000, however, hypervirulent strains like North American pulsed-field gel electrophoresis type 1 (NAP-1) (also described as PCR ribotype 027) that produced large amounts of toxin emerged. Subsequently, antibiotic failure rates significantly increased, particularly for metronidazole (16%–38%). Up to 30% of US CDI are now NAP-1 and the incidence, morbidity, and colectomy rates for CDI have increased. In a recent randomized trial, treatment with metronidazole or vancomycin resulted in equivalent cure rates (90% vs. 98%) for patients with mild CDI, but vancomycin had a superior cure rate compared to metronidazole in severe CDI (97% vs. 76%) (Zar et al., 2007). Another randomized trial found that fidaxomicin had equivalent cure rates compared to vancomycin with significantly fewer recurrences. This has led to a revision in the recent clinical practice guidelines, with vancomycin and fidaxomicin being recommended as the first-line agents for initial CDI rather than metronidazole (McDonald et al. 2018).

By far the most significant addition to the medical armamentarium for CDI since 2000 has been the use of fecal microbiota transplant (FMT). FMT is not a new concept. Fecal preparations were first recorded in Chinese medicine. Franz Paullini, a seventeenth-century German physician, wrote a textbook on the medical uses of human and animal feces. Veterinarians have been using FMT successfully for decades for a variety of gastrointestinal ailments. The first use of FMT in modern surgical practice for CDI was described in 1958 by Eiseman et al., where four patients with pseudomembranous colitis were successfully treated with fecal enemas (Eiseman et al., 1958). Sporadic use of FMT was reported over the next several decades in small nonrandomized studies. In 2013, the first randomized trial was conducted comparing vancomycin only, vancomycin with bowel lavage, and vancomycin with bowel lavage and FMT in patients with recurrent CDI (Van Nood et al., 2013). Although this was a small study, the cure rate for the FMT group was far superior to the other two groups. This and other randomized studies support a role for FMT in selected patients with recurrent CDI. For immunocompromised patients or those with severe CDI, the role for FMT is as yet unclear but there are some promising nonrandomized studies. In addition, the collection, storage, dosing, and route of FMT administration have yet to be standardized or fully regulated.

Indications for operative intervention for CDI include toxic megacolon, perforation, and septic shock with multiorgan failure unresponsive to medical therapy. For fulminant CDI, total colectomy conferred a survival advantage compared to medical management in a two-center study (Lamontagne et al., 2007). Patients older than 75 years who were immunocompetent, with a leukocytosis greater than 20,000/mm^3 or lactate between 2.2 and 4.9 mmol/L, benefited the most from operative intervention compared to medical management in this study.

Recently, diverting loop ileostomy with intraoperative colonic lavage combined with postoperative antegrade vancomycin enemas via ileostomy has been described in a retrospective study as a less morbid but effective alternative technique to total colectomy, with a lower mortality rate compared to historical controls (Neal et al., 2011). More recently, the outcomes of total colectomy (n = 77) and loop ileostomy (n = 21) with postoperative vancomycin enemas were retrospectively compared in a multicenter trial. The adjusted mortality was found to be significantly lower in the loop ileostomy patients (17.2% vs. 39.7%). It is worth noting that 3 of 21 (14%) loop ileostomy patients underwent total colectomy as a second procedure (Ferrada et al., 2017). Due to the lack of prospective randomized studies, the superiority of either surgical strategy has not been definitively shown.

In only 40 years, there have been significant advances in the recognition, diagnosis, and treatment of CDI. The benefits of FMT have only begun to be apparent. Monoclonal antibodies, vaccines, and colonization with non-toxigenic *C. difficile* strains are just some of the novel therapeutics being developed. Antibiotic stewardship remains paramount, but the emergence of hypervirulent strains has ensured that in this primarily medically treated disease, surgery still has an important role.

ANNOTATED REFERENCES FOR *CLOSTRIDIUM DIFFICILE* INFECTION

1. Bartlett JG, Chang TQ, Gurwith M, Gorbach SL, Onderdonk AB. Antibiotic-associated pseudomembranous colitis due to toxin-producing clostridia. *N Engl J Med.* 1978;298(10):531–534.

   This was the first study to correctly identify Clostridium difficile *as the pathogen in pseudomembranous colitis. In both cell cultures and a hamster animal model, stool isolates from patients were shown to be cytotoxic. This effect was neutralized by anti-Clostridial antibodies and the exact Clostridial species,* difficile, *was identified.*

2. Alonso R, Muñoz C, Pelaez T, Cercenado E, Rodriguez-Creixems M, Bouza E. Rapid detection of toxigenic *Clostridium difficile* strains by a nested PCR of the toxin B gene. *Clin Microbiol Infect.* 1997 Feb;3(1):145–147.

   PCR was introduced in this study as method of identifying toxin B in patients suspected to have CDI. PCR was compared to the standard cytotoxicity assay for more than 50 C. difficile *strains had 100% sensitivity, specificity, positive predictive value, and negative predictive value. This was a significant step forward for the diagnosis of CDI because PCR was much faster than the standard assay.*

3. Eastwood K, Else P, Charlett A, Wilcox M. Comparison of nine commercially available *Clostridium difficile* toxin detection assays, a real-time PCR assay for *C. difficile* tcdB, and a glutamate dehydrogenase detection assay to cytotoxin testing and cytotoxigenic culture methods. *J Clin Microbiol.* 2009;47(10)3211–3217.

   A study to evaluate traditional and modern diagnostic techniques for CDI. Six hundred diarrheal samples were tested. The gold standard traditional assays were compared to PCR, a GDH detection assay, and nine commercial EIA toxin assays. The optimum rapid single test was found to be PCR, as this had the highest negative predictive value. This study confirmed the value of PCR as a rapid and accurate way of diagnosing CDI.

4. McDonald LC, Gerding DN, Johnson S, et al. Clinical Practice Guidelines for *Clostridium difficile* Infection in Adults and Children: 2017 Update by the Infectious Diseases Society of America (IDSA) and Society for Health care Epidemiology of America (SHEA). *Clin Infect Dis.* 2018;66(7):987–994.

   The 2017 updated guidelines for the diagnosis, treatment, and prevention of CDI in adults and children. For the first time, metronidazole was no longer a recommended first-line agent, in favor of vancomycin or fidaxomicin. In addition, the recommended diagnostic algorithm for CDI included PCR alone or as a confirmatory test for GDH detection or EIA toxin assay where there were clinical symptoms suggested CDI.

5. Zar FA, Bakkanagari SR, Moorthi KM, Davis MB. A comparison of vancomycin and metronidazole for the treatment of *Clostridium difficile*-associated diarrhea, stratified by disease severity. *Clin Infect Dis*. 2007;45(3):302–307.

   This study presented the increasing incidence and severity of CDI and the issues related to failure of treatment with metronidazole. In this study vancomycin was compared to metronidazole in a prospective, randomized trial. Findings showed that metronidazole and vancomycin were equally effective for the treatment of mild CDI, but vancomycin was superior for treating patients with severe disease. This laid the foundation for the most recent clinical practice guidelines by McDonald et al.

6. Eiseman B, Silen W, Bascom GS, Kauvar AJ. Fecal enema as an adjunct in the treatment of pseudomembranous enterocolitis. *Surgery*. 1958;44(5):854–859.

   A case series that involved only four patients was the first published use of FMT to treat pseudomembranous colitis. It marks the genesis of FMT in modern practice.

7. Lamontagne F, Labbe AC, Hacek O, et al. Impact of emergency colectomy on survival of patients with fulminant *Clostridium difficile* colitis during an epidemic caused by a hyper-virulent strain. *Ann Surg*. 2007;245(2):267–272.

   A retrospective study of 165 cases of severe CDI in two Canadian centers during an outbreak of hypervirulent C. difficile. This showed that for critically ill patients with CDI, surgical management was superior to medical management with a 78% reduction in the odds of death.

8. Neal MD, Alverdy JC, Hall DE, Simmons RL, Zuckerbraun BS. Diverting loop ileostomy and colonic lavage: An alternative to total abdominal colectomy for the treatment of severe, complicated *Clostridium difficile*–associated disease. *Ann Surg*. 2011;254(3):423–427.

   A comparison of 42 cases of severe CDI treated with diverting ileostomy, lavage, and vancomycin enemas to historical controls treated with total colectomy at the same institution. It introduced an alternative option for surgical management in severe CDI that was minimally invasive and preserved the colon.

9. Ferrada P, Callcut R, Zielinski MD, et al.; EAST Multi-Institutional Trials Committee. Loop ileostomy versus total colectomy as surgical treatment for *Clostridium difficile*-associated disease: An Eastern Association for the Surgery of Trauma Multicenter Trial. *J Trauma Acute Care Surg*. 2017;83(1):36–40.

   A retrospective trial comparing colectomy and loop ileostomy with postoperative vancomycin enemas. This multicenter study was able to reproduce the result of Neal et al. and showed a significant reduction in mortality in severe CDI patients treated with loop ileostomy versus total colectomy. This trial was not randomized but was a big step forward in solidifying the place of loop ileostomy and vancomycin enemas in the surgical management of severe CDI.

DUODENAL INFUSION OF DONOR FECES FOR RECURRENT *CLOSTRIDIUM* DIFFICILE

van Nood E, Vrieze A, Nieuwdorp M, Fuentes S, Zoetendal EG, de Vos WM, Visser CE, Kuijper EJ, Bartelsman JF, Tijssen JG, Speelman P, Dijkgraaf MG, and Keller JJ,
N Engl J Med. 2013;368:407–415

ABSTRACT

Background Recurrent *Clostridium difficile* infection is difficult to treat, and failure rates for antibiotic therapy are high. We studied the effect of duodenal infusion of donor feces in patients with recurrent *C. difficile* infection.

Methods We randomly assigned patients to receive one of three therapies: an initial vancomycin regimen (500 mg orally four times per day for 4 days) followed by bowel lavage and subsequent infusion of a solution of donor feces through a nasoduodenal tube, a standard vancomycin regimen (500 mg orally four times per day for 14 days), or a standard vancomycin regimen with bowel lavage. The primary endpoint was the resolution of diarrhea associated with *C. difficile* infection without relapse after 10 weeks.

Results The study was stopped after an interim analysis. Of 16 patients in the infusion group, 13 (81%) had resolution of *C. difficile*–associated diarrhea after the first infusion. The three remaining patients received a second infusion with feces from a different donor, with resolution in two patients. Resolution of *C. difficile* infection occurred in 4 of 13 patients (31%) receiving vancomycin alone and in 3 of 13 patients (23%) receiving vancomycin with bowel lavage (P < 0.001 for both comparisons with the infusion group). No significant differences in adverse events among the three study groups were observed except for mild diarrhea and abdominal cramping in the infusion group on the infusion day. After donor-feces infusion, patients showed increased fecal bacterial diversity, similar to that in healthy donors, with an increase in *Bacteroides* species and *Clostridium* clusters IV and XIVa, and a decrease in *Proteobacteria* species.

Conclusions The infusion of donor feces was significantly more effective for the treatment of recurrent *C. difficile* infection than the use of vancomycin. (Funded by the Netherlands Organization for Health Research and Development and the Netherlands Organization for Scientific Research; Netherlands Trial Register number, NTR1177.)

Editor Notes

Assessment: This was a small, randomized, open-label trial of fecal transplantation versus standard care in patient who had relapsing *C. difficile* infections (manifested as diarrhea with positive stool test for *C. difficile* toxin) after at least one course of adequate antibiotic therapy. The proposed mechanism underlying fecal transplantation is reestablishment of a normal colonic microbiota as a host defense against *C. difficile*. Forty-three patients with recurrent *C. difficile* infections were randomized to either donor-feces infusion (17 patients) after 4 days of vancomycin and bowel lavage, vancomycin alone for 14 days (13 patients), or vancomycin for 14 days and bowel lavage (13 patients). The study was terminated after interim efficacy analysis due to a significantly better cure rate in the group that were infused with donor feces. Donor feces infusion cured 94%, whereas only 31% or 23% of the other treatment arms were cured. The primary endpoint was cure without relapse within 10 weeks. Eighteen patients who had a relapse after initial antibiotic treatment were cured with off-protocol donor feces infusion.

Limitations: The study implies that donor feces was infused into the duodenum, but the methodology only states that a nasogastric tube was used. It is unclear whether the infusion was intragastric or not, as gastric acid could impact viability of bacteria.

Conclusions: This study demonstrates the superiority of infusing donor feces into the gastrointestinal tract over antibiotic management. The logistics of infusing relatively large amounts of fresh donor feces has now been shown to be manageable.

CHAPTER 16

Acute Cholecystitis

Review by Contributor: Narong Kulvatunyou

Given that gallbladder surgery is the most common general surgical procedure, a discussion on landmark papers about acute cholecystitis (AC) should start with a description of the natural history of incidental gallstones as well as the approximated prevalence of the potential AC. In 2018, we can estimate that at least 13 million Americans potentially harbored gallstones (Everhart et al., 1999). Of those, 1%–3% annually will develop gallbladder-related complications every year (i.e., biliary colic, AC, pancreatitis, or choledocholithiasis) that require a cholecystectomy (Friedman, 1993). Even though existing studies do not tell us exactly what percentage of these complications are AC, we can estimate that between 130,000 to 390,000 cholecystectomies are performed annually. Additionally, according to a population-based study using the National Inpatient Sample (NIS) database, the incidence and costs (i.e., hospital charges not including physician fees) associated with AC went up from 1997 to 2012. The number of AC patients discharged from the hospital increased from 183,570 in 1997 to 272,130 in 2012. Likewise, the costs grew significantly from $14,608 in 1997 to $43,152 in 2012. The most interesting finding was also the shift in the age group with the highest admission rate for AC. Between 1997 and 2012, it went from 65–84 years old to 18–44 years old (Wadhwa et al., 2017).

A definitive diagnosis of AC can be challenging. One can choose to use a systematically defined Tokyo Guideline (TG) that divides symptoms into local signs (right upper quadrant pain/tenderness, Murphy sign), systemic signs (fever, leukocytosis), and a confirmatory test (ultrasound, a computed tomography [CT] scan, or a nuclear scan [HIDA]). According to the updated TG13 (Yokoe et al., 2013), AC diagnosis can be made with about 92% sensitivity and 96% specificity using TG13. However, the significant change from TG07 to TG13 guideline was the heavy reliance on confirmatory diagnostic tests for a definitive diagnosis of AC; it is important to note that the literature is still very unclear about which test modality has the highest sensitivity and specificity and should be used to diagnose AC.

Most clinicians, including emergency room physicians and surgeons, still rely heavily on an ultrasound as the first line to diagnose AC. It is easy to use, easily accessible, and avoids radiation exposure. Nonetheless, according to a meta-analysis study (Kiewiet et al., 2011), the accuracy of the ultrasound is at best 81% sensitivity and 83% specificity. However, this particular study analysis had a significant limitation due to the high heterogeneity of the different studies under review. Clearly, "verification bias" is the most confounding limitation for any study on the accuracy of any particular diagnostic test. A verification bias exists when only patients with positive test results undergo surgery while those with negative test results do not. When the standard reference for diagnosing AC is a pathology report and patients with negative test results do not undergo surgery, the true incidence of false negatives is unknown. Interestingly, when the verification bias was removed, the ultrasound sensitivity dropped to only 38% but specificity remained at 90% (Kulvatunyou et al., 2012). This low accuracy of the ultrasound then begs the question if one should rely on ultrasound to exclude the diagnosis of AC.

Upon a diagnosis of AC, most patients will at some point (see below regarding timing) need to undergo a cholecystectomy. The choice between a laparoscopic versus an open cholecystectomy now seems rather obvious and intuitive to the modern-day surgeon but the actual level I evidence to support such a claim is surprisingly lacking. There have been only four randomized controlled trials containing only 310 patients (Coccolini et al., 2015) that compared the laparoscopic to the open cholecystectomy. Despite findings that supported our assumption that the laparoscopic approach would lead to a lower wound infection rate and a shorter hospital length of stay (HLOS), the pooled study sample size remained rather small and underpowered, especially in regard to analyzing the incidence of bile duct injuries that were not reported in any of the studies.

Similarly, it seems rather commonsensical now that early cholecystectomy would benefit patients with AC in terms of relieving their pain and suffering, as well as shortening their convalescent period, but in the late 1990s and early 2000s, this was controversial and there was a heated discussion in publications. The debate ended with the largest multicenter randomized controlled trial (The ACDC trial) (Gutt et al., 2013) from Germany. In this study, more than 600 patients demonstrated that the "early" (mean 0.6 days) surgery in comparison to "delayed" surgery (mean 25 days) had significant overall benefits in term of overall morbidity (12% vs. 33%, $P < 0.001$), HLOS (5.4 days vs. 19 days, $P < 0.001$), and costs (2919 Euro vs. 4262 Euro, $P < 0.001$) with no effects on the conversion rate. The one small criticism of this study was that patients' duration of symptoms was not recorded before admission. This question was later addressed by another study from Switzerland (Roulin et al., 2016) that randomized patients who specifically presented with symptoms >72 hours to either an "early" or "delayed" cholecystectomy. This study also demonstrated the benefits of the "early" group in terms of morbidity, HLOS, and costs. The majority of morbidity in the "delayed" group was recurrent symptoms that required patients to undergo surgery sooner than originally planned.

In summary, AC is a common surgical disease that requires early laparoscopic chole-cystectomy once a definitive diagnosis has been made. An ideal confirmatory imaging study remains unknown and more studies are needed. Since AC has a significant health care and cost burden, the question remains whether a patient who presents to an emergency department (ED) with symptomatic gallstones but without an obvious diagnosis of AC should be offered surgical intervention sooner than the traditional discharge from ED and be referred to and followed-up in an outpatient surgical clinic.

ANNOTATED REFERENCES FOR ACUTE CHOLECYSTITIS

1. Everhart JE, Khare M, Hill M, Maurer KR. Prevalence and ethnic differences in gallbladder disease in the United States. *Gastroenterology.* 1999;117:632–639.

   This was the largest (n = 14,000) and the most contemporary screen available (1988–1994) using an ultrasound done by the National Health and Nutrition Examination Survey (NHANES III). It demonstrated the prevalence of gallstones in the United States affects 11 million people. If it is extrapolated to the 2018 US population census, that would be an equivalent of 13 million patients today who have gallstones. The study also concluded there was no ethnic difference except an increased prevalence among Mexican American women compared to white women; however, the study only identified three ethnicities: white, black, and Mexican American.

2. Friedman GD. Natural history of asymptomatic and symptomatic gallstones. *Am J Surg.* 1993;165:399–404.

   This was a review paper of the natural history of silent gallstones, a common clinical question often dealt with by a general surgeon. The author is an authority on this topic as he has published one of a few longitudinal studies looking at the natural history of silent gallstones. Although the author acknowledged the difficulty in most studies of classifying a patient's symptoms, the estimated probability of patients with gallstones who will go on to require cholecystectomy will be 1%–3% annually. The probability stays the same throughout the years, but it may be affected by other prognostic risk factors that have never been studied. However, the probability goes down after about 15 years.

3. Wadhwa V, Jobanputra Y, Garg SK et al. Nationwide trends of hospital admission for acute cholecystitis in the United States. *Gastroenterol Rep.* 2017;5(1):36–42.

   This was a population-based study of patients who were admitted and discharged with a diagnosis of AC from the hospital using the National Inpatient Sample (NIS) database from 1997–2012. The incidence and costs during that time span had increased, while the age group with the highest admission shifted from 65–84 to 18–44 years old.

4. Yokoe M, Takada T, Strasberg SM et al. TG13 diagnostic criteria and severity grading of acute cholecystitis. *J Hepatobiliary Pancreatic Sci.* 2013;20:35–46.

   This was an update to the TG of 2007 for the diagnosis and management of AC. Many Westerners were not very familiar with this guideline. Essentially, this updated article reiterated that the definitive diagnosis of AC could not be done without a definitive imaging study. However, the choice or the efficacy of an imaging study continued to be debated and was not answered by this review.

5. Kiewiet JJ, Leeuwenburg MM, Bipat S et al. A systematic review and meta-analysis of diagnostic performance imaging in acute cholecystitis. *Radiology* 2011;264:708–720.

   The authors performed a meta-analysis of the accuracy of diagnostic tests (cholescintigraphy [no longer used today], ultrasound, CT scan, and MRI). There were 57 studies in total, mostly cholescintigraphy, but there were 26 ultrasound, 3 MRI, and only 1 CT scan studies. Ultrasound had a summarized 81% sensitivity and 83% specificity, and MRI had comparable 85% sensitivity and 81% specificity; however, there was significant variability of prevalence as well as heterogeneity among studies, which limited the legitimacy of the study conclusions.

6. Kulvatunyou N, Joseph B, Gries L et al. A prospective cohort study of 200 acute care gallbladder surgeries: The same disease but a different approach. *J Trauma Acute Care Surg.* 2012;73:1039–1045.

*The authors studied 200 consecutive patients who presented to the emergency depart-
ment with right upper quadrant pain with suspected AC diagnosis. All patients
underwent an ultrasound study, and all patients underwent surgical removal of their
gallbladders. The prevalence of AC in the study was 32%, and using the pathology
report as the standard of reference for AC, the ultrasound had the reported sensitivity
of a mere 38% and specificity of 90%, somewhat different from most of the radiology
literature. This was due to the removal of a verification bias in which all patients, with
or without positive test for AC, still underwent surgery, with the final pathology report
as a gold standard.*

7. Coccolini F, Catena F, Pisano M et al. Open versus laparoscopic cholecystectomy in acute cholecystitis. Systematic review and meta-analysis. *Inter J Surg.*
   2015;18:196–204.

   *The authors performed a meta-analysis that included four randomized (n = 310) con-
   trolled trials and six other studies (n = 1064) and concluded that laparoscopic cholecystectomy decreased morbidity in terms of wound infection, pneumonia, and HLOS
   without a significant increase in operative time or blood loss. Despite pooling of all
   studies, the overall sample size remained underpowered, particularly for the incidence
   of bile duct injuries.*

8. Roulin D, Saadi A, Di Mare L, Demartines N, Halkic N. Early versus delayed
   cholecystectomy for acute cholecystitis, are the 72 hours still the rule? A randomized trial.
   Ann Surg. 2016;264:717–722.

   *The authors performed a single-center RCT of "early" versus "delayed" cholecystectomy
   for acute cholecystitis with the specific requirement that patients must have symptoms for
   72 hours or greater. The conclusion remained the same with benefits in terms of morbidity,
   HLOS, and costs favoring the early group.*

Landmark Article of 21st Century

ACUTE CHOLECYSTITIS: EARLY VERSUS DELAYED CHOLECYSTECTOMY, A MULTICENTER RANDOMIZED TRIAL

Gutt CN, Encke J, Köninger J, Harnoss JC, Weigand K, Kipfmüller K, Schunter O,
Götze T, Golling MT, Menges M, Klar E, Feilhauer K, Zoller WG, Ridwelski K,
Ackmann S, Baron A, Schön MR, Seitz HK, Daniel D, Stremmel W, and Büchler MW,
Ann Surg. 2013;258:385–393

ABSTRACT

Objective   Acute cholecystitis is a common disease, and laparoscopic surgery is the
standard of care.

Background   Optimal timing of surgery for acute cholecystitis remains controversial:
either early surgery shortly after hospital admission or delayed elective surgery after a
conservative treatment with antibiotics.

Methods   The ACDC (Acute Cholecystitis—early laparoscopic surgery versus
antibiotic therapy and Delayed elective Cholecystectomy) study is a randomized,

prospective, open-label, parallel group trial. Patients were randomly assigned to receive immediate surgery within 24 hours of hospital admission (group ILC) or initial antibiotic treatment, followed by delayed laparoscopic cholecystectomy at days 7–45 (group DLC). For infection, all patients were treated with moxifloxacin for at least 48 hours. Primary endpoint was occurrence of predefined relevant morbidity within 75 days. Secondary endpoints were as follows: (1) 75-day morbidity using a scoring system; (2) conversion rate; (3) change of antibiotic therapy; (4) mortality; (5) costs; and (6) length of hospital stay.

Results Morbidity rate was significantly lower in group ILC (304 patients) than in group DLC (314 patients): 11.8% versus 34.4%. Conversion rate to open surgery and mortality did not differ significantly between groups. Mean length of hospital stay (5.4 days vs. 10.0 days; P < 0.001) and total hospital costs (€2919 vs. €4262; P < 0.001) were significantly lower in group ILC.

Conclusions In this large, randomized trial, laparoscopic cholecystectomy within 24 hours of hospital admission was shown to be superior to the conservative approach concerning morbidity and costs. Therefore, we believe that immediate laparoscopic cholecystectomy should become therapy of choice for acute cholecystitis in operable patients.

Editor Notes

Assessment: This large prospective randomized controlled trial (n = 618 at 35 centers in Germany and Slovenia over 4 years) demonstrated that in patients with acute cholecystitis, early laparoscopic cholecystectomy (defined as less than 24 hours after admission) significantly reduced morbidity, hospital stay, and total hospital costs when compared to delayed laparoscopic cholecystectomy performed at day 7–45. Serious adverse events occurred almost three times as often in the delayed intervention group (28 patients in the early group vs. 85 in delayed). Hospital costs were 46% higher in the delayed surgery patients. There were no differences in conversion rates to open operations or mortality.

Limitations: The patients in the delayed intervention group appeared to be somewhat sicker, with an increased incidence at baseline of cancer, respiratory insufficiency, and congestive heart failure. There was no delineation of the amount of time prior to admission that the patients had symptoms. Obviously, there was no blinding as to the intervention group. Highest risk patients with ASA IV- and V were excluded along with those with a perforated gallbladder.

Conclusions: This study confirms the superiority of early intervention over delayed treatment in patients with acute cholecystitis and solidifies this management scheme as the standard of care in clinically stable patients.

CHAPTER 17

Acute Cholangitis

Review by Contributor: Chad G. Ball

Acute cholangitis is defined as acute inflammation and infection of the biliary tree. Although this diagnosis was initially described in the days of the Greek empire, its more contemporary history surrounds the clinical diagnosis and symptomatology described by Jean-Martin Charcot in 1877 (i.e., right upper quadrant pain, fever, and jaundice). This triad, known as "hepatic fever," underwent further elaboration in 1959 when Benedict Reynolds added mental status deterioration and hypotension to create his iconic pentad. Historically this condition was associated with a mortality rate greater than 55% given that standard therapy required exploration of the common bile duct via surgical intervention. With the ascension of endoscopic retrograde cholangiopancreatography in 1992, combined with the assessment and treatment pathways discussed below, acute cholangitis-associated mortality has now decreased to less than 4%.

Acute cholangitis is most commonly a consequence of biliary obstruction followed by bacterial overgrowth within bile itself (Kimura et al., 2007, 2013). The dominant cause of acute cholangitis is choledocholithiasis, followed by benign biliary stenosis and cancer. Interestingly, a recent report that included 794 patients did not show a significant difference between the incidence of gallstones (50.6%) and malignancies (49.4%) as the main source of obstruction (Higuchi et al., 2013). This likely reflects an aging populous. Regardless of the cause or site, obstruction of the biliary tree (most commonly of the common bile duct) leads to biliary hypertension and a reduction in the flow of bile into the intestine. This diminishes the physical barrier flushing action of the bile itself. The associated decrease in the bile salt delivery to the intestine also causes a decrease in the bile salt-mediated bacteriostatic and bactericidal activity and therefore leads to colonic bacterial overgrowth. The overgrowth typically disturbs protective bacterial flora and promotes local inflammation, injury, and subsequent increased rates of bacterial translocation into the portal circulation (i.e., which is also enhanced by biliary pressures greater than 15 mmHg). The increasing bacterial load is also infrequently cleared by the liver because of weakened hepatic tight junctions and increased ductal permeability. This scenario facilitates the translocation of bacteria and their products directly into the systemic vascular system. This entire process is clearly and highly dependent upon contamination of normally aseptic bile. It is also supported by data that reports 16% of patients undergoing a nonbiliary operation, 72% with acute cholangitis, 44% with chronic cholangitis, 50% with acute biliary obstruction, and 90% of patients with choledocholithiasis and jaundice have positive biliary cultures (Kimura et al., 2007, 2013). This is also directly related to the observation that following mechanical biliary interventions (percutaneous and/or endoscopic biliary access/tubes), most (75%) patients display at least intermittent bacteremia.

Patients with cholangitis may present with a wide variety of symptoms from non-specific findings to severe infection and fatal septic shock. Morbidity and mortality are minimized only via early diagnosis and treatment. Given that Charcot's triad (jaundice, fever, and right upper quadrant peritonitis) has a high specificity (>90%), but is observed in only 18.5% of patients, a high level of suspicion for the diagnosis is essential (Kiriyama et al., 2012).

This reality is reinforced by the initial TG that summarize the diagnosis must include at least (1) signs of systemic inflammation (i.e., fever), (2) cholestasis, and (3) specific findings on imaging (Kiriyama et al., 2012). Current recommendations also grade the severity of cholangitis (I [mild = diagnosis of exclusion], II [moderate = systemic inflammation without organ dysfunction], or III [severe = concurrent dysfunction of at least 1 organ system]). Despite this grading system, most patients (54%) present with grade I disease (only 11% develop grade III).

The treatment of acute cholangitis has shown dramatic improvement over the past decade with a current mortality of less than 30% (i.e., sepsis leading to multiorgan failure) (Kiriyama et al., 2012). Patients should receive general medical therapy including NPO, intravenous fluids, antibiotics, and analgesia. The selection of antimicrobials is particularly important due to increasing antimicrobial resistance (Gomi et al., 2018). Fundamental principles include broad initial coverage followed by early de-escalation as soon as the infecting isolates are confirmed. The appropriate duration of antimicrobial therapy is eloquently updated in the most recent Tokyo 2018 guidelines (Gomi et al., 2018). In addition to general critical care, various techniques for biliary decompression are also mandated (Lai et al., 1992). Approaches include endoscopic, percutaneous, and/or operative approaches based on the etiology of the cholangitis and patient physiology (Lau et al., 1991; Lee et al.,2002). Medical treatment may be sufficient in selected cases of grade I, but biliary drainage should be considered for all nonresponders (Miura et al., 2013). This scenario often incorporates postoperative patients. Patients with grade II disease require early endoscopic, percutaneous, or emergent operative (T-tube) biliary drainage. These drainage procedures may be definitive for patients with gallstone-associated cholangitis (Miura et al., 2013). Although it remains controversial if patients with cancer should undergo a definitive resection concurrent to their emergent decompression procedure, this is generally not recommended due to a lack of complete staging, higher postoperative complications, and known hospital volume-outcome relationships. Patients with cancer should be stabilized, undergo emergency drainage, and be referred for definitive treatment to a high volume hepatopancreatic biliary service (HPB) center. In the most critically ill patients, a multidisciplinary team of endoscopists, intensive care physicians, and sometimes HPB surgeons should participate with the acute care surgery team in the management of these patients. The type of biliary drainage selected by the surgeon is particularly important. Patients with hilar cholangiocarcinoma most often benefit from a percutaneous technique (percutaneous transhepatic catheter [PTC] as opposed to endoscopic). Endoscopic retrograde cholangio-pancreatography (ERCP)-based attempts at drainage of hilar cholangiocarcinoma are notorious for failing to achieve adequate drainage within the proximal liver, and subsequently often develop significant cholangitis due to instrumentation of the biliary system during this attempt. These patients *must* also receive high-fidelity cholangiographic information either prior to MRCP, or concurrent with the insertion of the PTC (i.e., via the PTC itself) to define resectability and reconstruction options. Patients with any periampullary malignancy should undergo ERCP-based stenting as the initial choice.

Patients with grade III cholangitis require admission to the intensive care unit for physiologic support in addition to general medical treatment (Miura et al., 2013). Urgent endoscopic, percutaneous, or surgical biliary drainage must also be performed. Considering that these patients are often physiologically unstable, the most rapid and least invasive procedure should be selected (operative intervention should be the last resort given the high associated mortality). Once the cholangitis has resolved, definitive treatment of the etiology (i.e., laparoscopic cholecystectomy for cholelithiasis, resection for cancer) is indicated.

Although the presentation of acute cholangitis can be variable for the acute care surgeon, the previously discussed pathways and principles will generally guide diagnosis and therapy in most cases. The specifics of antimicrobial utility and treatment are most recently outlined in the 2018 Tokyo guidelines for acute cholangitis and cholecystitis.

ANNOTATED REFERENCES FOR ACUTE CHOLANGITIS

1. Kimura Y, Takada T, Strasberg SM et al. TG13 current terminology, etiology, and epidemiology of acute cholangitis and cholecystitis. *J Hepatobiliary Pancreat Sci.* 2013;20(1):8–23.

   This global panel of experts has unified the lexicon and epidemiology for acute cholangitis. This important step allows clinicians and researchers alike to move forward with deeper and more organized scientific investigation to improve the care of patients with acute cholangitis.

2. Higuchi R, Takada T, Strasberg SM et al. TG13 miscellaneous etiology of cholangitis and cholecystitis. *J Hepatobiliary Pancreat Sci.* 2013;20(1):97–105.

   The panel describes the various etiologies and unified classification systems of acute cholangitis that allow a clinician to advance a directed diagnostic evaluation and subsequent appropriate intervention(s).

3. Kimura Y, Takada T, Kawarada Y et al. Definitions, pathophysiology, and epidemiology of acute cholangitis and cholecystitis: Tokyo Guidelines. *J Hepatobiliary Pancreat Surg.* 2007;14(1):15–26.

   This orginal version of the Tokyo Guidelines on acute cholangitis and cholecystitis set the foundation for subsequent revisions and a dramatic improvement in communication, research, and patient care.

4. Kiriyama S, Takada T, Strasberg SM et al. New diagnostic criteria and severity assessment of acute cholangitis in revised Tokyo Guidelines. *J Hepatobiliary Pancreat Sci.* 2012;19(5):548–556.

This manuscript represents the first update to the original 2007 Tokyo Guidelines and, more specifically, enhances the diagnostic and severity criteria for acute cholangitis.

5. Gomi H, Solomkin JS, Schlossberg D et al. Tokyo Guidelines 2018: Antimcrobial therapy for acute cholangitis and cholecystitis. *J Hepatobiliary Pancreat Sci.* 2018;25(1):3–16.

This most recent 2018 update consolidates all previous scientific and clinical approaches. Novel data include a deep discussion of the appropriate interval for antimicrobial therapy for acute cholangitis and cholecystitis, as well as a review of the recommendation of no prophylactic antimicrobial therapy for elective endoscopic retrograde cholangiopancreatography.

6. Lai EC, Mok FP, Tan ES et al. Endoscopic biliary drainage for severe acute cholangitis. *N Engl J Med.* 1992;326(24):1582–1586.

This original manuscript discusses the safety, efficacy, and mortality benefits of endoscopic biliary drainage in patients with severe acute cholangitis.

7. Lau WY, Chu KW, Yuen WK, Poon GP, Hwang JS, Li AK. Operative choledochoscopy in patients with acute cholangitis: A prospective, randomized study. *Br J Surg.* 1991;78(10):1226–1229.

This randomized trial evaluated the role and safety of operative choledochoscopy in patients requiring emergency surgery for severe acute cholangitis.

8. Lee DW, Chan AC, Lam YH et al. Biliary decompression by nasobiliary catheter or biliary stent in acute suppurative cholangitis: A prospective randomized trial. *Gastrointest Endosc.* 2002;56(3):361–365.

This publication discussed the comparative efficacy of endoscopic techniques (nasobiliary catheter vs. indwelling stent) for biliary decompression in patient with severe acute cholangitis.

9. Miura F, Takada T, Strasberg SM et al. TG13 flowchart for the management of acute cholangitis and cholecystitis. *J Hepatobiliary Pancreat Sci.* 2013;20(1):47–54.

This publication outlines a proposed "best practices" pathway for the management of acute cholangitis by a renowned and well-regarded guideline panel.

TG13: UPDATED TOKYO GUIDELINES FOR THE MANAGEMENT OF ACUTE CHOLANGITIS AND CHOLECYSTITIS

Takada T, Strasberg SM, Solomkin JS, Pitt HA, Gomi H, Yoshida M, Mayumi T, Miura F, Gouma DJ, Garden OJ, Büchler MW, Kiriyama S, Yokoe M, Kimura Y, Tsuyuguchi T, Itoi T, Gabata T, Higuchi R, Okamoto K, Hata J, Murata A, Kusachi S, Windsor JA, Supe AN, Lee S, Chen XP, Yamashita Y, Hirata K, Inui K, and Sumiyama Y; Tokyo Guidelines Revision Committee, *J Hepatobiliary Pancreat Sci.* 2013;20(1):1–7

ABSTRACT

Background   In 2007, the Tokyo Guidelines for the Management of acute cholangitis and Cholecystitis (TG07) were first published in the *Journal of Hepato-Biliary-Pancreatic Surgery*. The fundamental policy of TG07 was to achieve the objectives of

TG07 through the development of consensus among specialists in this field throughout the world. Considering such a situation, validation and feedback from the clinicians' viewpoints were indispensable. What had been pointed out from clinical practice was the low diagnostic sensitivity of TG07 for acute cholangitis and the presence of divergence between severity assessment and clinical judgment for acute cholangitis.

Methods   In June 2010, we set up the Tokyo Guidelines Revision Committee (TGRC) for the revision of TG07 and started the validation of TG07. We also set up new diagnostic criteria and severity assessment criteria by retrospectively analyzing cases of acute cholangitis and cholecystitis, including cases of noninflammatory biliary disease, collected from multiple institutions.

Results   TGRC held a total of 35 meetings as well as international email exchanges with co-authors abroad. On June 9 and September 6, 2011, and on April 11, 2012, we held three International Meetings for the Clinical Assessment and Revision of Tokyo Guidelines. Through these meetings, the final draft of the updated Tokyo Guidelines (TG13) was prepared on the basis of the evidence from retrospective multicenter analyses. To be specific, discussion took place involving the revised new diagnostic criteria, the new severity assessment criteria, new flowcharts of the management of acute cholangitis and cholecystitis, recommended medical care for which new evidence had been added, new recommendations for gallbladder drainage and antimicrobial therapy, and the role of surgical intervention. Management bundles for acute cholangitis and cholecystitis were introduced for effective dissemination with the level of evidence and the grade of recommendations. GRADE systems were utilized to provide the level of evidence and the grade of recommendations.

Conclusions   TG13 improved the diagnostic sensitivity for acute cholangitis and cholecystitis and presented criteria with extremely low false positive rates adapted for clinical practice. Furthermore, severity assessment criteria adapted for clinical use, flowcharts, and many new diagnostic and therapeutic modalities were presented. The bundles for the management of acute cholangitis and cholecystitis are presented in a separate section in TG13.

Editor Notes

Assessment: This manuscript is an update of the 2013 Tokyo Guidelines focusing on antimicrobial therapy in acute cholangitis and cholecystitis. Recommendations include: (i) bile cultures should be obtained at the initiation of any procedures that are beyond the lowest severity (Grade C recommendation); (ii) antibiotics should target the usual biliary pathogens found in the community (Grade D); (iii) duration of antibiotics should be 4–7 days in the routine setting (Grade C), or until clinical resolution of sepsis in the setting of perforation or abscess (Grade D).

Limitations: These recommendations are based upon low- to modest-quality studies and permit only low-level recommendations. There is little new material defined in the guidelines. Prophylactic antibiotics for ERCP are no longer recommended.

Conclusions: This international group of experts has attempted to compile the best available data to make intelligent recommendations regarding the optimal care of patients with acute cholangitis and cholecystitis.

CHAPTER 18

Acute Pancreatitis

Review by Contributors: Umar F. Bhatti and Hasan B. Alam

Herophilus was the first to appreciate the pancreas in the early medieval period. Rufus devised the name, which in the Greek language meant "all flesh." Gladen proposed that the pancreas served as a protective cushion to the underlying vasculature, and this false belief was first challenged in the 1600s when Wirsüng discovered the pancreatic duct. Physiology of the pancreas was better understood by the nineteenth century, and in the 1880s, Fitz demonstrated the clinical features of acute pancreatitis (AP). He thought that it stemmed from gastroduodenitis. Senn was first to suggest a surgical intervention to manage AP, albeit the dawn of the twentieth century saw mixed views and the pancreas was regarded as an organ ill-disposed to surgery. Today, the optimum treatment for AP is subject to debate (Lankisch, 2010).

AP is the most frequent gastrointestinal cause of hospital admissions in the United States, affecting 13 to 45/100,000 individuals annually. It is distributed equally between males and females; however, the gender demographic varies significantly with etiology—alcoholism being the most common risk factor in males and gallstones in females. Recently, there has been an increase in incidence among the pediatric population (Yadav and Lowenfels, 2013).

Abdominal pain that radiates to the back, serum amylase/lipase level greater than three times the upper limit, and evidence of pancreatitis on abdominal imagining are the three most important diagnostic features. Presence of any two of these establishes a diagnosis (Tenner et al. 2013). Although the levels of both amylase and lipase are raised in the serum, the lipase level is not only superior for ruling out the disease, but also provides a larger diagnostic window due to its longer half-life. Prognostic indices like the Ranson criteria, the Acute Physiology and Chronic Health Evaluation II (APACHE II), and the Bedside Index of Severity in Acute Pancreatitis (BISAP) are commonly used to evaluate severity. While all scoring systems have limitations, BISAP is regarded as a reliable and easy-to-use tool to classify disease severity (Papachristou et al., 2010). Ultrasonography is valuable in cases with gallstone etiology. Since necrosis takes time to become obvious, CT and MRI have limited utility in the first 48 to 72 hours of symptom onset unless the diagnosis is uncertain. Contrast-enhanced CT is performed in patients with severe pancreatitis to rule out acute necrotizing pancreatitis. Use of MRI is emerging due to its ability to better identify gallstones and characterize the contents of fluid collections seen on CT.

AP is an inflammatory pathology mediated by autodigestion of the pancreas due to abnormal activation of pancreatic enzymes—most notably trypsinogen. Based on the presence or absence of necrosis, the Atlanta classification divides AP into two distinct subtypes: interstitial edematous pancreatitis and necrotizing pancreatitis (Sarr, 2013). Regardless of the severity of disease, critical to the management of AP is the assessment of hemodynamic status and early intravenous fluid resuscitation with crystalloids to account for fluid losses due to third spacing. Pain is managed with intravenous analgesics. If tolerated well, an oral low-fat soft or solid diet is initiated. Parenteral modes of nutrition are reserved in cases where enteral routes are inadequate to meet the caloric requirement. Early nasoenteric tube feeding in patients that are at high risk of complications does not provide additive benefit over oral feeds (Bakker et al., 2014). Patients require intensive care due to increased susceptibility to complications like shock and multiorgan failure (MOF).

Since the etiology is not bacterial, use of antibiotics is generally not indicated. Antibiotic prophylaxis does not prevent progression in severe acute necrotizing pancreatitis and treatment with antibiotics does not improve outcomes in AP (Dellinger et al., 2007). An early cholecystectomy (within 48 hours of admission) is ideal for mild biliary pancreatitis because it is associated with decreased length of stay (LOS). According to the Pancreatitis of Biliary Origin, Optimal Timing of Cholecystectomy (PONCHO) trial for mild biliary pancreatitis, same-admission cholecystectomy (within 1 day of randomization) is superior to interval cholecystectomy (within 27 days of randomization) because of the decreased risk of mortality or readmissions for biliary complications (5% in same-admission vs. 17% in interval) (da Costa et al., 2015). However, implementing this approach can be challenging because it warrants a shift from elective to acute care surgery, which requires different skill set and infrastructure.

Endoscopic retrograde cholangiopancreatography (ERCP) with stent placement is useful in cases of biliary pancreatitis with concomitant cholangitis. In patients with mild to moderate biliary AP, postoperative ERCP is superior to preoperative ERCP due to shorter LOS and lower total expenditure (Chang et al., 2000). Symptomatic parapancreatic fluid collections like pseudocysts or walled-off pancreatic necrosis should be drained endoscopically when anatomically feasible.

A discord exists regarding the management of acute necrotizing pancreatitis (20% of the total cases) which carries a high risk of death (8%–39%). A secondary infection of necrotic tissue in patients with necrotizing pancreatitis (5% of all cases of AP) almost always warrants an intervention. Efforts are made to first wall off the necrotic debris by delaying the intervention for 4 weeks. While open necrosectomy is traditionally the standard for treating necrotizing pancreatitis with infectious necrosis, a minimally invasive step-up approach has been shown to decrease the rate of major complications like MOF, death, and the incidence of long-term complications like new-onset diabetes and incisional hernias according to a well-designed randomized trial (van Santvoort et al., 2010). This is in part because the drainage of infected debris in the step-up approach eliminates the infectious nidus and the minimally invasive technique elicits significantly less surgical trauma. In addition to better outcomes, it is believed that the step-up approach can reduce the annual health care costs in the United States by $185 million, which makes it a very compelling alternative to the more invasive open necrosectomy.

ANNOTATED REFERENCES FOR ACUTE PANCREATITIS

1. Lankisch PG. Treatment of acute pancreatitis: An attempted historical review. *Pancreatology.* 2010;10(2–3):134–141.

   This article is a fine attempt at a historical review of treatment of acute pancreatitis. It sheds light on how the past research impacts our current understanding of the topic. The author utilizes the well-known online medical libraries and their personal library collected over a period of 40 years as a pancreatologist to produce this excellent report.

2. Yadav D, Lowenfels AB. The epidemiology of pancreatitis and pancreatic cancer. *Gastroenterology.* 2013;144(6):1252–1261.

   The authors detail the descriptive epidemiology of pancreatic disease demonstrating the incidence, prevalence, and trends of acute pancreatitis with respect to patient demographics. The authors also elucidate the etiology of acute pancreatitis and provide insight on disease progression and mortality.

3. Tenner S, Baillie J, DeWitt J et al. American College of Gastroenterology guideline: Management of acute pancreatitis. *Am J Gastroenterol.* 2013;108(9):1400–1415;1416.

   ACGE guidelines on the management of patients with AP. These guidelines take into account the recent advances and development in the understanding of diagnosis, etiology, and management of AP.

4. Papachristou GI, Muddana V, Yadav D et al. Comparison of BISAP, Ranson's, APACHE-II, and CTSI scores in predicting organ failure, complications, and mortality in acute pancreatitis. *Am J Gastroenterol.* 2010;105(2):435–441;quiz 442.

   The authors perform a detailed comparison of various prognostic scoring systems for AP, including the more recent BISAP score. They deduce that the BISAP score is more reliable and easier to use because it has fewer components; however, it does not improve the predictive accuracy when compared to the conventional scoring systems like APACHE II and Ranson's score. The study emphasizes the need for devising novel models of scoring to improve the accuracy of predicting the severity of AP.

5. Sarr MG. 2012 revision of the Atlanta classification of acute pancreatitis. *Pol Arch Med Wewn.* 2013;123(3):118–124.

   An excellent account on the revised Atlanta classification of acute pancreatitis that features the changes from the older classification.

6. Bakker OJ, van Brunschot S, van Santvoort HC et al. Early versus on-demand nasoenteric tube feeding in acute pancreatitis. *N Engl J Med.* 2014;371(21):1983–1993.

   In this randomized controlled trial, the authors compared the outcomes of an early (within 24 hours of randomization) nasoenteric tube feeding to the outcomes of an oral diet initiated 72 hours after presentation and found that contrary to popular belief, nasoenteric tube feeding has no additive benefit over oral feeding in reducing the rate of infection or death in patients with AP who are at a high risk of complications.

7. Dellinger EP, Tellado JM, Soto NE et al. Early antibiotic treatment for severe acute necrotizing pancreatitis: A randomized, double-blind, placebo-controlled study. *Ann Surg.* 2007;245(5):674–683.

The authors conducted a double-blinded, randomized, placebo-controlled trial to study the role of antibiotic treatment and prophylaxis in 100 patients with clinically severe acute necrotizing pancreatitis. The study was conducted at 32 centers in North America and Europe. It was concluded that treatment with meropenem does not confer an advantage over placebo in reducing the risk of developing pancreatic or peripancreatic infections, mortality, or requirement of surgical intervention. It was also concluded that there is no benefit of antibiotic prophylaxis in patients with acute necrotizing pancreatitis.

8. Da Costa DW, Bouwense SA, Schepers NJ et al. Same-Admission versus Interval Cholecystectomy for Mild Gallstone Pancreatitis (PONCHO): A multicentre randomised controlled trial. *Lancet.* 2015;386.10000:1261–1268.

In this multicenter, parallel-group, assessor-masked, randomized controlled trial, the authors investigated the optimal timing of cholecystectomy for mild biliary pancreatitis. Same-admission cholecystectomy was associated with significantly lower risk of mortality and biliary complications (same-admission vs. interval cholecystectomy; 5% vs. 17%, p=0.002). The risk of recurrent pancreatitis and biliary colic was also significantly lower with same-admission cholecystectomy.

9. Chang L, Lo S, Stabile BE et al. Preoperative versus postoperative endoscopic retrograde cholangiopancreatography in mild to moderate gallstone pancreatitis: A prospective randomized trial. *Ann Surg.* 2000;231(1):82–87.

A randomized control trial was conducted on patients with mild to moderate biliary pancreatitis to see whether preoperative ERCP has an advantage over selective postoperative ERCP. It was concluded that in cases with mild to moderate pancreatitis without concomitant cholangitis, postoperative ERCP not only reduces the LOS and total cost of treatment but also decreases unnecessary ERCPs that would otherwise be performed preoperatively.

Landmark Article of 21st Century

A STEP-UP APPROACH OR OPEN NECROSECTOMY FOR NECROTIZING PANCREATITIS

van Santvoort HC, Besselink MG, Bakker OJ, Hofker HS, Boermeester MA, Dejong CH, van Goor H, Schaapherder AF, van Eijck CH, Bollen TL, van Ramshorst B, Nieuwenhuijs VB, Timmer R, Laméris JS, Kruyt PM, Manusama ER, van der Harst E, van der Schelling GP, Karsten T, Hesselink EJ, van Laarhoven CJ, Rosman C, Bosscha K, de Wit RJ, Houdijk AP, van Leeuwen MS, Buskens E, and Gooszen HG; Dutch Pancreatitis Study Group, *N Engl J Med.* 2010;362:1491–1502

ABSTRACT

Background Necrotizing pancreatitis with infected necrotic tissue is associated with a high rate of complications and death. Standard treatment is open necrosectomy. The outcome may be improved by a minimally invasive step-up approach.

Methods In this multicenter study, we randomly assigned 88 patients with necrotizing pancreatitis and suspected or confirmed infected necrotic tissue to undergo primary open necrosectomy or a step-up approach to treatment. The step-up approach consisted of percutaneous drainage followed, if necessary, by minimally invasive retroperitoneal necrosectomy. The primary endpoint was a composite of major complications (new-onset multiple-organ failure or multiple systemic complications, perforation of a visceral organ or enterocutaneous fistula, or bleeding) or death.

Results   The primary endpoint occurred in 31 of 45 patients (69%) assigned to open necrosectomy and in 17 of 43 patients (40%) assigned to the step-up approach (risk ratio with the step-up approach, 0.57; 95% confidence interval, 0.38−0.87; P = 0.006). Of the patients assigned to the step-up approach, 35% were treated with percutaneous drainage only. New-onset multiple-organ failure occurred less often in patients assigned to the step-up approach than in those assigned to open necrosectomy (12% vs. 40%, P = 0.002). The rate of death did not differ significantly between groups (19% vs. 16%, P = 0.70). Patients assigned to the step-up approach had a lower rate of incisional hernias (7% vs. 24%, P = 0.03) and new-onset diabetes (16% vs. 38%, P = 0.02).

Conclusions   A minimally invasive step-up approach, as compared with open necrosectomy, reduced the rate of the composite endpoint of major complications or death among patients with necrotizing pancreatitis and infected necrotic tissue. (Current Controlled Trials Number: ISRCTN13975868.)

Original Author Commentary: Hjalmar C. van Santvoort

Around 30% of patients with necrotizing pancreatitis develop secondary bacterial infection of the pancreatic and peripancreatic necrosis (van Santvoort et al., 2011). Infected necrosis causes sepsis with associated multiple-organ failure and is therefore an indication for invasive intervention (Working Group IAP/APA Acute Pancreatitis Guidelines, 2013). The historical treatment was primary open necrosectomy: a laparotomy with complete debridement of the infected necrosis. Open necrosectomy was associated with a high risk of complications (34%–95%) and death (11%–39%) (Beger et al., 1988; Traverso and Kozarek, 2005). The alternative "step-up approach" aims at reducing the pro-inflammatory response of major surgery by control of the source of infection rather than complete removal of the infected necrosis. The first step is percutaneous or endoscopic catheter drainage to mitigate sepsis; this may postpone or even obviate surgical necrosectomy. If drainage does not lead to clinical improvement, the next step is video-assisted retroperitoneal debridement (VARD) (Horvath et al., 2001).

In the 2010 PANTER trial, 88 patients from 19 hospitals of the Dutch Pancreatitis Study Group with (suspected) infected necrotizing pancreatitis were randomized to primary open necrosectomy (n = 45) or the step-up approach (n = 43) (van Santvoort et al. 2010). The step-up approach reduced the primary endpoint of major complications (i.e., multiple-organ failure, bleeding, enteric perforations) and death (69% vs. 40%, P = 0.006). Of the patients assigned to the step-up approach, 35% were treated with catheter drainage only. Patients assigned to the step-up approach also had a lower rate of incisional hernias (7% vs. 24%, P = 0.03) and new-onset diabetes (16% vs. 38%, P = 0.02).

Patients with infected necrotizing pancreatitis should be treated with a step-up approach consisting of catheter drainage, followed, if necessary, by minimally invasive necrosectomy.

References

Beger HG, Buchler M, Bittner R, Oettinger W, Block S, Nevalainen T. Necrosectomy and postoperative local lavage in patients with necrotizing pancreatitis: Results of a prospective clinical trial. *World J Surg*. 1988;12:255–262.

Horvath KD, Kao LS, Ali A, Wherry KL, Pellegrini CA, Sinanan MN. Laparoscopic assisted percutaneous drainage of infected pancreatic necrosis. *Surg Endosc*. 2001 Jul;15(7):677–682.

Traverso LW, Kozarek RA. Pancreatic necrosectomy: Definitions and technique. *J Gastrointest Surg*. 2005;9:436–439.

van Santvoort HC, Bakker OJ, Bollen TL et al. Dutch Pancreatitis Study Group. A conservative and minimally invasive approach to necrotizing pancreatitis improves outcome. *Gastroenterology*. 2011 Oct;141(4):1254–1263.

van Santvoort HC, Besselink MG, Bakker OJ et al. A step-up approach or open necrosectomy for necrotizing pancreatitis. *N Engl J Med*. 2010 Apr 22;362(16):1491–502.

Working Group IAP/APA Acute Pancreatitis Guidelines. IAP/APA evidence-based guidelines for the management of acute pancreatitis. *Pancreatology*. 2013 Jul–Aug;13(4 Suppl 2).

CHAPTER 19

Pancreatic Pseudocyst

Review by Contributor: Matthew J. Martin

There is a well-defined subset of patients with acute pancreatitis who will develop local complications including necrosis, infection, or peripancreatic fluid collections that prompt a surgical referral. It is critical for the surgeon to have a thorough understanding of this disease process and a well-developed algorithm to select from the myriad of currently available diagnostic and interventional options. This is particularly important when dealing with pancreatic pseudocysts (PS) due to the history of highly variable and confusing terminology, definitions, and classification systems for pancreatitis and peripancreatic fluid collections that have been used in the literature and that continue to be used in clinical practice.

TERMINOLOGY AND CLASSIFICATION

The term "pseudocyst" has been poorly defined in previous published literature, has been applied to a wide variety of pathologies that are not true PS, and continues to be utilized by radiologists and other specialties as a "catchall" term for any well-formed peripancreatic fluid collection. Thus, the first step in the evaluation process should be an accurate determination of whether the pathology truly is a PS. The recently revised Atlanta classification system divides acute pancreatitis into necrotizing or interstitial edematous variants and then uses 4 weeks as the cutoff between an early versus "mature" associated fluid collection. PS is diagnosed as a persistent mature fluid collection (>4 weeks) in association with interstitial edematous pancreatitis (IEP). Most importantly, the term "pseudocyst" should not be utilized in necrotizing pancreatitis (NP)-associated fluid collections, which are now termed "walled off necrosis" (WON). Arguably the most important aspect of maintaining this 4-week cutoff in the definition is to minimize attempts at early unnecessary and often nontherapeutic interventions for peripancreatic fluid collections, and particularly for PS. The most important epidemiologic aspect of PS is the fact that most will be asymptomatic or minimally symptomatic and 70%–90% will resolve spontaneously and not require any intervention.

CLINICAL EVALUATION

Patients with a possible PS who have no prior history of acute/chronic pancreatitis episodes or symptoms (or trauma) should prompt consideration of an alternative diagnosis of cystic neoplasm of the pancreas. However, up to 15% of PS have no clearly identified antecedent pancreatitis episode or trauma and a significant percent of pancreatic cystic neoplasms may initially present as an episode of acute pancreatitis. There are essentially no symptoms or exam findings that are specific to PS and the majority of patients will have either minimal or no symptoms. If symptoms are present, they most commonly will feature vague upper abdominal and/or back pain, bloating, early satiety or pain shortly after meals, or less commonly, symptoms of gastric outlet obstruction. Elevated serum amylase levels are seen in approximately 50% of patients with PS and are often mistakenly attributed to "recurrent pancreatitis."

DIAGNOSTIC IMAGING FOR PS

Abdominal radiologic imaging with CT and/or MRI has become the standard for evaluating the patient with a known or suspected PS and for surveilling patients to determine resolution versus persistence. CT scan is highly accurate for identifying pancreatic necrosis and for differentiating a true PS from necrotizing pancreatitis with walled-off necrosis. MRI and endoscopic ultrasound may also be particularly useful in delineating ductal anatomy and distinguishing a PS from a cystic neoplasm.

MANAGEMENT AND INTERVENTIONS

The most important distinction in selecting the optimal management strategy for PS is the presence or absence of associated symptomatology. The 2013 evidence-based guidelines from the American College of Gastroenterology state: "Asymptomatic PS do not warrant intervention regardless of size, location, and/or extension (moderate recommendation, high quality of evidence)." However, there are exceptions to this rule such as the inability rule out a cystic neoplasm, rapidly enlarging PS, and patients in high-risk occupations or locations. In addition to the lower likelihood of spontaneous resolution, the risk of complications such as rupture or infection are higher in larger lesions (>/=10 cm) and therefore the decision for intervention should be individualized. For symptomatic PS or those associated with pancreatic or pancreatic–ductal pathology that requires intervention, there are now a wide variety of options that range from minimally invasive endoscopic or percutaneous interventions to major open surgery. Image-guided percutaneous drainage (PD) is among the least invasive options for PS but is associated with higher rates of recurrence and pancreatic fistula. In a large national study of over 14,000 patients, PD was independently associated with increased complications, PS recurrence, and mortality.

Advanced endoscopic interventions have been among the most important advances in treating large or symptomatic PS and have now largely supplanted surgery. These can include internal (via transpapillary stenting) versus transmural (via stomach or duodenum) drainage procedures. Transpapillary drainage is only appropriate for PS with a clear and patent ductal communication; otherwise transmural drainage into the stomach or duodenum is the procedure of choice. This relies on the placement of stents or pigtail catheters to maintain the communication and should be left in place for at least 6 weeks. Although surgical intervention for PS has become much less common, it will continue to have a role in patients who are not candidates or who fail endoscopic/percutaneous intervention and in patients who require resection and/or reconstruction for pancreatic ductal disruption. The two standard surgical procedures for PS involve creating an anastomosis between the cyst wall and the abutting segment of the gastrointestinal tract with either cystogastrostomy or cystojejunostomy. Although traditionally performed via open surgery, these procedures can now be readily performed via minimally invasive techniques including laparoscopic and robotic-assisted. A landmark randomized trial in 2013, compared endoscopic versus surgical drainage among 40 patients with PS. They found no difference in success rates or complications, but the endoscopic approach had shorter lengths of stay, improved physical and mental health scores, and lower costs versus surgery. A subsequent large systematic literature review compared the three approaches of percutaneous, endoscopic, and surgery for PS and demonstrated that surgery was superior to percutaneous drainage and endoscopic drainage was superior to both. Although this data strongly supports endoscopic drainage as the initial preferred approach versus open surgery, further data comparing endoscopy to minimally invasive surgical approaches is needed. Finally, among patients with complex pancreatic ductal pathology such as significant structuring or the "disconnected duct" syndrome, the optimal intervention approach should be focused on the underlying anatomic abnormality and not on the PS itself. These cases typically require more complex surgical interventions including pancreatic resection and ductal reconstruction, which should be referred to an experienced pancreatic surgeon and center.

ANNOTATED REFERENCES FOR PANCREATIC PSEUDOCYST

1. Zhao X, Feng T, Ji W. Endoscopic versus surgical treatment for pancreatic pseudocyst. *Dig Endosc*. 2016;28:83–91.

   Systematic literature review and meta-analysis that combined five comparative studies with 255 patients. Patients who underwent surgical pseudocyst drainage had a significantly higher success rate compared to endoscopic drainage. However, there were no differences in complications or in rates of recurrence and need for reinterventions. Endoscopy was associated with shorter lengths of stay and lower costs versus surgery.

2. Teoh AY, Dhir V, Jin ZD, Kida M, Seo DW, Ho KY. Systematic review comparing endoscopic, percutaneous, and surgical pancreatic pseudocyst drainage. *World J Gastrointest Endosc*. 2016;8:310–318.

   Systematic literature review and meta-analysis that combined ten comparative studies, including three randomized trials. Surgical drainage was associated with lower adverse events and mortality compared to percutaneous PS drainage. However, surgical and endoscopic drainage had comparable success and complication rates, but endoscopic drainage was associated with shorter hospital stays, lower costs, and improved quality-of-life scores.

3. Gurusamy KS, Pallari E, Hawkins N, Pereira SP, Davidson BR. Management strategies for pancreatic pseudocysts. *Cochrane Database Syst Rev*. 2016;4:CD011392.

   A Cochrane Database systematic review and meta-analysis including four randomized trials with 177 total patients. Identified that all of the trials were at significant risk of bias and overall data quality was low or very low for all outcomes. Endoscopic drainage with endoscopic ultrasound and nasocystic drainage were associated with the best outcomes versus endoscopic drainage or surgical drainage.

4. Nealon WH, Bhutani M, Riall TS, Raju G, Ozkan O, Neilan R. A unifying concept: Pancreatic ductal anatomy both predicts and determines the major complications resulting from pancreatitis. *J Am Coll Surg.* 2009;208:790–799; discussion 9–801.

   Retrospective review of 563 patients with PS managed at a single center and using a grading system for the ductal anatomy developed by the authors. Demonstrated the importance of assessing and grading the ductal anatomy and any pathology as the assigned grade (grade I–IV) was a strong predictor of outcomes and of the need for interventions or advanced surgical reconstruction.

5. Matsuoka L, Alexopoulos SP. Surgical management of pancreatic pseudocysts. *Gastrointest Endosc Clin North Am.* 2018;28:131–141.

   Excellent overview and up-to-date review of management strategies for complicated PS, including open and minimally invasive surgical techniques. Also highlights the continued need for surgical intervention in patients with complicated PS, failure of less invasive interventions, and in patients with chronic pancreatitis and ductal anomalies.

6. Varadarajulu S, Christein JD, Tamhane A, Drelichman ER, Wilcox CM. Prospective randomized trial comparing EUS and EGD for transmural drainage of pancreatic pseudocysts (with videos). *Gastrointest Endosc.* 2008;68:1102–1111.

   Prospective randomized study of 30 patients with PS greater than 4 cm in size and who were referred for possible endoscopic drainage. Patients were randomized to standard endoscopic drainage versus drainage with EUS assistance. Standard endoscopic drainage was successful in only 33%, with the remainder requiring crossover to EUS drainage. There were no differences in recurrence or complication rates, but overall successful drainage was superior with EUS.

7. Loveday BP, Mittal A, Phillips A, Windsor JA. Minimally invasive management of pancreatic abscess, pseudocyst, and necrosis: A systematic review of current guidelines. *World J Surg.* 2008;32:2383–2394.

   Systematic review of existing guidelines for pancreatic abscess, infected PS, and infected necrosis from major medical organizations and societies. Sixteen guidelines were identified and analyzed. Percutaneous drainage was recommended by 50% of the guidelines for abscess or infected PS. Endoscopic drainage was recommended by 44% of guidelines and 10 of 16 did not include levels of evidence to support their recommendations. This highlighted the significant lack of consensus and concordance of published guidelines for infected pancreatic fluid collections.

8. Kahaleh M, Shami VM, Conaway MR, et al. Endoscopic ultrasound drainage of pancreatic pseudocyst: A prospective comparison with conventional endoscopic drainage. *Endoscopy.* 2006;38:355–359.

   Prospective study including 99 patients who underwent endoscopic drainage of PS using a standardized algorithm with 1- and 6-month follow-up data. Patients underwent either conventional endoscopic drainage (CED) or endoscopic ultrasound-assisted drainage (EUS). Short- and long-term success rates were 84%–94%, with no difference between groups. Complication rates were equivalent (18% vs. 19%) between the two groups concluding that either approach is acceptable.

9. Foster BR, Jensen KK, Bakis G, Shaaban AM, Coakley FV. Revised Atlanta classification for acute pancreatitis: A pictorial essay. *Radiographics.* 2016;36:675–687.

   Excellent review article of the updated and revised Atlanta classification system for acute pancreatitis. This included the clear definition of PS as a sterile fluid collection that has persisted for at least 4 weeks after the index episode and distinguishes it from walled-off necrosis that is associated with necrotizing pancreatitis. Includes example images of classic radiographic appearances of each of these lesions.

Landmark Article of 21st Century

EQUAL EFFICACY OF ENDOSCOPIC AND SURGICAL CYSTOGASTROSTOMY FOR PANCREATIC PSEUDOCYST DRAINAGE IN A RANDOMIZED TRIAL

Varadarajulu S, Bang JY, Sutton BS, Trevino JM, Christein JD, and Wilcox CM, *Gastroenterology.* 2013;145(3):583–590

ABSTRACT

Background and Aims Although surgery is the standard technique for drainage of pancreatic pseudocysts, use of endoscopic methods is increasing. We performed a single-center, open-label, randomized trial to compare endoscopic and surgical cystogastrostomy for pancreatic pseudocyst drainage.

Methods Patients with pancreatic pseudocysts underwent endoscopic (n = 20) or surgical cystogastrostomy (n = 20). The primary endpoint was pseudocyst recurrence after a 24-month follow-up period. Secondary endpoints were treatment success or failure, complications, re-interventions, length of hospital stay, physical and mental health scores, and total costs.

Results At the end of the follow-up period, none of the patients who received endoscopic therapy had a pseudocyst recurrence, compared with one patient treated surgically. There were no differences in treatment successes, complications, or re-interventions between the groups. However, the length of hospital stay was shorter for patients who underwent endoscopic cystogastrostomy (median 2 days vs. 6 days in the surgery group; $P < 0.001$). Although there were no differences in physical component scores and mental health component scores (MCS) between groups at baseline on the Medical Outcomes Study 36-Item Short-Form General Survey questionnaire, longitudinal analysis showed significantly better physical component scores ($P = 0.019$) and mental health component scores ($P = 0.025$) for the endoscopy treatment group. The total mean cost was lower for patients managed by endoscopy than surgery ($7011 vs. $15,052; $P = 0.003$).

Conclusions In a randomized trial comparing endoscopic and surgical cystogastrostomy for pancreatic pseudocyst drainage, none of the patients in the endoscopy group had pseudocyst recurrence during the follow-up period, therefore there is no evidence that surgical cystogastrostomy is superior. However, endoscopic treatment was associated with shorter hospital stays, better physical and mental health of patients, and lower cost.

Editor Notes

Assessment: This study compared endoscopic with surgical cystogastrostomy for pancreatic pseudocyst drainage in a small (n = 20/group), randomized, unblinded clinical trial at a single center over 1 year. There was no difference found in the primary endpoint, time to recurrence at 24 months, as no patient recurred in the endoscopy group and only one recurred in the surgery group. There was a statistically significant reduction in hospital stay (80%) and costs (50%) in the endoscopy group, and patients were more physically and emotionally satisfied.

Limitations: Small study subject to beta error. The study did not achieve its primary endpoint, time to recurrence, which was an illogical measure but was used to predict group size. It was unclear how the estimate of the effect of endoscopy was derived so as to determine the subsequent sample. A single surgeon performed all the procedures, which may have influenced length of stay based on the individual patient care protocols.

Conclusions: This paper changed our treatment algorithm, placing endoscopic drainage of pancreatic pseudocysts as the first or primary modality. The technique of endoscopic drainage appears to be highly effective, while at the same time less morbid, with lower associated patient costs than surgical intervention.

CHAPTER 20

Hepatic Abscess

Review by Contributor: Krista L. Kaups

Hepatic abscess has been recognized as a pathologic entity for many years, but historically as either a nearly uniformly fatal occurrence or as an autopsy finding. The etiologies, diagnostic modalities available, pathogens responsible, and outcomes have changed markedly in the last 100 years accompanied by even more marked alterations in treatment strategies.

Hepatic abscess results from bacterial (pyogenic), fungal, or amebic infection. Although the incidence of pyogenic abscess in the United States, Canada, and Europe is relatively low (1–3 cases annually per 100,000 population), the incidence is significantly higher in other parts of the world, particularly Asia, with an incidence of 18 annual cases per 100,000 population reported in Taiwan.

Pyogenic abscesses develop either due to a spread through the biliary system (cholangitis), via the portal system from appendicitis or diverticulitis, direct extension from adjacent processes (e.g., gallbladder), hematogenous spread that occurs with septicemia, or direct injuries from trauma (blunt, penetrating, or iatrogenic). In descriptions published in the first half of the twentieth century, portal vein spread from perforated appendicitis was a common mechanism, but biliary obstruction related to either gallstone disease or strictures of benign or malignant origin, predominates now. Also contributing are the widespread use of biliary interventional techniques and transplantation (Keefer, 1934; Huang et al., 1996; Lardière-Deguelte et al., 2015).

Risk factors for pyogenic abscess include diabetes mellitus, hepatobiliary or pancreatic disease, underlying malignancy, age >55 years, and male gender. Mortality is also associated with these factors but also with larger abscess size and rupture and the presence of jaundice, septic shock, and organ failure.

Diagnosis previously relied on relatively nonspecific signs and symptoms of fever, chills, right upper quadrant pain, and malaise. Presently, an estimated 90% of abscesses are diagnosed by imaging, with the remainder recognized intraoperatively. Both ultrasound and CT scan are highly sensitive and may also help to delineate the underlying cause of the abscess. MRI and MRCP may also be useful.

The microbiologic flora has also changed over time. In the earlier studies, *Escherichia coli* was the most common organism cultured, followed by *Streptococcus* and

Staphylococcus. In recent studies, *E. coli* has decreased and drug-resistant, virulent *K. pneumoniae* have increased markedly in both Asian and Western series. And, in contrast with the management of pyogenic abscess prior to antibiotic availability, multidrug-resistant bacteria are appearing more frequently, reported at 11%–40% in certain patient populations. Fungal species, most commonly Candida, are also being cultured, particularly in immunocompromised patients.

Contemporary management of hepatic abscess involves obtaining blood cultures and prompt administration of broad-spectrum antibiotics. Small abscesses can potentially be managed with antibiotics, but intervention promotes more rapid resolution. Percutaneous drainage, rather than aspiration, should be performed unless an associated need for surgical intervention is present (e.g., cholecystitis or perforated diverticulitis). The presence of bile in the drainage indicates a biliary source, which should be addressed.

In much of the world, hepatic abscess is most commonly due to *Entamoeba histolytica*. An estimated 1%–5% of the 50 million people infected annually will develop amebic hepatic abscesses. Patients often have a history of travel to endemic areas but may not always have had colitis. The affected population is younger and more often male than patients with pyogenic abscess. In addition, the development of the hepatic abscess may be significantly delayed, in some cases for years. The primary treatment is medical (metronidazole) but it is estimated that up to 15% of patients will require intervention and that 20% may have simultaneous bacterial infection. Percutaneous needle aspiration is useful for sampling, but percutaneous drainage has greater overall success at resolution and should particularly be considered for large abscesses and those determined to be at risk for rupture (Lodhi et al., 2004; Cai et al., 2014).

Important challenges remain in managing patients with hepatic abscesses. Despite significant improvements in treatment with prompt diagnosis facilitated by imaging, the aggressive use of broad-spectrum antibiotics, and the availability of percutaneous drainage, mortality remains relatively high and is reported at 5%–20%. These changes in management have also led to new challenges, including the emergence of multidrug-resistant bacteria, an increase in biliary stricture-related abscesses occurring after pancreaticoduodenal surgery and hepatic transplants, as well as the occurrence of fungal abscesses. Mortality is associated with the presence of malignant disease, septic shock, and comorbid conditions including immunocompromise are likely contributors.

The incidence of hepatic abscess also appears to be increasing, although it is not entirely clear how much of the increase is due to improvements in, and more readily available, imaging. However, the extensive use of biliary interventions, including endoscopic sphincterotomy, are likely contributing to the greater incidence. Furthermore, patients who have undergone hepatic transplantation are at particular risk of biliary ischemia and stricture as well as being immunocompromised. It has also been theorized that the frequent use of angioembolization to support nonoperative management of hepatic trauma results in ischemia which may then become seeded. And despite the utility of imaging studies, the source of infection remains cryptogenic for a certain percentage of patients.

Note: Despite the numerous studies and relatively large-scale comparison studies, essentially no large-scale randomized trials have been published. However, the advancement of treatment and improvement in mortality have served to validate the changes in management.

ANNOTATED REFERENCES FOR HEPATIC ABSCESS

1. Keefer CS. Liver abscess: Review of eighty-five cases. *N Engl J Med*. 1934;211:21.

   The author presents one of the earliest series of cases and reviews the etiologies and diagnosis of hepatic abscess based on history, signs, and symptoms. He also describes the means of infection, which is used in contemporary analyses, including pylephlebitis, primary process in the portal area without pylephlebitis, direct extension to the liver, extension through the biliary system, and from generalized sepsis. Suppurative appendicitis is one of the predominant causes, but in this pre-antibiotic era other associated conditions included otitis media and tonsillitis. Amebic and hydatid disease were also recognized.

2. Ochsner A, De Bakey ME, Murray S. Pyogenic abscess of the liver. II. An analysis of 47 cases with a review of the literature. *Am. J. Surg*. 1938;40:292.

   An early review, totaling 186 cases from a single institution, from well-known surgeons describing diagnosis and management in a pre-antibiotic era. Operative strategies include "prophylactic" treatment of pylephlebitis, with ligation of the ileocolic or even the superior mesenteric vein, to prevent suppurative spread via the portal system. Drainage procedures strongly emphasize avoidance of contaminating either the pleural or peritoneal cavities and advocate extraperitoneal or retroperitoneal approaches, which are described. Overall mortality rates are 70%–80%; 50%–65% in patients having operative drainage.

3. Joseph WL, Kahn AM, Longmire WP. Pyogenic liver abscess: Changing patterns in approach. *Am J Surg*. 1968;115:63–68.

   Thirty years later, the most common etiologies for hepatic abscess were intraperitoneal disease or septicemia as well as biliary obstruction. Antibiotics are now an important part of the treatment and transperitoneal drainage, rather than being condemned, is the treatment of choice. Percutaneous aspiration is "not recommended." Mortality remained high at >50% but was less than 20% in patients undergoing operative intervention.

4. Huang CJ, Pitt HA, Lipsett PA et al. Pyogenic hepatic abscess. Changing trends over 42 years. *Ann Surg*. 1996;223(5):600–607; discussion 607–9.

   Patients treated from 1952–1972, at a single institution, were compared to those from 1973–1993. The overall incidence of hepatic abscess increased, with an increased association with biliary obstruction and malignancy. The bacterial spectrum shifted and mortality decreased from 65% to 31%. Percutaneous drainage has become an accepted intervention with surgical drainage for failure.

5. Rajak CL, Gupta S, Jain S et al. *Am J Roentgenol*. 1998;170(4):1035–1039.

   A trial of 50 patients with hepatic abscess, including both amebic and pyogenic, which did not resolve with medical management, randomized to percutaneous needle aspiration versus percutaneous drainage. Needle aspiration was limited to two attempts. Catheter drainage was curative in all; however, the average time to resolution was the same in both groups.

6. Lodhi S, Sarwari AR, Muzammil M, Salam A, Smego RA. Features distinguishing amoebic from pyogenic liver abscess: A review of 577 adult cases. *Trop Med Int Health.* 2004;9:718–723.

Multivariate analysis in a retrospective review of 577 patients with hepatic abscesses demonstrated that age >50 years, pulmonary findings on examination, multiple abscesses, and amebic serology titers <1:256 IU were predictive of pyogenic rather than amebic infection.

7. Tan YM, Chung AY, Chow PK et al. An appraisal of surgical and percutaneous drainage for pyogenic liver abscesses larger than 5 cm. *Ann Surg.* 2005;241(3):485–490.

Surgical drainage is recommended over percutaneous drainage for hepatic abscess greater than 5 cm. Mortality rates are 4.5% for surgical drainage versus 2.8% for percutaneous drainage.

8. Cai YL, Xiong XZ, Lu J et al. Percutaneous needle aspiration versus catheter drainage in the management of liver abscess: A systematic review and meta-analysis. *HPB (Oxford).* 2014;17(3):195–201.

Five randomized controlled trials with 306 patients with both pyogenic and amebic hepatic abscesses were included in a meta-analysis of percutaneous needle aspiration versus percutaneous drainage techniques. The authors concluded that both methods were safe, overall mortality was low, and that percutaneous drainage was more likely to be successful.

9. Lardière-Deguelte S, Ragot E, Amroun K et al. Hepatic abscess: Diagnosis and management. *J Visc Surg.* 2015;152:231–243.

A contemporary and relatively comprehensive review of the topic of hepatic abscess including those occurring post-trauma and post-transplant.

10. Lo JZW, Leow JJJ, Ng PLF et al. Predictors of therapy failure in a series of 741 adult pyogenic liver abscesses. *J Hepatobiliary Pancreat Sci.* 2015;22:156–165.

The authors compare their experience from 2001–2011 with that from 1994–1997 and also examine worldwide data and trends. The incidence of hepatic abscess is increasing, as is bacterial resistance. Risk factors for antibiotic treatment failure were age >55 years, multiple abscesses, malignant etiology, and patients who had undergone endoscopic intervention.

PREDICTORS OF THERAPY FAILURE IN A SERIES OF 741 ADULT PYOGENIC LIVER ABSCESSES

Lo JZ, Leow JJ, Ng PL, Lee HQ, Mohd Noor NA, Low JK, Junnarkar SP, and Woon WW, *Hepatobiliary Pancreat Sci.* 2015;22:156–165

ABSTRACT

Background   Adult pyogenic liver abscess (PLA) is a major hepatobiliary infection. We aim to identify risk factors associated with therapy failure.

Methods   Retrospective study of 741 PLA patients (2001–2011) and comparison with earlier data (1994–1997). Risk factors associated with therapy failure were identified with multivariate analysis.

Results   Incidence of PLA is 86/100,000 admissions, with average size 5.75 cm. Sixty-eight percent of PLA were secondary to *Klebsiella pneumoniae* and there is increasing extended-spectrum beta-lactamase (ESBL) resistance. Compared with the 1990s, there is an increasing annual incidence (from 18 to 67). Elderly age ($\geq$55 years old), presence of multiple abscesses, malignancy as etiology, and patients who underwent endoscopic intervention are independent predictors for failure of antibiotics-only therapy, while average intravenous antibiotics duration and average abscess size are not. Eastern Cooperative Oncology Group (ECOG) performance status $\geq$2, preexisting hypertension, and hyperbilirubinemia are independent predictors for failure of percutaneous therapy, while the presence of multiple abscesses and average abscess size are not.

Conclusion   There is an increasing PLA incidence with increasing ESBL resistance. Percutaneous drainage should be considered early for elderly patients ($\geq$55 years old), those with multiple abscesses, malignancy as etiology, or who required endoscopic intervention. We should have a low threshold for surgical intervention for patients with ECOG performance status $\geq$2, comorbidity of hypertension, or hyperbilirubinemia.

Editor Notes

Assessment: This paper was a large review of adult pyogenic liver abscess in Singapore. Two time periods were compared: 3 years (1994–1997) to a subsequent 10 years (2001–2011). Risk factors were identified using multivariate analysis. Age over 55, presence of multiple abscesses, malignancy as etiology, and patients who underwent endoscopic intervention were independent predictors for failure of antibiotics treatment. Most (68%) of liver abscesses were due to *K. pneumoniae*, and there was an increased extended spectra beta-lactamase resistance over time. Those individuals with poor performance status or underlying hyperbilirubinemia more commonly required surgical intervention for failure of percutaneous drainage.

Limitations: This was a 10-year retrospective review from a single large center comparing results from two different time periods. No denominator was reported, meaning neither the change in the reporting population in Singapore nor the closure or increase of hospital beds in the region is known. A change in incidence of liver abscess therefore cannot be determined. The conclusions are not based on the actual data but rather upon expert opinion.

Conclusions: Pyogenic liver abscess appears to be increasing in both overall incidence and patterns of antibiotic resistance. The authors recommend that patients 55 and older with multiple abscesses, malignancy as etiology, and those who require endoscopic intervention should be considered for percutaneous drainage. These patients appear to be more likely to fail treatment with antibiotics alone.

CHAPTER 21

Cirrhosis in Surgery

Review by Contributor: Eric J. Ley

In Greek mythology, Prometheus defied the gods by stealing fire for all of humanity. As punishment, Zeus bound him to a rock so an eagle could feed on his liver each day while the liver would grow back during the night. The acute care surgeon might inquire about the amazing technical skills of that eagle who could operate with only a beak, but the myth continues that Hercules rescued Prometheus by killing the bird, leaving the source of the eagle's skills forever unanswered.

Unlike the liver injury with Prometheus, cirrhosis is chronic liver damage from a number of sources that causes irreversible fibrosis and leads to portal hypertension, ascites, spontaneous bacterial peritonitis, hepatic encephalopathy, variceal hemorrhage, coagulopathy, hepatorenal syndrome, and hepatocellular carcinoma. The major causes of cirrhosis include chronic hepatitis B virus (HBV) and hepatitis C virus (HCV) infection, alcoholism, and nonalcoholic steatohepatitis. Cirrhosis is the eighth leading cause of death in the United States and the thirteenth leading cause of death globally. A diagnosis of compensated cirrhosis is associated with a risk of death that is 4.7 times the general population, and decompensated cirrhosis is associated with a risk that is 9.7 times as high. The average life expectancy of a patient with compensated cirrhosis is 10–13 years, and the average life expectancy may be as low as 2 years for decompensated cirrhosis (Ge et al., 2016).

Managing the diverse complications related to cirrhosis may require expertise from several Hercules-like specialists. Gastroesophageal varices develop in more than one-third of patients with cirrhosis and lead to significant morbidity. The management of gastroesophageal varices includes hemorrhage prevention with beta-blockers and endoscopic ligation. In the face of an acute bleed, resuscitation, blood transfusions, and endoscopy should be utilized to treat variceal hemorrhage. Transjugular intrahepatic portosystemic shunt (TIPS) is indicated in patients with uncontrolled bleeding varices or when bleeding recurs despite combined pharmacological and endoscopic therapy. Balloon tamponade should be used as a temporizing measure for a maximum of 24 hours in patients with uncontrollable bleeding for whom a more definitive therapy such as TIPS or endoscopic therapy is planned. Patients with cirrhosis who survive an episode of active variceal hemorrhage should receive therapy to prevent recurrence of variceal hemorrhage. Patients who are otherwise transplant candidates should be referred to a transplant center for evaluation (Garcia-Tsao et al., 2007). Portacaval shunting, which was commonly performed to reduce portal hypertension, has virtually disappeared in modern-day surgery.

Cirrhotic patients with spontaneous bacterial peritonitis who received early as compared to delayed paracentesis had lower mortality (13% vs. 27%, P = 0.007) and each hour delay in paracentesis was associated with a 3.3% increase in mortality. Paracentesis performed less than 12 hours from admission may improve survival (Kim et al., 2014). In contrast to many cirrhotic complications, portal vein thrombosis can be a consequence of the progression of liver disease and may not be responsible for further progression of liver disease (Nery et al., 2015). This longitudinal study noted the cumulative incidence of portal vein thrombosis in patients with cirrhosis was 4.6%, 8.2%, and 10.7% at 1, 3, and 5 years. Although patients with more severe liver disease were at a higher risk for developing portal vein thrombosis, the progression of liver disease such as the development of ascites, reduced portal blood flow velocity, or other variables for liver decompensation were independent of the presence of portal vein thrombosis.

The annual incidence of hepatocellular carcinoma is 5% for those in the United States who have cirrhosis. The median survival among patients with limited hepatocellular carcinoma is approximately 2 years, and the median survival among those with advanced hepatocellular carcinoma is approximately 6 months. For cirrhotic patients with unresectable hepatocellular carcinomas, liver transplantation is an effective treatment when guided by the Milan criteria (single tumor less than 5 cm or three tumors or fewer, each less than 3 cm) (Clavien et al., 2012). Importantly, a phase 3 trial demonstrated a 97.5% cure rate for patients with hepatitis C and class A cirrhosis after 24 weeks of treatment. Eradication of the hepatitis C virus with antiviral therapy reduces the risk for hepatocellular carcinoma (Poordad et al., 2014).

For cirrhotic patients who require elective non-hepatic surgery, operative repair has traditionally been considered high risk. The most significant challenge is deciding when, or if, to operate. To guide the decision are two grading systems that quantify the severity of liver disease. The Child-Turcotte-Pugh (CTP) score is computed by rating the severity of five contributing factors (total bilirubin, serum albumin, prothrombin time, ascites, and encephalopathy) on a scale of 1–3 with the resulting score ranging from 5 to 15. Scores are then grouped into one of three grades from A to C. The Model for End-Stage Liver Disease (MELD) score was primarily developed to rate severity of end-stage liver disease among candidates for liver transplantation by predicting 90-day mortality, but is now widely used in many settings. The score is derived from incorporating international normalized ratio (INR), serum creatinine (Cr), total bilirubin, and now also serum sodium (Na). Of note, the two most heavily weighted variables in the MELD scoring system are the INR and the creatinine. The MELD score can guide the mortality risk for elective surgical procedures. Thirty-day mortality ranges from 5.7% for MELD score less than 8 to more than 50% for MELD score greater than 20 (Teh et al., 2007).

Cirrhotic patients with ascites have a high rate of umbilical hernias due to the increased intra-abdominal pressure from ascites, weakness of the abdominal fascia and muscle wasting, and/or an umbilical vein dilating the fascial opening due to portal hypertension. Umbilical hernia repair was one of the first procedures advocated for elective repair in select patients with cirrhosis although initial efforts noted that surgical management resulted in wound complications and recurrence. On the other hand, conservative management was associated with a high rate of incarceration and readmission, leading to higher mortality when managed with emergent surgical treatment (Marsman et al., 2007). This Marsman paper questioned the typical thinking that it is better to manage cirrhotic patients with ascites conservatively, as surgical treatment was too risky. Similarly, the incidence of cholelithiasis is higher in cirrhotic patients and historically laparoscopic cholecystectomy was contraindicated. Increasingly, laparoscopic cholecystectomy is now considered safe in select cirrhotic patients, with an expected conversion rate of 11% and mortality of 4.3% (Quillin et al., 2013). Management of colorectal cancer in cirrhotic patients has also evolved. Although operative intervention for colorectal cancer in cirrhotic patients is associated with increased mortality, no difference in anastomotic leakage was observed. Importantly, cirrhosis does not impact oncological outcomes and should not be considered as a contraindication to curative treatment of colon cancer (Sabbagh et al., 2016). For trauma patients with cirrhosis, especially those with traumatic brain injury, mortality is significantly higher. Each unit increase in the MELD score is associated with an 18% increase in the odds for mortality, and any trauma patient with cirrhosis should be considered for ICU admission (Inaba et al., 2011).

ANNOTATED REFERENCES FOR CIRRHOSIS IN SURGERY

1. Teh SH, Nagorney DM, Stevens SR et al. Risk factors for mortality after surgery in patients with cirrhosis. *Gastroenterology*. 2007;132(4):1261–1269.

   For patients undergoing elective surgical procedures, the relationship between MELD score and mortality was assessed to determine whether surgery should be delayed until after liver transplantation. Thirty-day mortality ranged from 5.7% for MELD score less than 8 to more than 50% for MELD score greater than 20, suggesting that in select cirrhotic patients elective surgery is safe.

2. Quillin RC, Burns JM, Pineda JA et al. Laparoscopic cholecystectomy in the cirrhotic patient: Predictors of outcome. *Surgery*. 2013;153(5):634–640.

   Laparoscopic cholecystectomy was considered safe in select cirrhotic patients who had a mean MELD score of 11 ± 5. The conversion to open surgery rate was 11%, and serum albumin, MELD score, and blood loss predicted conversion. Mortality was 4.3% and was predicted by INR, Child-Turcotte-Pugh score, and intraoperative blood and platelet transfusions.

3. Sabbagh C, Chatelain D, Nguyen-Khac E, Rebibo L, Joly JP, Regimbeau JM. Management of colorectal cancer in patients with cirrhosis: A retrospective, case-matched study of short- and long-term outcomes. *Dig Liver Dis*. 2016;48(4):429–434.

   This study provided short- and long-term outcomes in cirrhotic patients with colorectal cancer and found a higher postoperative complication rate (57.5% vs. 26.5%, respectively; p =0.002) but no difference in anastomotic leakage. The 3-year survival was higher in Child A cirrhosis (71% vs. 92%, p =0.03) and Child B cirrhosis (69% vs. 100%, p =0.04) compared to non-cirrhotic patients. Cirrhosis had no impact on oncological outcomes and should not be considered as a contraindication to curative treatment of colon cancer.

4. Clavien PA, Lesurtel M, Bossuyt PM, Gores GJ, Langer B, Perrier A; OLT for HCC Consensus Group. Recommendations for liver transplantation for hepatocellular carcinoma: An international consensus conference report. *Lancet Oncol.* 2012;13(1):e11–e22.

   Liver transplantation is an effective treatment for small unresectable hepatocellular carcinomas in cirrhotic patients with the Milan criteria (single tumor less than 5 cm or three tumors or fewer, each less than 3 cm) have an excellent outcome. The 37 recommendations presented cover the most controversial topics surrounding liver transplantation for hepatocellular carcinoma.

5. Poordad F, Hezode C, Trinh R et al. ABT-450/r-ombitasvir and dasabuvir with ribavirin for hepatitis C with cirrhosis. *N Engl J Med.* 2014;370(21):1973–1982.

   This phase 3 trial demonstrated a 97.5% cure rate for patients with hepatitis C and class A cirrhosis after 24 weeks of treatment.

6. Inaba K, Barmparas G, Resnick S et al. The Model for End-Stage Liver Disease score: An independent prognostic factor of mortality in injured cirrhotic patients. *Arch Surg.* 2011;146(9):1074–1078.

   Cirrhotic trauma patients were reviewed to determine how MELD score altered survival after trauma. The overall mortality rate was 14.7%; the patients who died had a higher MELD score than survivors (14.1 vs. 11.2; P <0.001). Each unit increase in the MELD score was associated with an 18% increase in the odds for mortality.

7. Garcia-Tsao G, Sanyal AJ, Grace ND, Carey W; Practice Guidelines Committee of the American Association for the Study of Liver Diseases. Prevention and management of gastroesophageal varices and variceal hemorrhage in cirrhosis. *Hepatology.* 2007;46(3):922–938.

   Expert opinion is provided for the prevention and management of gastroesophageal varices due to cirrhosis in a format intended for health care providers.

8. Kim JJ, Tsukamoto MM, Mathur AK et al. Delayed paracentesis is associated with increased in-hospital mortality in patients with spontaneous bacterial peritonitis. *Am J Gastroenterol.* 2014;109(9):1436–1442.

   Cirrhotic patients with spontaneous bacterial peritonitis who received early versus delayed paracentesis had lower mortality (13% vs. 27%, P =0.007), and each hour delay in paracentesis was associated with a 3.3% increase in mortality. Paracentesis performed less than 12 hours from admission may improve survival.

9. Nery F, Chevret S, Condat B et al.; Groupe d'Etude et de Traitement du Carcinome Hépatocellulaire. Causes and consequences of portal vein thrombosis in 1,243 patients with cirrhosis: Results of a longitudinal study. *Hepatology.* 2015;61(2):660–667.

   In cirrhosis, portal vein thrombosis could be a cause or a consequence of the progression of liver disease. There is no evidence that the development of portal vein thrombosis is responsible for further progression of liver disease.

10. Ge PS, Runyon BA. Treatment of patients with cirrhosis. *N Engl J Med.* 2016;375(8): 767–777.

    This article reviews the treatment of patients with cirrhosis with a focus on recent developments. Recommendations are based on clinical trials or current expert opinion.

Landmark Article of 21st Century

MANAGEMENT IN PATIENTS WITH LIVER CIRRHOSIS AND AN UMBILICAL HERNIA

Marsman HA, Heisterkamp J, Halm JA, Tilanus HW, Metselaar HJ, and Kazemier G, *Surgery.* 2007;142:372–375

ABSTRACT

Background   Optimal management in patients with umbilical hernias and liver cirrhosis with ascites is still under debate. The objective of this study was to compare the outcome in our series of operative versus conservative treatment of these patients.

Methods   In the period between 1990 and 2004, 34 patients with an umbilical hernia combined with liver cirrhosis and ascites were identified from our hospital database. In 17 patients, treatment consisted of elective hernia repair and 13 were managed conservatively. Four patients underwent hernia repair during liver transplantation.

Results   Elective hernia repair was successful without complications and recurrence in 12 out of 17 patients. Complications occurred in 3 of these 17 patients, consisting of wound-related problems and recurrence in 4 out 17. Success rate of the initial conservative management was only 23%; hospital admittance for incarcerations occurred in 10 of 13 patients, of which 6 required hernia repair in an emergency setting. Two patients of the initially conservatively managed group died from complications of the umbilical hernia. In the 4 patients who underwent hernia correction during liver transplantation, no complications occurred and 1 patient had a recurrence.

Conclusions   Conservative management of umbilical hernias in patients with liver cirrhosis and ascites leads to a high rate of incarcerations with subsequent hernia repair in an emergency setting, whereas elective repair can be performed with less morbidity and is therefore advocated.

> **Editor Notes**
>
> **Assessment:** Patients with cirrhosis of the liver have historically been considered to have a prohibitive risk for surgery. In this retrospective review, 34 patients with cirrhosis underwent umbilical hernia repair. Those undergoing elective procedures did remarkably well despite high MELD scores (23), while those undergoing nonoperative management faired much more poorly. The patient's age and MELD score were very similar. Complication rates in the elective surgery group were 14% versus 75% with conservative care (p = 0.002).

Limitations: No standardized protocol for patient management or operative technique was utilized. The study stretched over 14 years and was a single-center experience. Selection of patients for nonoperative management rather than early elective intervention may have influenced the management plan and therefore the operative risks. Recurrence rate was quite high (25%).

Conclusions: This small retrospective review supported the notion that elective surgical management of cirrhotic patients can be performed with a low morbidity and has superior outcomes to the nonoperative approach with subsequent emergent procedure in these complex patients.

CHAPTER **22**

Management of Internal Hemorrhoids

Review by Contributor: Elizabeth R. Benjamin

Hemorrhoids result from disruption of the anal cushions and are a common problem, equally affecting men and women. Internal hemorrhoids occur just proximal to the dentate line and are largely painless, most commonly present with bleeding, and can be mild (grade I), with reversible prolapse (grade II), manually reducible (grade III), or unable to be reduced (grade IV). Treatment options are driven by clinical symptoms and grade. Clinical practice guidelines, published by the American Society of Colon and Rectal Surgeons, are available to guide management (Davis et al., 2018).

DIAGNOSIS

Hemorrhoids are visible on physical examination, but the diagnosis is most commonly made based on clinical history. The most common presenting symptoms include painless bleeding, pruritis, and tissue prolapse with defecation, and the history is best focused on the duration and severity of these symptoms. The history should include an evaluation of contributing factors including bowel habits, constipation, and fiber intake. In evaluating a patient for symptoms of internal hemorrhoids, it is imperative to also address potential alternate diagnoses including cancer, inflammatory bowel disease, colitis, diverticular disease, or angiodysplasia. The diagnosis of hemorrhoids is one of the most common reasons for missed cancer diagnosis. Family history is a critical element of the risk stratification, and endoscopy should be liberally utilized.

MEDICAL AND CONSERVATIVE MANAGEMENT

The mainstay of medical management for hemorrhoid disease remains dietary and habit modification. Increased fiber and fluid intake to improve symptoms of constipation, and limiting straining and commode time are recommended. In a meta-analysis including 378 participants, the use of fiber was associated with a 0.47 (95% CI 0.32 to 0.68) risk reduction in disease progression and symptoms (Alonso-Coello et al., 2005). Few other medication options for hemorrhoid disease exist; however, evolving data exist on the use of phlebotonics, suggesting that they may be associated with overall symptom improvement and a reduction in bleeding (Alonso-Coello et al., 2006; Perera et al., 2012).

Several office procedures exist to address the symptoms of progressive hemorrhoid disease including rubber band ligation, sclerotherapy, and infrared coagulation. Although these treatments may require repeat therapy, they can be offered to temporize symptoms and delay need for definitive treatment in patients with grade II and III disease. Sclerotherapy involves submucosal injection of a sclerosing agent into the apex of the hemorrhoid and relies on subsequent fibrosis to fix the tissue in place and prevent prolapse; however, this modality lacks effectiveness and durability. Rubber band ligation is the most common and effective office procedure performed for the treatment of hemorrhoid disease. In performing this technique, the proximal aspect of the hemorrhoidal tissue is grasped and the rubber bands are applied to the base of the tissue, effectively strangulating the hemorrhoid. In a review of 750 cases of symptomatic grade III or lower hemorrhoids treated with rubber band ligation over an 8-year period, immediate resolution (87%) or symptomatic improvement (6%) was achieved in 93% of patients. Over 85% of patients had 2-year follow-up with a symptomatic recurrence rate of only 11%, and overall a minimal side effect profile from the procedure (El Nakeeb et al., 2008).

SURGICAL MANAGEMENT

Surgical management is the gold standard in the treatment of severe hemorrhoids, and several options including excisional hemorrhoidectomy, ligasure hemorrhoidectomy, stapled hemorrhoidopexy, and hemorrhoidal artery ligation are described. In comparison to office-based procedures, however, surgical management is more invasive and carries a higher rate of complications.

In a multicenter randomized trial comparing rubber band ligation with hemorrhoid artery ligation in patients with grade II and III hemorrhoid disease, hemorrhoid artery ligation was more effective at preventing recurrence (30% vs. 49%, $p = 0.0005$); however, it was also associated with a higher degree of post-procedure pain and complications (Brown et al., 2016). Considering that many of the patients who underwent rubber band ligation went on to have additional banding procedures to treat their hemorrhoids, these data support reserving surgical intervention for those patients who are unable to tolerate or fail office procedures or those who have complex or high-grade disease.

The traditional hemorrhoidectomy involves an elliptical incision, excision of the hemorrhoidal tissue, and closure of the mucosa over the defect. The stapled hemorrhoidopexy has been introduced as an alternative procedure. This procedure circumferentially excises the tissue above the hemorrhoidal cushion, reapproximating the mucosa using a staple line to pexy the tissue and prevent prolapse. Due to the promising initial reports with this technique, a multicenter randomized trial was conducted to compare the short- and long-term outcomes of excisional hemorrhoidectomy and stapled hemorrhoidopexy (Watson et al., 2016). The two procedures had similar short-term complication rates, and patients who underwent the stapled hemorrhoidopexy procedure reported lower levels of pain. However, despite early superiority of the stapled procedure, at 12- and 24-month follow-up, patients treated with traditional excisional hemorrhoidectomy reported lower symptom scores and lower rates of recurrence.

Following surgical intervention for hemorrhoid disease, the most common complications include bleeding, urinary retention, and postoperative pain. Several adjuncts have been introduced postoperatively to minimize narcotic requirement and reduce post-procedure discomfort. In a randomized controlled trial, Amoli et al. showed that application of diltiazem cream significantly reduced the postoperative pain and narcotic analgesia use after hemorrhoid surgery (Amoli et al., 2011). Similar results have been found with in a randomized controlled trial with bupivacaine injection versus placebo post hemorrhoidectomy. Use of bupivacaine was associated with a higher percentage of patients opioid-free at 12–72 hours, longer time to first opioid consumption, and overall improved patient satisfaction (Gorfine et al., 2011).

Hemorrhoids are a common problem and most effectively treated with an approach tailored to the grade and degree of symptomatology. Presentation with painless bleeding is commonly related to hemorrhoid disease; however, a thorough history with liberal use of additional studies are needed to rule out malignant pathology in the appropriate setting. Diet and behavior modifications are the mainstay of initial management, followed by office procedures such as rubber band ligation. Progressive or recurrent disease may be treated operatively with surgical excision of the hemorrhoid and postoperative nonnarcotic adjuncts such as bupivacaine or diltiazem cream for pain control.

ANNOTATED REFERENCES FOR MANAGEMENT OF INTERNAL HEMORRHOIDS

1. Davis BR, Lee-Kong SA, Migaly J, Feingold DL, Steele SR. The American Society of Colon and Rectal Surgeons Clinical Practice Guidelines for the Management of Hemorrhoids. *Dis Colon Rectum.* 2018;61(3):284–292.

   Serially updated guidelines outlining management options and supportive data for the treatment of hemorrhoid disease. This manuscript provides recommendation grades and presents summarized data on contemporary treatment modalities.

2. Alonso-Coello P, Guyatt G, Heels-Ansdell D et al. Laxatives for the treatment of hemorrhoids. *Cochrane Database Syst Rev.* 2005(4):CD004649.

   Cochrane Review including seven randomized trials evaluating the use of fiber dietary supplements for the treatment of hemorrhoids. Fiber is a relatively commonly recommended treatment with a desirable side effect profile, and this review supports its use as one of the few effective medical adjuncts to be used in the noninvasive treatment of hemorrhoid disease.

3. Perera N, Liolitsa D, Iype S et al. Phlebotonics for haemorrhoids. *Cochrane Database Syst Rev.* 2012(8):CD004322.

   Although strong data on the use of phlebotonics is lacking, there is sufficient evidence to suggest that they may be a beneficial adjunct in the treatment of hemorrhoids.

4. Alonso-Coello P, Zhou Q, Martinez-Zapata MJ et al. Meta-analysis of flavonoids for the treatment of haemorrhoids. *Br J Surg.* 2006;93(8):909–920.

   The mainstay of medical management for hemorrhoid disease remains dietary and habit modification. It is recommended to increase fiber and fluid intake to improve symptoms of constipation, and limiting straining and commode time. In a meta-analysis including 378 participants, the use of fiber was associated with a 0.47 (95% CI 0.32 to 0.68) risk reduction in disease progression and symptoms.

5. El Nakeeb AM, Fikry AA, Omar WH et al. Rubber band ligation for 750 cases of symptomatic hemorrhoids out of 2200 cases. *World J Gastroenterol.* 2008;14(42):6525–6530.

    Clear and concise review of one of the most common office procedures performed for mild to moderate hemorrhoid disease. Given the potential complications and pain with operative intervention, understanding the low side effect profile and effective use of rubber band ligation as an office procedure encourages a step-up approach to the treatment of hemorrhoid disease.

6. Brown SR, Tiernan JP, Watson AJM et al. Haemorrhoidal artery ligation versus rubber band ligation for the management of symptomatic second-degree and third-degree haemorrhoids (HubBLe): A multicentre, open-label, randomised controlled trial. *Lancet.* 2016;388(10042):356–364.

    In patients with severe or refractory disease, rubber band ligation is insufficient for durable treatment and surgical treatment becomes necessary. Although several techniques for surgical treatment exist, this manuscript introduces the need for transition to surgical management in select cases.

7. Watson AJ, Hudson J, Wood J et al. Comparison of stapled haemorrhoidopexy with traditional excisional surgery for haemorrhoidal disease (eTHoS): A pragmatic, multicentre, randomised controlled trial. *Lancet.* 2016;388(10058):2375–2385.

    Stapled hemorrhoidopexy gained popularity and was considered an alternative management option for severe hemorrhoid disease. In this randomized study, the increased complications and decreased effectiveness of this procedure are described. Although there may be specific cases in which this procedure is a desired choice, this analysis supports traditional excision over stapled pexy in the operative management of hemorrhoid disease.

8. Amoli HA, Notash AY, Shahandashti FJ, Kenari AY, Ashraf H. A randomized, prospective, double-blind, placebo-controlled trial of the effect of topical diltiazem on posthaemorrhoidectomy pain. *Colorectal Dis.* 2011;13(3):328–332.

    The use of topical diltiazem has a positive effect on postoperative pain after hemorrhoid excision surgery, while carrying a minimal side effect profile.

9. Gorfine SR, Onel E, Patou G, Krivokapic ZV. Bupivacaine extended-release liposome injection for prolonged postsurgical analgesia in patients undergoing hemorrhoidectomy: A multicenter, randomized, double-blind, placebo-controlled trial. *Dis Colon Rectum.* 2011;54(12):1552–1559.

    In the era of narcotics overuse and abuse, adjuncts to decrease narcotic usage are of extreme importance. Similar to the previous article, the use of alternative therapy, especially in the early postoperative period, results in significant improvement in pain profiles, narcotic use, and patient satisfaction.

COMPARISON OF STAPLED HAEMORRHOIDOPEXY WITH TRADITIONAL EXCISIONAL SURGERY FOR HAEMORRHOIDAL DISEASE (eTHoS): A PRAGMATIC, MULTICENTRE, RANDOMISED CONTROLLED TRIAL

Watson AJ, Hudson J, Wood J, Kilonzo M, Brown SR, McDonald A, Norrie J, Bruhn H, and Cook JA; eTHoS study group, *Lancet.* 2016;388(10058):2375–2385

ABSTRACT

Background   Two commonly performed surgical interventions are available for severe (grade II–IV) hemorrhoids: traditional excisional surgery and stapled hemorrhoidopexy. Uncertainty exists as to which is most effective. The eTHoS trial was designed to establish the clinical effectiveness and cost effectiveness of stapled hemorrhoidopexy compared with traditional excisional surgery.

Methods   The eTHoS trial was a large, open-label, multicenter, parallel-group, pragmatic randomized controlled trial done in adult participants (aged 18 years or older) referred to hospital for surgical treatment for grade II–IV hemorrhoids. Participants were randomly assigned (1:1) to receive either traditional excisional surgery or stapled hemorrhoidopexy. Randomization was minimized according to baseline EuroQol 5 dimensions 3 level score (EQ-5D-3L), hemorrhoid grade, sex, and center with an automated system to stapled hemorrhoidopexy or traditional excisional surgery. The primary outcome was area under the quality-of-life curve (area under the curve [AUC]) measured with the EQ-5D-3L descriptive system over 24 months, assessed according to the randomized groups. The primary outcome measure was analyzed using linear regression with adjustment for the minimization variables. This trial is registered with the ISRCTN registry, number ISRCTN80061723.

Findings   Between January 13, 2011 and August 1, 2014, 777 patients were randomized (389 to receive stapled hemorrhoidopexy and 388 to receive traditional excisional surgery). Stapled hemorrhoidopexy was less painful than traditional excisional surgery in the short term, and surgical complication rates were similar between groups. The EQ-5D-3L AUC score was higher in the traditional excisional surgery group than the stapled hemorrhoidopexy group over 24 months; mean difference -0.073 (95% CI -0.140 to -0.006; $p = 0.0342$). EQ-5D-3L was higher for stapled hemorrhoidopexy in the first 6 weeks after surgery; the traditional excisional surgery group had significantly better quality-of-life scores than the stapled hemorrhoidopexy group. Twenty-four (7%) of 338 participants who received stapled hemorrhoidopexy and 33 (9%) of 352 participants who received traditional excisional surgery had serious adverse events.

Interpretation   As part of a tailored management plan for hemorrhoids, traditional excisional surgery should be considered over stapled hemorrhoidopexy as the surgical treatment of choice.

Funding   National Institute for Health Research Health Technology Assessment Program.

Editor Notes

Assessment: This large multicenter trial from the United Kingdom randomized patients with grade II–IV internal hemorrhoids to undergo conventional excisional hemorrhoidectomy or stapled hemorrhoidectomy. The primary study outcomes were quality-of-life measures and disease recurrence at 24 months, both of which solidly favored conventional excisional surgery.

Limitations: This trial was not blinded and therefore patients and clinicians were aware of the operative group. The techniques were performed by surgeons with variable experience with the stapled hemorrhoidectomy technique. The large number of centers and surgeons employing the two techniques is a strength and a weakness of this trial. This investigation included grade II hemorrhoids (22% of the study population), with history of failure of other methods of resolution, but these mild hemorrhoids would make good outcomes more likely in both groups. Finally, there was a significant loss to follow-up in the two groups at 24 months (about 15% and 25%).

Conclusions: This important trial provided meaningful data on the benefits of excisional hemorrhoidectomy for internal hemorrhoids, leading to a high quality of life and a low recurrence rate.

CHAPTER 23

Fissure-in-Ano and Fistula-in-Ano

Review by Contributors: Clarence E. Clark, III and Jacquelyn Seymour Turner

ANAL FISSURE

The relationship between the neuromuscular physiology of the anus and the presence of an anal fissure often drives operative and nonoperative management strategies in modern day medicine. An example of this concept starts with the findings by Farouk et al. (1994) who showed that hypertonia of the internal anal sphincter may be relevant to the pathogenesis of untreated anal fissure. In addition, Klosterhalfen et al. (1989) revealed that posterior midline fissures have poor blood flow, thus explaining why one sees chronic tears more commonly in this location. Furthermore, the consistency of bowel movements with straining has been implicated as a risk factor for the development of an anal fissure. Paralleling and following these reports, numerous articles advocating medical and surgical therapies target these physiologic derangements to promote healing.

One such example is the use of bran and sitz baths as first-line therapy for acute fissure-in-ano. Jensen et al. (1986) compared bran with sitz baths to topical ointments and showed warm sitz baths plus an intake of unprocessed bran improved healing rates and resolution of symptoms for an acute first episode of posterior anal fissure. For those who have failed medical management, sphincterotomy has been the mainstay of surgical management for decades. The approach to sphincterotomy was defined more clearly by Abcarian et al. (1980) when they compared lateral internal sphincterotomy (LIS) to posterior midline sphincterotomy. Dr. Abcarian, a pioneer in colorectal surgery, showed the importance of lateral internal sphincterotomy regarding not only healing but also in avoiding complications related to posterior defects. In addition, his report concluded that fissurectomy with midline sphincterotomy should be reserved for patients in whom local fistulization has complicated anal fissure.

Last, for those who are poor candidates for sphincterotomy as it relates to the development of postoperative fecal incontinence, the use of onabotulinumtoxin A (Botox) has emerged as an alternative therapy. Mentes et al. (2003) reported early recovery and fewer complications when Botox was compared to sphincterotomy. Their study also defined the time frame of 6 months for repeat treatment, used commonly today for those who have refractory disease after first treatment. The contributions of these works have provided insight into the pathophysiology of this disease and guided management to date.

ANAL FISTULA

Fistula-in-ano is a challenging anorectal disease to manage. Identifying the anatomy of the tract is particularly important for obtaining operative cure and minimizing fecal incontinence. In most cases, the external opening may be obvious to find. However, the internal opening is often more difficult to locate. Goodsall noted the difficulty of finding the internal opening in a 1900 publication. Here, Goodsall noted that anterior fistulae have a radial tract toward the anal canal that is used to predict the internal opening. Posterior fistulae have curvilinear projection to the posterior midline, predicting a posterior midline internal opening (Goodsall et al., 1990). However, Cirocco et al. evaluated the accuracy of Goodsall's rule. The posterior external opening followed Goodsall's rule 90% of the time. However, Goodsall's rule was not predictive of anterior fistulae which followed the rule 49% of the time. Cirocco et al. found that many of the anterior fistula also had midline openings (71%) like posterior fistulae (Cirocco and Reilly, 1992).

Once the external opening, internal opening, and tract are identified, treatment is dependent on the type of fistula, best classified by Dr. Parks, another pioneer in the field of proctology. Intersphincteric fistulae are the most common type (45%–70%). These fistulae originate in the anal canal, pass though the internal sphincter muscle and the intersphincteric plane, and terminate in the perianal skin. This type is the only one that does not involve the external sphincter muscle (Parks et al., 1976). Since this fistula does not traverse the external sphincter, a fistulotomy (fileting the fistula tract open over a probe) can be performed with minimal risk in developing fecal incontinence (Swerdlow et al., 1958). Transsphincteric is the next most common type of anal fistula (23%–30%). This fistula originates in the anal canal and crosses both the internal and external anal sphincter muscles and then into the ischiorectal fossa, and terminates in the perianal skin. Less common is the suprasphincteric fistula (5%–20%). These fistulae pass into the intersphincteric plane and travel above the puborectalis muscle, then downward through the levator muscle into ischiorectal fossa. It is the most difficult to treat given that it involves the entire sphincter complex. This fistula is associated with lateral extent called a horseshoe abscess, forming a horseshoe tract (Parks et al., 1976). The internal opening of a horseshoe fistula is often posterior midline. Dr. Hanley pioneered a procedure which involves a partial fistulotomy (or fistulectomy with chronic well-formed tracts) over the internal opening in the posterior midline to treat this type of fistula. The fistulotomy is then extended toward the coccyx, dividing the anococcygeal ligament to get into the deep postanal space. If necessary, perianal counter-incisions are made to completely drain the tract. This wound is then left to heal by secondary intention (Hanley et al., 1976).

Extrasphincteric fistulae are the least common type of fistula (2%–5%). Extrasphincteric fistulae include a tract that passes from the perianal skin through the ischiorectal fossa and levator ani muscle and terminates in the rectal wall. This fistula does not have a cryptoglandular origin. These fistulae can be caused by trauma, cancer, inflammatory bowel disease, pelvic inflammation, or iatrogenic breaks through the levator ani muscle. Treatment of this type of fistula includes treating the underlying cause (Parks et al., 1976).

Fistulectomy is mainly a historical procedure that was used for fistulae that involved a significant amount of anal sphincter muscle such as transsphincteric and supra-sphincteric fistulae. However, fistulectomy was noted to cause fecal incontinence and thus has been replaced by endorectal advancement flap (ERAF). ERAF involves the mobilization of the mucosa, submucosa, and musculomucosa of the rectum for advancement over the internal opening where the flap is secured. It has a reported overall success rate of 63.6%, with a 77.1% success rate in patients with cryptoglandular disease (Sonoda et al., 2002). While fistulotomy remains the gold standard of treating fistula-in-ano, many techniques such as ERAF are evolving to improve surgical outcomes for this disease.

ANNOTATED REFERENCES FOR FISSURE-IN-ANO AND FISTULA-IN-ANO

1. Farouk R, Duthie GS, MacGregor AB, Bartolo DC. Sustained internal sphincter hypertonia in patients with chronic anal fissure. *Dis Colon Rectum.* 1994;37(5):424–429.

   Relaxing the internal sphincter is the mainstay of therapies for anal fissure. With that said, the early work of Farouk et al. to prove the hypothesis that internal sphincter hypertonia may be relevant to the pathogenesis of this disorder is critical to our understanding of this disease.

2. Klosterhalfen B, Vogel P, Rixen H, Mittermayer C. Topography of the inferior rectal artery: A possible cause of chronic, primary anal fissure. *Dis Colon Rectum.* 1989;32(1):43–52.

   Improving blood flow to the primary anal fissure is also a causative effect for the chronicity of this disease. In this article, the authors have shown that posterior midline fissures have poor blood flow, thus explaining the location often seen in this condition.

3. Jensen SL. Treatment of first episodes of acute anal fissure: Prospective randomised study of lignocaine ointment versus hydrocortisone ointment or warm sitz baths plus bran. *Br Med J (Clin Res Ed).* 1986;292(6529):1167–1169.

   Jensen trial comparing bran with sitz baths to topical ointments showed warm sitz baths plus an intake of unprocessed bran is the treatment of choice for an acute first episode of posterior anal fissure. This finding set the stage for the first-line therapy for this condition.

4. Abcarian H. Surgical correction of chronic anal fissure: Results of lateral internal sphincterotomy vs. fissurectomy–midline sphincterotomy. *Dis Colon Rectum.* 1980;23(1):31–36.

   To define the best approach to anal fissure, Abcarian, another pioneer in colorectal surgery, showed the importance of lateral sphincterotomy regarding not only healing but also in avoiding complications related to posterior defect. In addition, he concluded, fissurectomy-midline sphincterotomy should be reserved for patients in whom local fistulization has complicated anal fissure.

5. Mentes BB, Irkorucu O, Akin M et al. Comparison of botulinum toxin injection and lateral internal sphincterotomy for the treatment of chronic anal fissure. *DCR.* 2003;46(2)232–237.

Botox remains a key component to fissure management with the authors showing early recovery and fewer complications when compared to sphincterotomy. This paper also defined the key time component to healing and when a repeat injection should be considered for Botox therapy, which is at 6 months.

6. Parks AG, Gordon PH, Hardcastle JD. A classification of fistula-in-ano. *Br J Surg.* 1976;63:1–12.

These authors describe their classification of fistula-in-ano based on 400 patients treated for anorectal fistula over a 15-year time span. Patients with anorectal cancer, ulcerative colitis, and Crohn disease were excluded. The authors were able to group the fistulae into four broad categories based on the anatomic findings of the fistula tract: intersphincteric, transsphincteric, suprasphincteric, and extrasphincteric.

7. Goodsall DH, Miles WE. Ano-rectal fistula. In: *Diseases of the Anus and Rectum.* Goodsall DH, Miles WE (Eds) London: Longmans, Green and Co.; 1990:92–137.

8. Cirocco WC, Reilly JC. Challenging the predictive accuracy of Goodsall's rule for anal fistulas. *Dis Colon Rectum.* 1992;35:537–542.

These authors evaluated the external and internal opening of 216 patients to evaluate the accuracy of Goodsall's rule. There were 124 patients with posterior external opening and 92 patients with an anterior external opening. Fistulas with an anterior external anal opening were the most difficult to predict the internal opening, especially in women. Only 49% of anal fistulas with an anterior external opening obeyed the rule (57% in men and 31% in women). However, Goodsall's rule is accurate in predicting the internal opening in patients with posterior external anal openings (87% in men, 97% in women, and 90% overall).

9. Swerdlow H. Fistulotomy and fistulectomy for fistulas about the anus and rectum. *Am J Surg.* 1958;95:818–821.

The author describes the technique of fistulotomy and fistulectomy. The author also details when it is appropriate to use either of these techniques. Fistulotomy is the unroofing of a fistula over a probe in the tract. It is mainly used when there is little muscle involved. Fistulectomy was used as a two-stage procedure for fistulae that involve a significant portion of muscle. During the first stage, the fistula tract is meticulously cored out. A seton is then placed around the remaining muscle. During the second stage the muscle is incised 10–14 days later.

10. Hanley PH, Ray JE, Pennington EE, Grablowsky OM. Fistula-in-ano: A ten-year follow-up study of horseshoe-abscess fistula-in-ano. *Dis Colon Rectum.* 1976;19:507–515.

The authors of this paper report the results of a relatively new technique at the time of its publication. They reviewed 41 patients who underwent the Hanley procedure for horseshoe abscesses and fistulae over the span of 10 years. They detailed the procedure, which in summary includes a posterior midline fistulotomy or fistulectomy, depending on the chronicity of disease, to get into the postanal space. Counter-incisions were then made depending on how the fistula tracked. This technique minimizes the deformity of the anus and anal canal. The authors report that all 41 patients healed with this technique.

11. Sonoda T, Hull T, Piedmonte MR, Fazio VW. Outcomes of primary repair of anorectal and rectovaginal fistulas using the endorectal advancement flap. *Dis Colon Rectum.* 2002;45:1622–1628.

The authors of this paper evaluated 105 patients (male and female) over a 5-year period who underwent endorectal advancement flaps (ERAF) for anorectal and rectovaginal fistulas. They noted a 77.1 success rate in anorectal fistulae with a cryptoglandular etiology. There was a 50% success rate in anorectal fistulae in patients with Crohn's disease. Other factors such as posterior fistulae, age over 60, body surface area over 100, prior abscess drainage and seton placement, and fistulae that drained less than 3 months before repair were all associated with improved success rate of ERAF repair.

Landmark Article

A COMPARISON OF INJECTIONS OF BOTULINUM TOXIN AND TOPICAL NITROGLYCERIN OINTMENT FOR THE TREATMENT OF CHRONIC ANAL FISSURE

Brisinda G, Maria G, Bentivoglio AR, Cassetta E, Gui D, and Albanese A,
N Engl J Med. 1999;341:65–69

ABSTRACT

Background and Methods   Lateral internal sphincterotomy, the most common treatment for chronic anal fissure, may cause permanent injury to the anal sphincter, which can lead to fecal incontinence. We compared two nonsurgical treatments that avert the risk of fecal incontinence. We randomly assigned 50 adults with symptomatic chronic posterior anal fissures to receive treatment with either a total of 20 U of botulinum toxin injected into the internal anal sphincter on each side of the anterior midline or 0.2% nitroglycerin ointment applied twice daily for 6 weeks.

Results   After 2 months, the fissures were healed in 24 of the 25 patients (96%) in the botulinum toxin group and in 15 of the 25 (60%) in the nitroglycerin group ($P = 0.005$). No patient in either group had fecal incontinence. At some time during treatment, five patients in the nitroglycerin group had transient, moderate to severe headaches that were related to treatment. None of the patients in the botulinum toxin group reported adverse effects. Ten patients who did not have a response to the assigned treatment—one in the botulinum toxin group and nine in the nitroglycerin group—crossed over to the other treatment; the fissures subsequently healed in all 10 patients. There were no relapses during an average of about 15 months of follow-up.

Conclusions   Although treatment with either topical nitroglycerin or botulinum toxin is effective as an alternative to surgery for patients with chronic anal fissure, botulinum toxin is the more effective nonsurgical treatment.

Editor Notes

Assessment: This small prospective randomized study from Italy (25 patients in each group) examined the difference in anal fissure healing between botulinum toxin injected into the internal anal sphincter on each side of the anterior midline or 0.2% nitroglycerin ointment applied twice daily for 6 weeks. After 2 months, 96% of the patients in the botulinum toxin healed compared to 60% in the nitroglycerin ointment group. No patients in either group had incontinence, as surgical treatment such as lateral internal sphincterotomy may cause permanent injury to the anal sphincter, leading to fecal incontinence. From the nitroglycerin group, 9 of the 10 patients who failed crossed over into the botulinum toxin arm, with all anal fissures healing in these patients. There were no relapses in the 15-month follow-up.

Limitations: This study was simple in design and does not have many faults. One could argue that the dosage of nitroglycerin was not optimized, but the fact that 96% of the patients with anal fissures were well treated and healed at 15 months without relapse is difficult to criticize.

Conclusions: This study supports the concept that both botulinum toxin and nitroglycerin are effective alternatives to surgical therapy for patients with chronic anal fissures.

CHAPTER 24

Anorectal Infections and Abscesses

Review by Contributor: Nathaniel Holmes

Anorectal infections and abscesses have afflicted mankind since antiquity. Current descriptions of anorectal abscess are attributed to Hippocrates, but early references of treatment of anorectal disease can be found in ancient Egyptian medical papyrus dating back as early as 1600 BC. Anorectal abscess continues to be a very common problem, yet its true incidence is unknown. A review of hospital databases in England covering a period of 15 years revealed an incidence of 20 per 100,000 for patients presenting with anorectal abscess for the first time. This is short of the true incidence, as patients treated outside the National Health Service and those with recurrent disease are not included (Sahnan et al., 2017). In the United States, the estimated incidence of anorectal abscess approaches 100,000 cases per year. This is based on data extrapolated from hospital discharges as well as operating room data, and is widely viewed as an underestimation as it does not take into account patients who were treated in an ambulatory setting, physician's office, or those who spontaneously drained (Abcarian, 2011).

Anorectal suppuration begins in the anal crypts and advances to local tissues by way of an obstructed anal gland and duct. The sequence of events is described as inflammation which leads to occlusion of the duct allowing for bacterial overgrowth and abscess formation. This cryptoglandular origin of infection accounts for 90% of idiopathic anorectal abscess formation. The remaining 10% are the result of other disease factors such as Crohn disease, HIV, malignancy, and rarely, diverticulitis. Once suppuration begins, the infection follows the path of least resistance and will occupy one of the many potential spaces of the anorectum. Perianal abscess is the most common (42.7%), followed by ischiorectal (22.7%), intersphincteric (21.4%), and supralevator (7.33%) (Ramanujam et al., 1984). Adult males are twice as likely to present with anorectal abscess as adult females. The age range at presentation is 20–60 with an average age of 40. Pain and swelling is the hallmark clinical presentation. Pain out of proportion to physical findings may represent a deeper abscess. Examination under anesthesia may be required if pain precludes adequate evaluation. Imaging studies such as CT, MRI, or endorectal ultrasound may be helpful when physical exam is not possible or reveals no obvious finding and deeper perirectal abscess is suspected.

Incision and drainage remains the hallmark of treatment. This is a common procedure that may be performed in the emergency department, operating room, or physician's office. While this aspect of treatment is widely agreed upon, most other aspects of management are not. The use of postoperative antibiotics (Sozener et al., 2011), primary fistulotomy at the time of surgery (Cochran), and management of the open wound (Pearce et al., 2016) continue to be controversial. Once adequate surgical drainage has been effected, it is a common practice to pack the wound open with plain or iodoform gauze. This routine practice appears to have started over 60 years ago and has been attributed to Lister's use of carbolic acid dressings and later Johnson's development of iodoform gauze. The packing ritual often takes many forms. The wound is initially packed in the operating room and subsequently cared for by either the patient and family or by home nursing care. Packing is typically continued until the wound cavity is closed. Despite lack of evidence, packing the wound remains a routine practice. There are many suggested benefits of wound packing, including maintaining an open wound, allowing for drainage, and hemostasis as well as decreased rate of abscess recurrence and fistula formation. Supportive evidence for these claims is scarce at best. It has been shown to be safe and effective to treat perianal abscess with incision and drainage alone without the use of packing (Tonkin et al., 2004).

Wound packing may come with negative consequences. A multicenter study found packing to be painful and costly and did not demonstrate a decrease in the rate of abscess recurrence or fistula formation (Pearce et al., 2016). Passive drainage utilizing a Penrose, Malecot, or other drainage system has been advocated as an alternative to wound packing. In this system, the drain is left in place for up to 10 days or until no further drainage is appreciated (Beck et al., 1988).

Antibiotics alone as primary treatment for anorectal is abscess not recommended. However, it remains a common practice to routinely administer postoperative antibiotics to patients with anorectal abscess. Routine use of antibiotics has not been shown to improve wound healing, reduce abscess recurrence, or decrease fistula formation as some suggest. Unless there is significant cellulitis, systemic sepsis, or underlying immunocompromise, routine administration of oral or intravenous antibiotics is not recommended (Sozener et al., 2011).

Anorectal abscess is a common and costly condition. Our current management has not changed for six decades. Successful management of perianal abscess has been demonstrated without the use of packing. Routine packing of the perianal abscess cavity adds to the patient's burden with time off from work, home care, and pain. Celsus described incision and drainage of abscess in his medical text, *De Medicina*, 2000 years ago (Kockerling et al., 2013). His eloquent description of surgical drainage of the site, debridement of unhealthy tissue, and evacuation of all fluid continues to guide our treatment today. Celsus did not include packing the wound in his description but did suggest infusing the abscess cavity with honey. Perhaps we should revisit this practice, as the disinfectant properties of honey are well documented (Simon et al., 2009).

ANNOTATED REFERENCES FOR ANORECTAL INFECTIONS AND ABSCESSES

1. Pearce L, Newton K, Smith SR et al. Multicentre observational study of outcomes after drainage of acute perianal abscess. *Br J Surg*. 2016;103:1063–1068.

The authors set out to measure the impact of internal dressing (packing) by measuring number of dressings, frequency of healing at 4 weeks, 8 weeks, and 6 months, frequency of abscess recurrence, postoperative fistula-in-ano, and return to work or activities of daily living. They found that packing is painful and costly and did not improve outcome.

2. Tonkin DM, Murphy E, Brooke-Smith M et al. Perianal abscess: A pilot study comparing packing with no packing of the abscess cavity. *Dis Colon Rectum.* 2004;47(9):1510–1514.

In this pilot study, authors compared packing with no packing. Abscess recurrence and fistula rates were similar in both groups and they concluded that packing the abscess cavity offers no clinical advantage.

3. Abcarian H. Anorectal infection: Abscess-fistula. *Clin Colon Rectal Surg.* 2011;24:14–21.

This is an in-depth review of the current diagnosis and management of anorectal infection.

4. Read DR, Abcarian H. A prospective survey of 474 patients with anorectal abscess. *Dis Colon Rectum.* 1979;22:566–568.

5. Sozener U, Gedik E, Kessaf Aslar A et al. Does adjuvant antibiotic treatment after drainage of anorectal abscess prevent development of anal fistulas? A randomized placebo-controlled, double blind, multicenter study. *Dis Colon Rectum.* 2011;54(8):923–929.

6. Sahnan K, Askari A, Adegbola SO et al. Natural history of anorectal sepsis. *Br J Surg.* 2017;104(13):1857–1865.

This is a retrospective review of a prospective database of the National Health Service in England. The authors review the Hospital Episode Statistics database to identify all patients presenting with new anorectal abscess. The aim is to identify factors predictive of fistula formation.

7. Malik A, Nelson RL, Tou S. Incision and drainage of perianal abscess with or without treatment of anal fistula. *Cochrane Database Syst Rev.* 2010;(7):CD006827.

This is a review of all randomized trials comparing incision and drainage of perianal abscess with or without concomitant fistula treatment. A meta-analysis of six trials showed a significant reduction in recurrence, persistent abscess/fistula, or repeat surgery in favor of fistula surgery at the time of incision and drainage with no increase in incontinence.

8. Kockerling F, Kockerling D, Lomas C. Cornelius Celsus—Ancient encyclopedist, surgeon-scientist, or master of surgery? *Langenbecks Arch of Surg.* 2013;389(4):609–616.

Interesting historical review of the work of the Roman nobleman Cornelius Celsus. His general encyclopedia included an eight-volume medical compendium with two volumes dedicated to surgery, and is praised as the "most significant medical document following the Hippocratic writings."

9. Simon A, Traynor K, Santos K, Blaser G, Bode U, Molan P. Medical honey for wound care—still the 'latest resort'? *Evid Based Complement Alternat Med.* 2009;6(2):165–173.

This is a fairly comprehensive review of the use of medical grade honey for wound care. They are quick to point out that the review is specific to Medihoney, a commercial grade honey licensed as a medical product. They review the pros and cons and discuss the mechanism of action as well as a comparison to antibiotics. In addition, they report the use of Medihoney in several clinical situations.

10. Beck DE, Fazio VW, Lavery IC, Jagelman DG, Weakley FL. Catheter drainage of ishiorectal abscesses. *South Med J.* 1988;81:444–446.

This is one of the early series evaluating the feasibility of treating perirectal abscess utilizing catheter drainage as an alternative to traditional incision and drainage. This retrospective review of 55 patients demonstrated that catheter drainage was safe and cost effective.

11. Ramanujam PS, Prasad ML, Abcarian H, Tan AB. Perianal abscesses and fistulas. A study of 1023 patients. *Dis Colon Rectum.* 1984;27(9):593–597.

A large study of over 1000 patients with anorectal abscess and fistula. Has a very good discussion of the various treatment options for each type of abscess/fistula and is one of the early works to espouse the use of primary fistulotomy in selected cases.

MULTICENTRE OBSERVATIONAL STUDY OF OUTCOMES AFTER DRAINAGE OF ACUTE PERIANAL ABSCESS

Pearce L, Newton K, Smith SR, Barrow P, Smith J, Hancock L, Kirwan CC, and Hill J; North West Research Collaborative, *Br J Surg.* 2016;103(8):1063–1068

ABSTRACT

Introduction   Management of perianal abscesses has remained largely unchanged for over 50 years. The evidence for postoperative wound packing is limited and may expose patients to painful procedures with no clinical benefit and at considerable increased cost.

Methods   Patients were recruited in 15 UK centers between December 2013 and October 2014. Outcome measures included number of dressing (pack) changes, healing, recurrence, return to work/normal function, postoperative fistula-in-ano and health utility scores (EQ-5D™). Pain was measured before, during, and after dressing change on a visual analog scale.

Results   Some 141 patients were recruited (median age 39 [range 18–86] years). The mean number of dressing changes in the first 3 weeks was 13 (range 0–21), equating to an annual cost to the National Health Service of €6,453,360 in England alone per annum. Some 43.8% of wounds were healed by 8 weeks after surgery and 86% of patients had returned to normal function. Some 7.6% of abscesses had recurred and 26.7% of patients developed a fistula-in-ano by 6 months following surgery. Patients reported a two- to threefold increase in pain scores during and after dressing changes.

Conclusion   Recurrent abscess is rare, and fistula occurs in one-quarter of the patients. Packing is painful and costly.

> **Editor Notes**
>
> **Assessment:** In this 10-month prospective observational study in the United Kingdom, the outcomes of patients with perianal abscesses after drainage and packing were recorded. Packing of perianal wounds increased wound pain two- to threefold. Recurrence was uncommon (7.6%), but many patients (26.7%) developed fistula-in-ano by 6 months.

Limitations: No CONSORT diagram is presented, so we have no idea what fraction of the total population of perianal abscesses in these 15 hospitals this represents. Only 141 patients were recruited in these centers, so one is left with a degree of uncertainty as to the generalizability of this study. This is basically a registry study with no specific intervention. It appears to reflect local custom and risks a high degree of variability. The use of packing has been previously explored and found to be unnecessary in these patients (after the initial hemostatic packing), so it is unclear why this study was conducted.

Conclusions: Not surprisingly, this study's primary finding was that packing is painful.

CHAPTER 25

Pilonidal Abscess

Review by Contributor: James C. Doherty

Pilonidal disease is a commonly encountered painful condition localized to the gluteal cleft of the sacrococcygeal area. The proposed pathophysiology of the disease is a foreign body reaction to hair follicles present in the skin of the natal cleft with associated formation of midline pits, inflammation, and secondary infection. The disease presents on a spectrum ranging from acute inflammation with extensive subcutaneous tracts and abscess formation to chronic inflammation with sinus formation and persistent drainage. Acute symptoms include intense pain of the sacrococcygeal area with or without associated drainage. Constitutional symptoms are rare. The intensity and location of the pain often results in significant limitation of physical activity.

Standard treatment of an initial presentation of acute pilonidal disease with abscess formation is incision and drainage with healing of the resulting wound by secondary intention. Incision and drainage alone does not guarantee successful long-term healing due to the frequent presence of multiple pits and lateral sinus tracts that contribute to impaired healing and recurrence. The addition of curettage of the abscess cavity to incision and drainage may improve healing and reduce recurrence rates (Vahedian et al., 2005). Shaving along the intergluteal fold and the surrounding region in conjunction with maintenance of adequate hygiene at the site is a standard postoperative adjunct that may also improve healing and limit recurrence (Al-Naami, 2005). Administration of antibiotics has not been shown to improve outcomes but should be considered in the presence of significant cellulitis, underlying immunosuppression, or concomitant systemic illness (Kronborg et al., 1985). In general, incision and drainage yields overall successful healing rates of approximately 60%, with the remaining patients requiring additional surgical intervention to treat residual pilonidal disease prior to definitive wound closure (Jensen and Harling, 1988).

Chronic pilonidal disease may manifest as recurrent abscesses, chronic sinus tracts, and/or persistent non-healing wounds with drainage. The basic principles of treatment are eradication of any remaining sinus tract(s), complete healing of the overlying skin, and prevention of recurrence. Fibrin glue and phenol injection therapies have shown success in the management of chronic pilonidal sinuses, but there is a lack of high-quality data to support the routine use of these techniques, and their utilization is limited to select patients at select centers with experience in these approaches (Calikoglu et al., 2017; Lund et al., 2017). A recent randomized controlled trial demonstrated comparable rates of healing between patients treated with standard excision with primary wound closure and patients treated with injection therapy with a novel mixture of a sclerosing agent with an herbal product (*Lawsonia inermis* powder) with known antimicrobial and wound healing properties (Salih et al., 2018). This treatment also was noted to be associated with decreased hospital stay, decreased work absence, decreased cost, and decreased perioperative pain. Nevertheless, despite these promising less-invasive modalities, the standard approach to chronic pilonidal disease in the twenty-first century remains surgical.

Surgical treatment of chronic pilonidal disease follows two general approaches: first, excision of all disease with healing of the resulting open wound by secondary intention, and second, excision of all disease with primary closure. The open wound approach also includes partial closure techniques such as marsupialization. A 2010 Cochrane systematic review concluded that there is no obvious advantage to open wound management versus primary closure (Al-Khamis et al., 2010). The evidence suggests lower recurrence rates when wounds are left open, but this potential benefit is offset by significantly longer healing times compared to primary surgical closure. The same review also concluded that there was a clear advantage to off-midline closure in comparison with midline closure (Al-Khamis et al., 2010). The off-midline approach has consistently demonstrated faster healing, lower complication rates, and lower recurrence rates. When primary closure is employed, drains are frequently placed to minimize fluid accumulation deep to the closure site. Drains may also be used to provide access for wound irrigation. The practice of drain placement on a case-by-case basis may reduce wound failure rates without contributing to any increase in infection rates.

Wound closure after excision of complex and/or recurrent pilonidal disease may require flap-based strategies to provide healthy tissue for wound coverage. A variety of flap techniques have been described (Vartanian et al., 2018). These include the rhomboid or Limberg flap, the Karydakis flap, the cleft–lift technique, the V–Y advancement flap, and Z–plasty techniques. All of these techniques require significant technical expertise and should be utilized only by experienced surgeons who are comfortable in their performance.

Incision and drainage remains the primary strategy for management of acute pilonidal abscess. Wounds that fail to heal adequately post-drainage or that develop recurrence of pilonidal disease require formal excision. Primary wound closure after excision may reduce the morbidity and economic impact associated with caring for a slow-healing chronic sacrococcygeal wound. When primary wound closure is undertaken, it should be done via an off-midline approach to optimize short- and long-term results of treatment.

ANNOTATED REFERENCES FOR PILONIDAL ABSCESS

1. Vahedian J, Nabavizadeh F, Nakhaee N, Vahedian M, Sadeghpour A. Comparison between drainage and curettage in the treatment of acute pilonidal disease. *Saudi Med J.* 2005;26:553–555.

In this randomized trial, the authors demonstrated that curettage of the abscess cavity and removal of inflammatory debris when added to incision and drainage was associated with significantly greater healing at 10 weeks (96% vs. 79%) and lower recurrence rate at 65 months (10% vs. 54%).

2. Al-Naami MY. Outpatient pilonidal sinotomy complemented with good wound and surrounding skin care. *Saudi Med J*. 2005;26:285–288.

This retrospective study looked at outcomes after pilonidal sinotomy and healing of resulting wound by secondary intention. Patients were managed with daily dressing changes and weekly shaving and achieved very low rates of both delayed healing (10%) and recurrence (2%).

3. Kronborg O, Christensen K, Zimmerman-Nielsen C. Chronic pilonidal disease: A randomized trial with a complete 3-year follow-up. *Br J Surg*. 1985;72:303–304.

This randomized study compared outcomes among three treatment groups: wounds managed with healing by secondary intention, wounds managed with primary closure, and wounds managed with primary closure with additional 2-week course of treatment with clindamycin. The addition of clindamycin failed to exert any effect upon wound healing times.

4. Jensen SL, Harling H. Prognosis after simple incision and drainage for a first-episode acute pilonidal abscess. *Br J Surg*. 1988;75:60–61.

This study followed patients undergoing simple incision and drainage of pilonidal abscess over a 3-year period. Fifty-eight percent achieved complete healing within 10 weeks. Nine percent of these patients developed recurrence during their prospective period of observation (median duration = 60 months). Patients who failed to heal primarily and required additional surgical intervention for definitive closure demonstrated more pits and lateral tracts compared to those with successful primary healing. This approach yielded an overall cure rate of 76% after 18 months.

5. Calikoglu I, Gulpinar K, Oztuna D et al. Phenol injection versus excision with open healing in pilonidal disease: A prospective randomized trial. *Dis Colon Rectum*. 2017;60(2):161–169.

This recent prospective randomized clinical study compared two groups of 70 patients with chronic pilonidal disease randomly assigned to either treatment with phenol injection or excision with open healing. The phenol group had decreased time to complete wound healing, decreased time to resume daily activities, and better pain control. Recurrence rates during a mean follow-up period of 39 months were similar between the two groups. The authors concluded that phenol injection was as effective as excision with open healing.

6. Lund J, Tou S, Doleman B, Williams JP. Fibrin glue for pilonidal disease. *Cochrane Database Syst Rev*. 2017;(1):CD011923.

This Cochrane review looked at four RCTs comparing flap procedures for treatment of pilonidal disease to fibrin glue monotherapy or to fibrin glue as an adjunct to those flap procedures. The RCTs were all small in size and subject to bias. The authors concluded that the existing evidence for the primary outcome measures of time to healing and adverse events is of very low quality, and larger randomized and blinded studies are needed to identify any benefit to fibrin glue as monotherapy or as an adjunct in the treatment of pilonidal sinus disease.

7. Salih AM, Kakamad FH, Salih RQ et al. Nonoperative management of pilonidal sinus disease: One more step toward the ideal management therapy—A randomized controlled trial. *Surgery.* 2018;164:66–70.

   This study showed that injection therapy with a mixture of a sclerosing agent with an herbal product resulted a rate of healing of pilonidal disease similar to that of conventional surgical treatment with excision and primary closure. The less invasive approach also was associated with significant cost savings and superior pain control compared to surgical treatment.

8. Vartanian E, Daniel JG, Lee SW, Patel K. Pilonidal disease: Classic and contemporary concepts for surgical management. *Ann Plastic Surg.* 2018;81(6):e12–e19.

   This recent review outlines the surgical approaches to the treatment of pilonidal disease including the various asymmetric flap closure techniques. Open healing is characterized as a widely used and reliable approach that achieves low recurrence rates and low morbidity at the expense of prolonged wound healing. The asymmetric flap techniques achieve more rapid wound closure with acceptable recurrence rates but are associated with more potential complications.

Landmark Article of 21st Century

HEALING BY PRIMARY VERSUS SECONDARY INTENTION AFTER SURGICAL TREATMENT FOR PILONIDAL SINUS

Al-Khamis A, McCallum I, King PM, and Bruce J, *Cochrane Database Syst Rev.* 2010;(1):CD006213

ABSTRACT

Background　Pilonidal sinus arises in the hair follicles in the buttock cleft. The estimated incidence is 26 per 100,000, people, affecting men twice as often as women. These chronic discharging wounds cause pain and impact upon quality of life. Surgical strategies center on excision of the sinus tracts followed by primary closure and healing by primary intention or leaving the wound open to heal by secondary intention. There is uncertainty as to whether open or closed surgical management is more effective.

Objectives　To determine the relative effects of open compared with closed surgical treatment for pilonidal sinus on the outcomes of time to healing, infection, and recurrence rate.

Search Methods　For this first update we searched the Wounds Group Specialised Register (24/9/09), the Cochrane Central Register of Controlled Trials (CENTRAL), the Cochrane Library (Issue 3, 2009), Ovid MEDLINE (1950, September, Week 3, 2009), Ovid MEDLINE(R) In-Process and Other Non-Indexed Citations (September 24, 2009), Ovid EMBASE (1980–2009, Week 38), and EBSCO CINAHL (1982, September Week 3, 2009).

Selection criteria   All randomized controlled trials (RCTs) comparing open with closed surgical treatment for pilonidal sinus. Exclusion criteria were non-RCTs, children aged younger than 14 years, and studies of pilonidal abscess.

Data collection and analysis   Data extraction and risk of bias assessment were conducted independently by three review authors (AA/IM/JB). Mean differences were used for continuous outcomes and relative risks with 95% confidence intervals (CI) for dichotomous outcomes.

Main Results   For this update, 8 additional trials were identified, giving a total of 26 included studies (n = 2530). Seventeen studies compared open wound healing with surgical closure. Healing times were faster after surgical closure compared with open healing. Surgical-site infection (SSI) rates did not differ between treatments; recurrence rates were lower in open healing than with primary closure (RR 0.60, 95% CI 0.42−0.87). Six studies compared surgical midline with off-midline closure. Healing times were faster after off-midline closure (MD 5.4 days, 95% CI 2.3−8.5). SSI rates were higher after midline closure (RR 3.72, 95% CI 1.86−7.42) and recurrence rates were higher after midline closure (Peto OR 4.54, 95% CI 2.30−8.96).

Conclusions   No clear benefit was shown for open healing over surgical closure. A clear benefit was shown in favor of off-midline rather than midline wound closure. When closure of pilonidal sinuses is the desired surgical option, off-midline closure should be the standard management.

Original Author Commentary: Julie Bruce

This study came about in 2006 after I was approached by Peter King, consultant general surgeon at Aberdeen Royal Infirmary, Scotland. King wanted to review wound healing after surgical management of pilonidal sinus disease. Iain McCallum, then a junior surgeon, had an interest in undertaking research. I had been awarded an MRC Fellowship to investigate surgical adverse events, therefore the topic was a good fit.

We registered the systematic review with the Cochrane Collaboration in 2006 and attended the introductory training on searching, critical appraisal, and meta-analysis. This was mandatory training for all new review teams. Unfortunately, we were deprived from visiting a more glamorous location, as the UK Cochrane workshop was held at the University of Aberdeen Medical School. McCallum and I learned of the pitfalls of different meta-analytical techniques, supported by the excellent team at the Wounds Group, led by Nicky Cullum (now Dame Cullum DBE) and Sally Bell-Syer. Eighteen clinical trials were included in the review, 12 studies comparing open healing with primary closure and six comparing healing after different midline and off-midline closure techniques.

We found a clear benefit for off-midline closure compared to midline closure on wound healing outcomes. McCallum suggested submitting the final review to the *BMJ*, which I felt was being somewhat ambitious but relented as staff in the Department of Public Health took bets on the fastest time for receiving a *BMJ* rejection email. Thanks to McCallum's enthusiasm and positivity, plus of course a great research study, we were delighted to be featured on the front cover and have an accompanying editorial. Not many surgeons have their first-ever research study published in the *BMJ* and it was great citation to add to my fellowship report.

However, the volume of published clinical trials of pilonidal sinus disease management was rapidly increasing and Bell-Syer soon requested a review update. McCallum had since left Aberdeen and had commenced a PhD at Newcastle. Our department ran a master's in Public Health Research and I submitted the topic as a potential project, although very few surgeons registered for training in public health. I was soon approached by Ahmed Al-Khamis, a trainee general surgeon who was looking for a master's project. Al-Khamis needed no encouragement; within weeks he had undertaken searches and immersed himself completely in the review, despite studying for MSc exams, overseas medical entrance exams, and higher surgical fellowship exams. The Cochrane process had since become even more stringent; however, within a year the review was completed and published.

The updated 2010 Cochrane review included 26 trials with 2530 participants. Healing times were faster after surgical closure compared with open healing, and surgical-site infection rates did not differ by type of wound closure. However, recurrence rates were lower after open healing than with primary closure (RR 0.60; 95 CI 0.42−0.87). Six studies compared surgical midline closure with off-midline closure and there was evidence of higher recurrence rates after midline closure (OR 4.54; CI 95% 2.30−8.96).

However, this review urgently needs updating. Cochrane reviews are for life unless you relinquish the topic to another research team! I am incredibly grateful to Al-Khamis and McCallum for their unfailing enthusiasm, hard work, and for being such great colleagues. McCallum is now a consultant colorectal surgeon at Northumbria NHS Trust, England and Al-Khamis has completed a colorectal fellowship in the United States and is assistant professor and colorectal and minimally invasive surgeon at Kuwait University School of Medicine.

CHAPTER 26

Incarcerated Inguinal Hernias

Review by Contributor: Esteban Varela

The first description of a surgical repair for an inguinal hernia was reported by Celsus. Unfortunately, this was undertaken via a non-anatomical approach. It was later that the accurate description of the inguinal anatomy was made by Galenus. He also described the inguinal herniation as a rupture of the peritoneum. It was not until late 1800s when Bassini described for the first time a tissue repair of the posterior wall of the inguinal canal. This was the first attempt to reconstruct the inguinal anatomy. Later, Shouldice perfected Bassini's repair by reconstructing this posterior wall with a running suture. Although there was tension associated to this repair, the technique resulted in significant decrease in postoperative hernia recurrence. This latter technique underwent multiple revisions such as the known McVay Cooper's ligament repair. Later, in the 1960s, Usher described the first inguinal hernia repair with the use of a polypropylene mesh. It was not until the 1980s, when Lichtenstein described the most popular open tension-free hernioplasty. This is still considered the standard of care for an anterior approach to an inguinal hernia repair. Soon thereafter, an open preperitoneal approach with the same prosthetic was also described by Nyhus which also facilitated the repair of recurrent inguinal hernias. Most recently, the laparoscopic trials have shown significant advantages in terms of postoperative pain, recurrence rates, and return to daily activities as compared to the most common open approaches (McCormack, Liem). Other studies have found open and laparoscopic techniques to have comparable outcomes (Bansal). Nevertheless, laparoscopic techniques offer the advantage of evaluating the various inguinal defects bilaterally, placement of a tension-free mesh, and access to the inguinal area through a virgin plane. However, these techniques are costly and technically more challenging. For primary elective repair, a prospective randomized multicenter study has shown that open technique using the Lichtenstein technique is superior to the laparoscopic technique in terms of recurrence and complication on a 2-year follow-up (Neumayer).

Inguinal hernias are relatively common within the general population (2%–4%). The demographics are largely represented by the older male population, with a lifetime risk of 27%, in the case of inguinal hernias and older females for femoral hernias. Nonincarcerated inguinal hernias typically present as a painful and recurrent inguinal bulging that increases in size in the standing position and that may reduce spontaneously during the supine position. The great majority of these inguinal hernias may be repaired on an elective basis via an open or laparoscopic approach.

The pathophysiology of an incarcerated inguinal hernia differs in its presentation, as it comprises a non-reducible intra-abdominal viscera which is most often omentum but can be small or large intestine along with subsequent venous stasis and edema. The contents may evolve to strangulating ischemia, which can lead to visceral gangrene and perforation. The clinical presentation of a painful and irreducible inguinal hernia represents a true surgical emergency given the patient's demographics and associated increased morbidity and mortality. This diagnosis requires immediate surgical intervention via an open or laparoscopic approach for visceral reduction and evaluation with temporary or permanent inguinal hernia defect repair. When clinically indicated, a plain abdominal x-ray may be consistent with a clinical presentation of small bowel obstruction. However, a computed tomography of the pelvis has better sensitivity and specificity, particularly in obese individuals, and may provide significant information regarding hernia location, presence of intra-abdominal fluid, and suggest visceral edema and/or ischemia. Nonetheless, the diagnosis is most commonly made on clinical examination. External hernia sac changes on examination such as erythema or ecchymosis are ominous signs of visceral strangulation and perforation.

The surgical approach and the use and type of mesh for the repair of an incarcerated or strangulated inguinal hernia is still an area of debate. To date, there are no quality prospective randomized trials to clarify this controversy. However, the type of surgical approach and repair depends on the facility's resources and the surgeon's training and skills. Nevertheless, there are critical aspects that the acute care surgeon should keep in mind.

First, the inguinal hernia contents must be reduced to its original intra-abdominal location, and second, the intra-abdominal viscera must be evaluated by either an open or laparoscopic approach. For incarcerated inguinal hernias, the hernia sac contents may be reduced manually under general anesthesia with muscle relaxation and/or paralysis. Evaluation of the intra-abdominal contents may be performed via an anterior or preperitoneal open inguinal incision, hernia sac laparoscopy, standard transabdominal or totally extraperitoneal laparoscopy or via a midline laparotomy (Karatepe, Sgourakis). Both extraperitoneal and transabdominal laparoscopic techniques have been found to be comparable (Wake). The advantage of performing a transabdominal laparoscopy approach is that it offers a way to reduce the hernia contents intra-abdominally while applying manual external pressure and allowing evaluation of the intra-abdominal viscera in question. Care must be taken at the time of intra-abdominal access and visceral manipulation in the presence of intestinal dilatation, as inadvertent injury may occur. Simple manual reduction of the viscera without evaluating its viability is related to increased morbidity and mortality.

If there is no contamination or bowel content spillage and the incarcerated viscera appears to be viable, the use of a permanent prosthetic mesh such as polypropylene is advisable and considered safe by either approach (Duan). If an anterior open approach is performed, a tension-free Lichtenstein hernioplasty with polypropylene mesh is still the preferred technique. Prospective randomized clinical trials in the face of primary and recurrent inguinal hernia repairs favor the use of heavyweight versus lightweight polypropylene material (Burgmans, Dedemadi).

In the case of gross contamination and bowel spillage within the hernia sac, and after proper reduction of the viscera, the surgeon may elect to perform a temporary tissue repair to approximate the hernia defect or use a temporary biologic-type mesh. Whichever approach is selected, these may require a deferred and definitive tension-free repair with polypropylene mesh at a later setting. In the case of patient's hemodynamic instability with signs of sepsis and significant visceral ischemia and bowel contamination, a "damage control" approach may be used as the last option for source control, which may include bowel resection, bowel discontinuity, and temporary inguinal or abdominal closure with plans for a "second look" for primary bowel anastomosis with inguinal hernia repair and definitive incisional closure.

In summary, incarcerated inguinal hernias are surgical emergencies which require immediate surgical intervention with visceral reduction and inspection. The acute care surgeon most exercise good judgment in terms of the available surgical approaches (open vs. laparoscopic), type of repair (tissue vs. prosthetic mesh), use and type of prosthetic (non-absorbable vs. biologic), as well as timing of repair (primary vs. deferred).

ANNOTATED REFERENCES FOR INCARCERATED INGUINAL HERNIAS

1. McCormack K, Scott NW, Go PM, Ross S, Grant AM. EU Hernia Trialists Collaboration. Laparoscopic techniques versus open techniques for inguinal hernia repair. *Cochrane Database Syst Rev.* 2003;(1):CD001785.

   This Cochrane review included an analysis of 41 prospective randomized trials comparing laparoscopic vs. open techniques for inguinal hernia repair involving 7161 participants. The rate of complications was higher with laparoscopic surgery with no differences in hernia recurrences or length of stay with either approach. Laparoscopic repair was associated with less pain and numbness.

2. Liem MS, van der Graaf Y, van Steensel CJ, Boelhouwer RU, Clevers GJ, Meijer WS, Stassen LP, Vente JP, Weidema WF, Schrijvers AJ, van Vroonhoven TJ. Comparison of conventional anterior surgery and laparoscopic surgery for inguinal-hernia repair. *N Engl J Med.* 1997;336(22):1541–1547.

   In this randomized, multicenter trial, 994 patients were assigned to conventional anterior or extraperitoneal laparoscopic approaches. Patients in the laparoscopic group had less infections and faster recovery. The authors concluded that laparoscopic repair was related to fewer recurrences than open repair.

3. Bansal VK, Misra MC, Babu D, Victor J, Kumar S, Sagar R, Rajeshwari S, Krishna A, Rewari V. A prospective, randomized comparison of long-term outcomes: Chronic groin pain and quality of life following totally extraperitoneal (TEP) and transabdominal preperitoneal (TAPP) laparoscopic inguinal hernia repair. *Surg Endosc.* 2013;27(7):2373–2382.

   The authors randomized 314 patients to undergo TEP or TAPP repairs for primary uncomplicated inguinal hernias. They concluded that both techniques were comparable in terms of chronic pain, quality of life and resumption of daily activities.

4. Neumayer L, Giobbie-Hurder A, Jonasson O, Fitzgibbons R Jr, Dunlop D, Gibbs J, Reda D, Henderson W; Veterans. Affairs Cooperative Studies Program 456 Investigators. Open mesh versus laparoscopic mesh repair of inguinal hernia. *N Engl J Med.* 2004;350(18):1819–1827.

In this large prospective clinical trial, 2164 veterans with inguinal hernias at 14 VA medical centers were randomized to open or laparoscopic repair with mesh. Recurrences and complications were higher in the laparoscopic group for primary hernias. However, the laparoscopic group had less pain postoperatively and returned faster to normal activities. Recurrence rates were noted to be similar for both techniques after repair for recurrent hernias. The author concluded the open technique was superior to the laparoscopic one for mesh repair of primary hernias.

5. Karatepe O, Adas G, Battal M, Gulcicek OB, Polat Y, Altiok M, Karahan S. The comparison of preperitoneal and Lichtenstein repair for incarcerated groin hernias: A randomised controlled trial. *Int J Surg.* 2008;6(3):189–192.

In this randomized trials, 45 patients were studied to receive an open preperitoneal vs. Lichtenstein mesh repairs for incarcerated inguinal hernias. Morbidity was associated with the use of the Lichtenstein approach if additional incisions were required. Thus the authors recommended the use of the preperitoneal approach for incarcerated hernias as this provides a wider access to the peritoneal cavity for visceral inspection.

6. Sgourakis G, Radtke A, Sotiropoulos GC, Dedemadi G, Karaliotas C, Fouzas I, Karaliotas C. Assessment of strangulated content of the spontaneously reduced inguinal hernia via hernia sac laparoscopy: Preliminary results of a prospective randomized study. *Surg Laparosc Endosc Percutan Tech.* 2009;19(2):133–137.

Patients with spontaneous reduction of an incarcerated inguinal hernia (n=41) were randomly assigned to receive a hernia sac laparoscopy vs. standard treatment with no laparoscopy. The authors indicated that sac laparoscopy appears to be an accurate and safe method to prevent unnecessary laparotomies and major morbidity.

7. Wake BL, McCormack K, Fraser C, Vale L, Perez J, Grant AM. Transabdominal preperitoneal (TAPP) vs. totally extraperitoneal (TEP) laparoscopic techniques for inguinal hernia repair. *Cochrane Database Syst Rev.* 2005;(1):CD004703.

This meta-analysis of randomized controlled trials comparing laparoscopic TAPP vs. TEP for inguinal hernia repair were included. There were no statistical differences between approaches in terms of complications, length of stay, return to activities, or recurrence rates. However, the authors noted insufficient quality data.

8. Duan SJ, Qiu SB, Ding NY, Liu HS, Zhang NS, Wei YT. Prosthetic mesh repair in the emergency management of acutely strangulated groin hernias with grade I bowel necrosis: A rational choice. *Am Surg.* 2018;84(2):215–219.

Prosthetic mesh repair vs. primary suture was randomized in 208 patients with acute strangulated inguinal hernias. Mortality and wound-related complications, such as wound infections, were significantly associated with the degree of bowel necrosis. It was concluded that the use of prosthetic mesh is as safe as primary repair in patients with non-infected strangulated bowel.

9. Burgmans JP, Voorbrood CE, Simmermacher RK, Schouten N, Smakman N, Clevers G, Davids PH, Verleisdonk EM, Hamaker ME, Lange JF, van Dalen T. Long-term results of a randomized double-blinded prospective trial of a lightweight (Ultrapro) versus a heavyweight mesh (Prolene) in laparoscopic total extraperitoneal inguinal hernia repair (TULP-trial). *Ann Surg.* 2016;263(5):862–866.

950 patients with primary reducible inguinal hernias were to receive TEP repair with light weight vs. heavy weight mesh. At 1- and 2-year follow-up, postoperative pain was significantly higher in the light weight mesh group. In addition, there were more hernia recurrences in the light weight group. The authors noted that the use of light weight mesh during TEP inguinal hernia repair offered no benefit at 2 years.

10. Dedemadi G, Sgourakis G, Karaliotas C, Christofides T, Kouraklis G, Karaliotas C. Comparison of laparoscopic and open tension-free repair of recurrent inguinal hernias: a prospective randomized study. *Surg Endosc.* 2006;20(7):1099–1104.

In this study, patients were randomly assigned to TEP, TAPP or open repair of recurrent inguinal hernias who had prior open standard repairs. Within the open group, the operative time was shorter, however postoperative pain and return to daily activities were longer in favor of laparoscopic approaches. They concluded that laparoscopic hernia repair should be the choice for recurrent hernias.

Landmark Article of 21st Century

OPEN MESH VERSUS LAPAROSCOPIC MESH REPAIR OF INGUINAL HERNIA

Neumayer L, Giobbie-Hurder A, Jonasson O, Fitzgibbons R Jr, Dunlop D, Gibbs J, Reda D, and Henderson W; Veterans Affairs Cooperative Studies Program 456 Investigators, *N Engl J Med.* 2004;350(18):1819–1827.

ABSTRACT

Background Repair of inguinal hernias in men is a common surgical procedure, but the most effective surgical technique is unknown.

Methods We randomly assigned men with inguinal hernias at 14 Veterans Affairs (VA) medical centers to either open mesh or laparoscopic mesh repair. The primary outcome was recurrence of hernias at 2 years. Secondary outcomes included complications and patient-centered outcomes.

Results Of the 2164 patients who were randomly assigned to one of the two procedures, 1983 underwent an operation; 2-year follow-up was completed in 1696 (85.5%). Recurrences were more common in the laparoscopic group (87 of 862 patients [10.1%]) than in the open group (41 of 834 patients [4.9%]; odds ratio, 2.2; 95% confidence interval, 1.5–3.2). The rate of complications was higher in the laparoscopic surgery group than in the open surgery group (39.0% vs. 33.4%; adjusted odds ratio, 1.3; 95% confidence interval, 1.1–1.6). The laparoscopic surgery group had less pain initially than the open surgery group on the day of surgery (difference in mean score on a visual analog scale, 10.2 mm; 95% confidence interval, 4.8–15.6) and at 2 weeks (6.1 mm; 95% confidence interval, 1.7–10.5) and returned to normal activities 1 day earlier (adjusted hazard ratio for a shorter time to return to normal activities, 1.2; 95% confidence interval, 1.1–1.3). In prespecified analyses, there was a significant interaction between the surgical approach (open or laparoscopic) and the type of hernia (primary or recurrent) (P = 0.012). Recurrence was significantly more common after laparoscopic repair than after open repair of primary hernias (10.1% vs. 4.0%), but rates of recurrence after repair of recurrent hernias were similar in the two groups (10.0% and 14.1%, respectively).

Conclusions   The open technique is superior to the laparoscopic technique for mesh repair of primary hernias.

Editor Notes

Assessment: Large randomized, multicenter study performed at 14 VA medical centers that assigned men with inguinal hernias to either open mesh (Lichenstein) or laparoscopic mesh repair. The primary outcome was recurrence at 2 years and the follow-up rate was high at 85.5%. Open repair recurrence rate was 4.9% compared to 10.1% in the laparoscopic group. The complication rate was the secondary outcomes, and it was 33.4% in the open group compared to 39% in the laparoscopic group. The laparoscopic group had less pain on the day of surgery as well at the 2-week follow up period. The return to normal activities was 1 day earlier in the laparoscopic group.

Limitations: The recurrences after primary hernia repair were from surgeons with less experience who used the laparoscopic technique. When comparing experienced surgeons, the recurrence rate was low (approximately 5%) in both groups. The study showed no difference between the two techniques of recurrent hernias. However, this was a post-hoc analysis and the number of patients with recurrent hernia operations was small, as less than 10% of the study population were operated on for recurrent hernias. Another limitation is that since this study was done at the VA, the men were older than the general population.

Conclusions: The open repair is superior to the laparoscopic technique for mesh repair of primary hernias. For recurrent hernias, the numbers were too small to show a difference.

CHAPTER 27

Incisional Hernias: When Do They Occur?

Review by Contributor: Jonathan Nguyen

Ventral hernias are a long-standing surgical disease and have been described as far back as ancient Egypt. These are weaknesses in the midline abdominal fascia that increase in size over time. Similarly, incisional hernias develop as a failure of the midline fascia to heal after an abdominal surgery and have been prevalent ever since surgeons have been cutting on the abdomen. Weaknesses in the abdominal wall, poor wound healing, obesity, and inadequate fascial bites during closure have all been suggested as contributors to hernia formation. Subsequent increases in intra-abdominal pressures then lead to outpouchings, and abdominal contents begin to fill the empty space. Unchecked, these hernias grow in diameter as continued pressure stretches the fascial defect.

Prevention of hernias from the initial surgery is critical, and as such, several authors have studied how to avoid hernia formation all together. Several modifiable risk factors have been identified that can contribute to postoperative hernia formation, including tobacco use, obesity, and diabetes. There is an association between rising BMI and the risk of wound infections, hernia recurrence, and mortality increases. Another risk factor is tobacco use, which inhibits wound healing and has been associated with increased risk of infections and dehiscence. Similarly, uncontrolled diabetes impairs wound healing and has increased complications. For these reasons, several experts advocate for weight loss, tobacco cessation, and glucose control prior to operating.

With the incisional hernia rate now reaching over 20%, surgical technique plays a crucial role in hernia prevention. In 1993, Israelsson and colleagues examined the relationship between the length of the incision and the suture length in a prospective non-randomized study. They found that maintaining a suture length to wound length ratio of >4 dramatically decreased the incidence of postoperative hernias (9% compared to 23.7%, p = 0.001) (Israelsson and Jonsson, 1993). Hodgson et al. continued to add to this body of literature and performed a meta-analysis to evaluate continuous and interrupted fascial closure. They identified 11 articles that described the type of closure and suture type (absorbable vs. nonabsorbable). The odds of a hernia after using a running suture closure was 0.73 versus interrupted, thus favoring a continuous closure. And while overall the use of nonabsorbable suture decreases the risk of hernia formation, the use of PDS versus Prolene did not have an increase in incisional hernias (Hodgson et al., 2000). Deerenberg's STITCH trial shook surgical dogma when they examined the use of smaller bites and travel. This was a prospective multicenter double-blinded study involving 560 patients. By using smaller bites, 5 mm instead of 10 mm, the rate of hernias decreased from 21% to 13% (p = 0.022) (Deerenberg et al., 2015). This group also had a longer closure time and used more suture. Retention stitches have also been suggested to decrease the hernia formation. Intuitively, this makes sense to us as surgeons as it adds additional strength to the closure; however, the data are mixed. There is no convincing literature to support the use of internal retention stitches, and at best, there are only limited data to support the use of external retention stitches in high-risk patients. Because of the multitude of risk factors contributing to hernia formation, some surgeons have begun prophylactic mesh placement as part of the routine closure. Borab et al. performed a meta-analysis including 2114 patients, 1152 of which had prophylactic mesh placement on closure. They demonstrated an 85% risk reduction in postop hernias (p = <0.00001), which seemingly strongly advocates for prophylactic mesh placement (Borab et al., 2017). Authors have further studied the use of prophylactic mesh placements in abdominal aortic aneurysm (AAA) repairs, 12-mm umbilical incisions for laparoscopic cholecystectomies, and colostomy sites. These were randomized controlled studies, and all show improvements in hernia rates with similar outcomes in complications and infections (Armañanzas et al., 2014; Muysoms et al., 2016; Brandsma et al., 2017). This has to be balanced with several points. Prophylactic mesh placement can increase the risk of chronic pain, seroma formation, and risk of infection. Furthermore, some critics suggest that good surgical techniques would decrease the hernia rate, and that prophylactic mesh placement increases operative time and costs without much benefit.

Once ventral hernias arise, they can be diagnosed by physical exam and CT scan. If the presence of a hernia on physical exam is unclear, further imaging should be obtained. This is because a large meta-analysis has demonstrated that up to 58% of incisional hernias may be missed on exam alone (Kroese et al., 2018). Complicated hernias occur with recurrent operations, infected fields, the classic swiss-cheese defects, and those with previous open abdomens. Closure of incisional hernias requires thoughtful and deliberate selection of technique. The open repair has been well established, and techniques like the Rive-Stoppa and component separation have proven very effective in closing large complex defects. The use of and location of mesh has always been hotly debated, as mesh can be placed as an onlay, inlay, underlay, or sublay. A recent meta-analysis by Holihan et al. (2016) identifies that a retrorectus (sublay) repair has decreased recurrence and infection rates. Thus, the growing trend is a primary closure with sublay mesh placement instead of an onlay or inlay repair. The acute abdomen poses a particularly difficult situation. These patients are sometimes at highest risk for hernia formation; however, an infected field or peritonitis prevents surgeons from placing a synthetic mesh. In these situations, surgeons have advocated for the use of biologic mesh; however, despite the growing types and usage of biologic meshes over the years, the evidence is still inconclusive about its value. At best, it bridges a gap temporarily but will ultimately leave the patient with a hernia months down the line. Argudo et al. (2014) studied the use of synthetic prophylactic mesh in patients with infected fields and peritonitis. They found that it dramatically reduced the incidence of hernias, however had a slight increase in wound complications and mortality attributed to patient selection. While it may be too soon to start placing mesh in every patient prophylactically, the study does demonstrate feasibility, and further investigation is needed.

As new technologies emerge, the way in which we tackle problems advances. As such, over the past decade, laparoscopic and robotic hernia repairs have grown in popularity. Initial experiences with laparoscopic intraperitoneal onlay mesh (IPOM) hernia repairs have shown similar outcomes compared to open repairs without the large wound complications. This procedure was performed by placing a large mesh intraperitoneally in order to cover or bridge all the defects. In 2016, Kokotovic et al. conducted a long-term study comparing outcomes of laparoscopic and open repairs. This large cohort study with good follow-up demonstrated that laparoscopic mesh repairs had the lowest recurrence rates (Kokotovic et al., 2016). Continued advancements in the field of robotics have allowed surgeons to replace transfascial tacks with intracorporeal suturing to decrease postop pain. Again, as surgeon skills and technology improved, the procedure evolved into a robotic sublay repair after the primary defect was sewn shut. This provided the strength of an open repair with the benefits of laparoscopic surgery (decreased pain, infection rate, and seroma formation). Now, surgeons are performing robotic totally extraperitoneal (TEP) hernia repairs, staying completely extraperitoneal, with promising results (Kokotovic et al., 2016; Baker et al., 2018; Kennedy et al., 2018). All of this must be weighed with risks and benefits. Eker et al. (2013) compared laparoscopic to open ventral hernias by performing a multi-institutional randomized control trial. They identified that the laparoscopic repair group had longer operative times and perioperative complications, including wound drainage, bowel perforations, and bladder injuries. The long term follow-up showed similar recurrence rates and pain scores.

Ventral hernias will continue to be an issue as long as surgeons are operating on the abdomen. Despite its long history, the selection and technique for repairing them is still evolving. Continued research into this field will bring about more innovations and ways to address an age-old problem.

ANNOTATED REFERENCES FOR INCISIONAL HERNIAS: WHEN DO THEY OCCUR?

1. Israelsson LA, Jonsson T. Suture length to wound length ratio and healing of midline laparotomy incisions. *Br J Surg*. 1993;80:1284–1286.

   A landmark article for its time, the authors demonstrate that suture length matters during the closure of a laparotomy. The authors advocate for a suture length to fascia defect ratio of >4. However, they accomplish this by comparing suture length to various laparotomy incision sizes. The argument could be made that smaller incisions are less likely to develop hernias.

2. Hodgson NC, Malthaner RA, Ostbye T. The search for an ideal method of abdominal fascial closure: A meta-analysis. *Ann Surg*. 2000;231:436–442.

   A well-done meta-analysis comparing continuous to interrupted fascial closure. They also compare suture material (absorbable to nonabsorbable). The culmination of 11 articles over 30 years reveals that continuous nonabsorbable closures have lower recurrence rates. However, in a subset analysis, they were unable to find a significant difference between PDS and Prolene closures.

3. Deerenberg EB, Harlaar JJ, Steyerberg EW et al. Small bites versus large bites for closure of abdominal midline incisions (STITCH): A double-blind, multicentre, randomised controlled trial. *Lancet*. 2015;386:1254–1260.

   Deerenberg et al. perform a well-designed prospective randomized study of 560 patients. They challenge the well-established notion that 1 cm bites and 1 cm travel is the optimal way to close fascia. This is done only for elective laparotomies however, and their conclusions may not apply to emergent operations.

4. Borab ZM, Shakir S, Lanni MA et al. Does prophylactic mesh placement in elective, midline laparotomy reduce the incidence of incisional hernia? A systematic review and meta-analysis. *Surgery*. 2017;161:1149–1163.

   Another meta-analysis that reviews the effectiveness of prophylactic mesh placement at the time of laparotomy. With over 2000 patients, 1152 receiving mesh, the authors find that prophylactic use of mesh decreases the rate of incisional hernia by 85% at 2-year follow-up. This group did have a higher rate of pain and operative time.

5. Armañanzas L, Ruiz-Tovar J, Arroyo A et al. Prophylactic mesh vs. suture in the closure of the umbilical trocar site after laparoscopic cholecystectomy in high-risk patients for incisional hernia. A randomized clinical trial. *J Am Coll Surg*. 2014;218:960–968.

   The authors performed a randomized study comparing closure of the 12-mm trocar site with nonabsorbable suture versus a mesh repair. The hernia rate was reduced from 31.9% to 4.3% with no significant change in complication rates.

6. Brandsma H-T, Hansson BM, Aufenacker TJ et al. Prophylactic mesh placement during formation of an end-colostomy reduces the rate of parastomal hernia. *Ann Surg*. 2017;265:663–669.

   Brandsma randomized patients undergoing elective end colostomies into mesh or no-mesh groups. The mesh was placed in a parastomal retro-rectus fashion. At 2 years, the hernia rate in the mesh group was 4.5% compared to 24.2% in the no-mesh group. This study only included 133 patients.

7. Muysoms FE, Detry O, Vierendeels T et al. Prevention of incisional hernias by prophylactic mesh-augmented reinforcement of midline laparotomies for abdominal aortic aneurysm treatment: A randomized controlled trial. *Ann Surg*. 2016;263:638–645.

   Patients who had their AAA repaired through a midline incision were randomized into a mesh or no-mesh closure. Of the 120 patients, patients without mesh had a 28% chance of hernia versus 0% in the mesh group.

8. Kroese LF, Sneiders D, Kleinrensink GJ, Muysoms F, Lange JF. Comparing different modalities for the diagnosis of incisional hernia: A systematic review. *Hernia*. 2018;22:229–242.

   A large meta-analysis was performed identifying 2986 patients who had either an ultrasound or CT scan of their hernia. Most notably, up to 58% of hernias were only identified on imaging, thus raising suspicion of our ability to palpate them on physical exam.

9. Holihan JL, Nguyen DH, Nguyen MT, Mo J, Kao LS, Liang MK. Mesh location in open ventral hernia repair: A systematic review and network meta-analysis. *World J Surg*. 2016;40:89–99.

   The authors examine the optimal mesh location during a ventral hernia repair. They identify that the sublay mesh placement has the lowest recurrence. Furthermore, the sublay mesh placement has the lowest rates of surgical-site infections.

10. Argudo N, Pereira JA, Sancho JJ, Membrilla E, Pons MJ, Grande L. Prophylactic synthetic mesh can be safely used to close emergency laparotomies, even in peritonitis. *Surgery.* 2014;156:1238–1244.

Argudo et al. prophylactically placed mesh in high-risk patients after laparotomies for peritonitis. This group had a significantly smaller risk of hernias (5.9% vs. 33%). This group did have fewer patients with contaminated surgical sites. In addition, they had a higher mortality and wound complications, though this was attributed to the patient population.

11. Kokotovic D, Bisgaard T, Helgstrand, F. Long-term recurrence and complications associated with elective incisional hernia repair. *JAMA.* 2016;316:1575–1582.

This prospective cohort study examined over 3000 patients who received elective incisional hernia repairs in Denmark. They found that the laparoscopic IPOM repair was superior to an open mesh repair, which was superior to an open primary suture repair. The caveat to this is that the laparoscopic group had higher long-term complications, which may offset its benefits.

12. Baker JJ, Öberg S, Andresen K, Rosenberg J. Decreased re-operation rate for recurrence after defect closure in laparoscopic ventral hernia repair with a permanent tack fixated mesh: A nationwide cohort study. *Hernia.* 2018;22(4):577–584.

The authors evaluated the utility of laparoscopic primary defect closure with mesh by comparing almost 1000 patients. The group that received defect closure in addition to mesh placement had a 50% reduction in recurrence (3.6% vs. 7.2%).

13. Kennedy M, Barrera K, Akelik A et al. Robotic TAPP ventral hernia repair: Early lessons learned at an inner city safety net hospital. *JSLS.* 2018;22.

Kennedy et al. describe their initial experience with robotic-assisted TAPP. They compared a robotic IPOM to a TAPP and find similar outcomes. Interestingly, their only complications arise in the IPOM group. This is an initial experience, and further investigation is required as their N = 63.

14. Eker HH, Hansson BM, Buunen M et al. Laparoscopic vs. open incisional hernia repair: A randomized clinical trial. *JAMA Surg.* 2013;148:259–263.

This multicenter study recruited 206 patients between 10 hospitals and randomized them into open or laparoscopic repairs. The laparoscopic group had higher perioperative complications without significant improvement in recurrence rates. The article suggests that there may not be a significant benefit to laparoscopic repairs.

SMALL BITES VERSUS LARGE BITES FOR CLOSURE OF ABDOMINAL MIDLINE INCISIONS (STITCH): A DOUBLE-BLIND, MULTICENTRE, RANDOMISED CONTROLLED TRIAL

Deerenberg EB, Harlaar JJ, Steyerberg EW, Lont HE, van Doorn HC, Heisterkamp J, Wijnhoven BP, Schouten WR, Cense HA, Stockmann HB, Berends FJ, Dijkhuizen FPH, Dwarkasing RS, Jairam AP, van Ramshorst GH, Kleinrensink GJ, Jeekel J, and Lange JF, *Lancet.* 2015;386(10000):1254–1260

ABSTRACT

Background Incisional hernia is a frequent complication of midline laparotomy and is associated with high morbidity, decreased quality of life, and high costs. We aimed to compare the large bites suture technique with the small bites technique for fascial closure of midline laparotomy incisions.

Methods   We did this prospective, multicenter, double-blind, randomized controlled trial at surgical and gynecological departments in 10 hospitals in the Netherlands. Patients aged 18 years or older who were scheduled to undergo elective abdominal surgery with midline laparotomy were randomly assigned (1:1) via a computer-generated randomization sequence to receive small tissue bites of 5 mm every 5 mm or large bites of 1 cm every 1 cm. Randomization was stratified by center and between surgeons and residents with a minimization procedure to ensure balanced allocation. Patients and study investigators were masked to group allocation. The primary outcome was the occurrence of incisional hernia; we postulated a reduced incidence in the small bites group. We analyzed patients by intention to treat. (This trial is registered at Clinicaltrials.gov, Number NCT01132209 and with the Nederlands Trial Register, Number NTR2052.)

Findings   Between October 20, 2009, and March 12, 2012, we randomly assigned 560 patients to the large bites group (n = 284) or the small bites group (n = 276). Follow-up ended on August 30, 2013; 545 (97%) patients completed follow-up and were included in the primary outcome analysis. Patients in the small bites group had fascial closures sutured with more stitches than those in the large bites group (mean number of stitches 45 [SD 12] vs. 25 [10]; p<0.0001), a higher ratio of suture length to wound length (5.0 [1.5] vs. 4.3 [1.4]; p<0.0001) and a longer closure time (14 [6] vs. 10 [4] min; p<0.0001). At 1-year follow-up, 57 (21%) of 277 patients in the large bites group and 35 (13%) of 268 patients in the small bites group had incisional hernia (p = 0.0220, covariate adjusted odds ratio 0.52, 95% CI 0.31–0.87; p = 0.0131). Rates of adverse events did not differ significantly between groups.

Interpretation   Our findings show that the small bites suture technique is more effective than the traditional large bites technique for prevention of incisional hernia in midline incisions and is not associated with a higher rate of adverse events. The small bites technique should become the standard closure technique for midline incisions.

Funding   Erasmus University Medical Center and Ethicon.

Editor Notes

Assessment: This was prospective, multicenter, double-blind, randomized control trial utilizing 10 hospitals in the Netherlands. Gynecological and surgical departments randomly assigned patients undergoing midline laparotomy to either receive small tissue bites of 5 mm every 5 mm or larger bites of 1 cm every 1 cm to close the fascia. This was ensured by the use of 31-mm versus a 48-mm needle. Randomization was stratified by center, surgeons, and residents with a minimization procedure to ensure balanced allocation. There were 560 patients randomized and

97% of the patients had completed a follow-up examination. The small bites group had significantly more suture bites placed (mean of 45 vs. 25) and took significantly longer to complete the fascial closure (14 min vs. 10 min). At 1-year follow-up, the incisional hernia rate was significantly higher in the large bite group compared to the small bite group (21% vs. 13%). Physical exam missed 47% of the 87 incisional hernias (identified on imaging studies).

Limitations: Incisional hernias are extremely common, even considering a mere 1-year follow up. The suture technique did not compare interrupted to running. The hernia rate that may occur over an extended time period was not determined by this study.

Conclusions: This study challenged the dogma that large fascial bites lead to a reduction in wound complications such as ventral hernia occurrence. Using sSmall bites for fascial in the fascia during closure (0.5 cm × 0.5 cm) were demonstrated to be more effective than larger bites (1 cm × 1 cm), resulting in significantly reducing lower incisional hernia rates at 1-year follow-up.

CHAPTER 28

Emergency Abdominal Surgery in the Transplant Population

Review by Contributors: Suresh Agarwal and Christopher Reed

The history of transplantation reflects a simultaneous improvement in surgical technique and immunology. With a better understanding of innate immunology and armed with tools to modify this response to antigen, Joseph Murray and J. Hartwell Harrison were first able to perform a successful allotransplant in 1954: a kidney transplant in identical twins. Although immunosuppression was not needed in this case, cortisone was utilized in transplants until 1959 when azathioprine was identified. Subsequently, the first pancreas transplant was performed by Richard Lillehei and William Kelly in 1966 and the first liver and heart transplants were performed in 1967 by Thomas Starzl and Christian Barnard, respectively. More powerful immunosuppressants, such as cyclosporin, rapamycin, and tacrolimus, discovered in the 1970s and 1980s, heralded an improved survival in allograft recipients as well as a more aggressive surgical approach. In 1981, Bruce Reitz performed the first heart-lung transplant; in 1983, the first lung transplant was performed by Joel Cooper, and, more recently (in the twenty-first century), hand and face transplants have found success.

Ever since immunosuppression was utilized to improve graft survival, the transplant population has presented an interesting dilemma in the management of patients requiring emergent or urgent surgery. Infection, often due to atypical organisms, has been a leading cause of morbidity and mortality in this group of patients. And understandably so; in order for the graft to survive, it must have protection from the host's innate immunologic barriers. However, due to the immunosuppressants that they must receive in order to protect the graft, patients often do not exhibit the classical signs and symptoms that are seen in the non-immunosuppressed patient.

As transplant patients receive steroids and other immune and inflammatory response modulators, they are prone to presenting late in the course of the disease process, often with large degrees of contamination despite having little to no outward signs of peritonitis or abdominal discomfort. Similarly, laboratory values are of limited utility, as leukocytosis may not predict infection as white blood cell counts may be elevated due to steroid usage or other regimen.

Regardless of the organ transplanted, the mortality for patients requiring abdominal surgery, particularly for perforation, remains high. Even in patients who do not require bowel resection, or in whom perforation does not occur, urgent or emergent operative management does have its risks. Cholecystectomy after transplantation carries a risk as high as 50% (Gupta et al., 2000). The largest series thus far reported, with 1054 patients or 4.42% of all cardiac transplant patients requiring cholecystectomy, still demonstrated a risk of 3.5% with a morbidity of 12%, both significantly higher than in the non-immunocompromised population (Kilic et al., 2013). Similarly, in complicated diverticulitis without perforation, the rate of death and complications in post-transplant patients far exceeds the general surgical population, with complications ranging from 7.7% to 75% and death ranging from 0% to 100% (Paul et al., 2009; Reshef et al., 2012; De'Angelis et al., 2016). The same can be seen in cases of small bowel obstruction necessitating operative intervention, with mortality ranging from 0% to 50% (Miller et al., 2006; Paul et al., 2009). It is only in appendicitis that we see mortality that is similar to the general population; 0%. Although the denominator of cases for this disease process remains small, it cannot account for the increased rate of complications compared to the general surgical population: 23.5%–33.3% (De'Angelis et al., 2016).

This backdrop of increased risk in operating on these patients makes Catena's paper examining gastrointestinal perforations following kidney transplantation even more interesting. The paper, published in 2008 in *Transplantation Proceedings*, remains the largest series examining abdominal perforations after solid organ transplant (Catena et al., 2008). With sources of perforation coming from, in descending order, the colon, the small intestines, the duodenum, and the stomach, the series had a complication rate of 53% and a mortality of 24%. The etiology of the perforations varied from infections (cytomegalovirus and *Helicobacter pylori*) to transplant related pathology (lymphoma) to causes similar to those found in the non-immuno-suppressed population such as diverticulitis or ischemia. The incidence of perforation remained at 3% over a 30-year period; however, half of the perforations occurred when the patients were exposed to the highest doses of immunosuppression, during the first year post-transplant. (De'Angelis' systematic review found similar results when it combined Catena's findings with those of others, including a mortality of 17.5%.) Diagnostic indications for surgery varied from chest x-ray to abdominal CT scan, with no patient going to the OR based upon physical exam findings in isolation (De'Angelis et al., 2016).

The increase in transplants over time has resulted in an increase in complications seen in this population, including in general surgical emergencies. A systematic review published in 2016 concludes that emergency abdominal surgery after transplantation is not a rare event. Despite the case reviews and reports that have been published there is no consensus on methods for prevention. Nor are there recommendations for management of immunosuppression during the postoperative period after these emergent operations (De'Angelis et al., 2016). Despite accumulating thousands of cases of transplantation and evaluating hundreds of cases of emergency abdominal surgery, the conclusions drawn must be limited, as they are based exclusively on retrospective studies and expert opinion. Graft failure rates, as a complication or endpoint, were not mentioned in most articles, and recommendations for surgical procedure or immunosuppression regimen in the postoperative period were also not strongly reinforced in most of the literature. However, one thing remains constant in the literature: that surgeons must remain vigilant in the face of immunosuppression, maintaining a high degree of suspicion with earlier operative therapy and less contamination leading to decreased morbidity and mortality.

ANNOTATED REFERENCES FOR EMERGENCY ABDOMINAL SURGERY IN THE TRANSPLANT POPULATION

1. Gupta D, Sakorafas GH, McGregor CG, Hamsen WS, Farnell MB. Management of biliary tract disease in heart and lung transplant patients. *Surgery.* 2000;128:641–649.

   Retrospective review of 178 thoracic transplant patients: 143 heart transplants, 30 lung transplants, and 5 heart-lung transplants. Of these, six required a cholecystectomy, with morbidity of 50% and a mortality of 50%.

2. Kilic A, Sheer A, Shah AS, Russell SD, Gourin CG, Lidor AO. Outcomes of cholecystectomy in US heart transplant recipients. *Ann Surg.* 2013;258:312–317.

   The largest retrospective review of heart transplant patients in a national registry: 23,854 patients. Of these, 1054 required cholecystectomy, with 12% reporting a complication and 3.5% reporting a death.

3. Reshef A, Stocchi L, Kiran RP et al. Case-matched comparison of perioperative outcomes after surgical treatment of sigmoid diverticulitis in solid organ transplant recipients verses immunocompromised patients. *Colorectal Dis.* 2012;14:1546–1552.

   This study examines the incidence and outcome of complicated diverticulitis comparing liver, kidney, and lung transplant patients separately with those who were immunosuppressed for other reasons. Although the overall incidence of diverticulitis was low in the three groups of patients, the mortality rate varied from 25% to 0% to 33%, respectively.

4. Paul S, Escareno CE, Clancy K, Jaklitsch MT, Bueno R, Lautz DB. Gastrointestinal complications after lung transplantation. *J Heart Lung Transplant.* 2009;28:475–479.

   These authors demonstrated a 100% mortality in the two lung transplant patients who had complicated diverticulitis.

5. De'Angelis N, Esposito F, Memeo R et al. Emergency abdominal surgery after solid organ transplantation: A systematic review. *World J Emerg Surg.* 2016;11:43–54.

   This systematic review is based upon case reviews and studies and includes large database reviews in their assessment. Although this increases the overall number of patients in each cohort that they assess, there is significant chance for overlap between studies. Cholecystectomy, gastrointestinal perforation, complicated diverticulitis, appendicitis, and small bowel obstruction are the emergent operations that are reviewed.

6. Miller CB, Malaisrie SC, Patel J, Garrity E, Vigneswaran WT, Gamelli RL. Intraabdominal complications after lung transplantation. *J Am Coll Surg.* 2006;203:653–660.

   This is a case series of two patients who had small bowel obstructions. The mortality rate was 50% in their cohort.

7. Catena F, Ansaloni L, Gazzotti F et al. Gastrointestinal perforations following kidney transplantation. *Transplant Proc*. 2008;40:1895–1896.

   These authors present the largest series of gastrointestinal perforation after transplantation. They exclusively examine kidney transplantation but break down the source of perforation as well as the pathological diagnosis in most cases.

Landmark Article of 21st Century

OUTCOMES OF CHOLECYSTECTOMY IN US HEART TRANSPLANT RECIPIENTS

Kilic A, Sheer A, Shah AS, Russell SD, Gourin CG, and Lidor AO, *Ann Surg*. 2013;258:312–317

ABSTRACT

Objective The aim of this study was to evaluate outcomes and predictors of in-hospital mortality after cholecystectomy in heart transplant (HTx) recipients.

Background There is a paucity of data on outcomes after cholecystectomy in HTx recipients.

Methods The Nationwide Inpatient Sample (NIS) database was used to identify HTx recipients who underwent cholecystectomy between 1998 and 2008. Multivariate logistic regression analysis was constructed using clinically relevant covariates (age, gender, Charlson comorbidity index, race, admission acuity, complicated gallstone disease, hospital teaching status, and open vs. laparoscopic approach) to identify predictors of in-hospital mortality.

Results A total of 1687 HTx recipients underwent cholecystectomy (open n = 420; laparoscopic n = 1267) during the study period. Mean age was 57.1 ± 12.5 years, and there were 1230 (72.9%) males. The majority of patients had acute cholecystitis (n = 1218; 72.2%) and were admitted urgently/emergently (n = 1028; 60.9%). Overall inpatient mortality occurred in 37 (2.2%) patients, with a higher mortality rate in open cholecystectomy compared with laparoscopic (6.2% vs. 0.9%; P = 0.009), and in urgent/emergent versus elective cases (3.6% vs. 0%; P = 0.04). Open or urgent/emergent cholecystectomies also had higher overall complication and respiratory failure rates as compared with laparoscopic or elective cases. Predictors of inpatient mortality in multivariable analysis included urgent/emergent admission, open cholecystectomy, and complicated gallstone disease (each P < 0.05).

Conclusions This is the largest reported study to date of cholecystectomy in HTx recipients. HTx patients appear to be at increased risk of inpatient mortality and morbidity after cholecystectomy as compared with the general population, and this rate is particularly high in those with a nonelective admission who undergo open cholecystectomy for complicated gallstone disease. Therefore, strong consideration should be given to prophylactic cholecystectomy in HTx recipients with asymptomatic and uncomplicated gallstone disease.

Editor Notes

Assessment: How to best manage the asymptomatic patient with gallstones is an ongoing debate. However the question now being asked is if prophylactic cholecystectomy should be done in recipients of heart transplants, as asymptomatic gallstones are much more common in this population. This was a retrospective study of heart transplant recipients who underwent cholecystectomy. The authors used the NIS database to determine the outcome and predictors of in-hospital mortality. The multivariate logistic regressions were done on 1687 patients over 10 years and reported that the outcome was affected by urgency and how the operation was performed (open vs. laproscopic). The mortality rate was 2.2%. As one would expect, patients who had open repair on an urgent basis did the worst, with higher complication rates such as respiratory failures and higher mortality.

Limitations: The comparison group in this study was historical reports of the general population. It would seem obvious that patients who underwent heart transplant would have more health problems, especially since they are immunosuppressed and have worse cardiopulmonary reserves. In the general population, the urgency of the operation and whether it is done open or laparoscopically also affects outcome. The overall mortality rate was 2.2%, and 72.2% of the patients in this study underwent cholecystectomy for acute disease. The average age was also older, at 57. Because in the general population the outcome is also worse after acute disease process necessitating urgent operation, the recommendation of prophylactic cholecystectomy has been heavily debated based on the same reasoning. Although the number of patients in this study was larger than previous reports, due to the lack of comparison data, the debates will most likely continue. Comparison to the general public by reviewing historical reports is not generally a strong methodology. Assuming that the rate of cholecystectomy in the heart transplant recipients is much higher, in order to recommend prophylactic cholecystectomy one would need the rate of mortality and morbidity of asymptomatic cholecystectomy in heart transplant recipients, which is not known.

Conclusions: The study concludes that the recipients of heart transplants are at higher risk of inpatient mortality and morbidity after cholecystectomy compared to the general population. Thus the authors recommend that consideration should be given to prophylactic cholecystectomy in recipients of heart transplants with asymptomatic and uncomplicated gallstone disease.

CHAPTER 29

Thoracic and Chest Disease

Review by Contributor: Lydia Lam

Thoracic and cardiac procedures remain largely in the hands of our cardiac and thoracic colleagues. However, a few things the acute care surgeon may be called upon for the surgical care of the patient will be discussed.

Pneumothorax or pleural effusions compromising respiratory status can be rapidly addressed. Chest tubes are placed with the classic teaching of larger tubes for fluid and smaller tubes for air. Extrapolating from recent trauma data, we know that size does not really matter. In a study by Inaba et al. (2012), prospective data was collected in patients requiring chest tubes from trauma and compared large versus small tubes with a total of 353 tubes placed in 293 patients. There were no differences in complications or additional procedures needed in the two groups and no difference in pain reported by patients. In Kulvatunyou et al. (2014), a comparison of a 14-Fr pigtail versus a 28-Fr chest tube for pneumothorax suggested that the pigtail was just as effective as a chest tube. Kulvatunyou et al. (2012) went on to suggest a 14-Fr pigtail be adequate to drain a hemothorax with good results, and the group further reported the same findings with a 7-year prospective study showing that pigtails were not inferior to chest tubes (Bauman et al., 2018).

Esophageal perforations have many etiologies including cancer, trauma, or just increased pressure from forceful coughing or retching. The management of esophageal perforations has changed drastically in the last 10 years. The gold standard is to require an open thoracotomy, possible repair, wide drainage, and buttressing with perfused tissue, and all this with tenuous results, as the esophageal blood supply is minimal. The morbidity and mortality rates of esophageal perforations are high. Endoscopic stents have changed the management of this disease with improved outcomes. Stents were first described for esophageal perforations as early as the nineteenth century but it was not until the 1990s that stents were modernized and their use in esophageal disease was more successful. In 2018, Watkins and Farivar (2018) reviewed the many endoluminal therapies that are available for esophageal perforations and leaks. Esophageal perforations need to be diagnosed and treated early for optimal outcome with source control and effective drainage. Endoscopic clips, stents, and vacuum therapy are discussed in this review. Regarding stents, the options of metal or plastics stents are available. Originally for patients unstable for surgery or palliation, its success led to all esophageal perforations for consideration. However, an operation may still be needed for patients with significant contamination for adequate drainage. Ten retrospective studies were reviewed and found clinical effectiveness ranged from 63%–89%, with the most common complication being stent migration. Mortality ranged from 0%–17%. Dasari et al. (2014) collected 27 case series that only included anastomotic leaks and benign esophageal perforations. Primary outcome was failure requiring surgery, with secondary outcomes including migration, reinterventions, strictures, procedure complications, and cost. The clinical success for stenting was 81%. No significant difference was seen from surgical procedure, and the authors concluded this to be safe and should be considered a treatment option with early diagnosis and limited contamination.

Many studies evaluating stents are case series, cohort studies, or retrospective reviews. In 2017, in a systematic literature review of these, the best evidence in a 10-year period was made for the leaking esophagus, specifically comparing stents to surgical exploration by Persson et al. (2017). After reviewing the articles extracted for stents and surgical treatment, only 17 papers from both groups were analyzed. The overall reported success of stents was 88%, with an in-hospital mortality rate of 7.3%. In contrast, the overall reported success rate of surgical exploration was 83%, with an in-hospital mortality rate of 17%. The authors concluded that a stent is a reasonable choice of therapy if the presentation is less than within 48 hours of injury and a careful treatment strategy is planned should the stent not control the leak. The emergency surgeon can help expedite the care of these patients, working closely with their endoscopic/thoracic colleagues to assure the optimal care for the patient.

Empyema management has also moved to the less invasive route. Empyema exists in three stages, where each stage gets progressively more scars and is more difficult to evacuate. Without appropriate debridement of the infectious material and release of the lung, respiratory status will fail and sepsis will progress. Open thoracotomy with decortication has been the mainstay, but minimally invasive procedures have since been taken seriously in the last 15 years. Video-assisted thoracoscopic surgery (VATS) has gained popularity in its use for the decortication of stage 2 and 3 empyema. Tong et al. (2010) looked retrospectively over a 10-year period at their institution on VATS versus open decortication for benign disease. To date, they have one of the largest numbers of patients included in a study. Three hundred twenty-six VATS and 94 open decortication patients were identified, with an 11.4% conversion to open rate on the VATS patients. The VATS group was found to have shorter operative time, hospital length of stay (LOS), fewer complications, and lower mortality.

As the stages of empyema has very different characteristics, Reichert et al. (2018) in 2018 specifically identified stage 3 empyema patients and compared the two therapeutic modalities. The patients were retrospectively collected over a 12-year period with 110 VATS patients and 107 thoracotomy patients. They found a longer operation time, and ICU stay was longer in the thoracotomy patients. However, complications, recurrence, and mortality did not show statistical differences between the two groups. In 2017, a meta-analysis of VATS versus open decortication with Pan et al. (2017) was able to compare five retrospective studies and found that VATS may be superior in operative time, postop complications, and pain. However, it did not show a difference between the two groups in relapse rate of the empyema. Similar to the esophageal perforations, there have been no randomized studies on this comparison.

As technology improves, treatment options have moved toward more minimally invasive options for patients. It is important that the acute care surgeon knows these options are available.

ANNOTATED REFERENCES FOR THORACIC AND CHEST DISEASES FOR THE ACUTE CARE SURGEON

1. Inaba K, Lustenberger T, Recinos G et al. Does size matter? A prospective analysis of 28–32 versus 36–40 French chest tube size in trauma. *J Trauma.* 2012;72:422–427.

   This study wanted to see if smaller chest tubes could be used instead of larger chest tubes for hemothorax in trauma. The data was prospectively collected, but the size of the tube was at the physician's discretion. The authors did not find a difference in the need for a second tube, further intervention, or unresolved pneumothorax. Interestingly, no difference in pain was reported by patients. The conclusion from the authors was tube size did not matter in drainage.

2. Kulvatunyou N, Erickson L, Vijayasekaran A et al. Randomized clinical trial of pigtail catheter versus chest tube in injured patients with uncomplicated traumatic pneumothorax. *BJS.* 2014;101:17–22.

   This was a randomized, prospective study evaluating the use of a 14-Fr pigtail instead of a chest tube for non-emergent placement in trauma patients for pneumothoraces. The authors wanted to also evaluate the pain associated with the tube placement. Forty patients were enrolled, with 20 in each group. Primary outcome was pain, while secondary was the successful of pneumothorax resolution. Conclusion was that pain was reduced with no difference in resolution of pneumothorax.

3. Kulvatunyou N, Joseph B, Friese RS et al. 14 French pigtail catheters placed by surgeons to drain blood on trauma patients: Is 14-Fr too small? *J Trauma Acute Care Surg.* 2012;6:1423–1427.

   The paper aimed to evaluate the drainage of hemothorax or hemopneumothorax due to trauma with a 14-Fr pigtail. The authors prospectively collected 36 pigtail patients over 2 years, while their chest tube patients were retrospectively identified in their trauma database. They found the pigtails went in later than the chest tube group but that the initial outputs were similar as well as the duration, complications, and failure rates. They concluded that their small group of pigtail patients did as well as their matched counterparts for hemo- and hemopneumothorax.

4. Bauman ZM, Kulvatunyou N, Joseph B et al. A prospective study of 7-year experience using percutaneous 14-fr pigtail catheters for a traumatic hemothorax/hemopneumothorax at a level-1 trauma center: Size still does not matter. *World J Surg.* 2018;42:107–113.

   The authors wanted to further compare pigtails to chest tube over a longer period. A prospective database maintained by a trauma attending was used. Four hundred ninety-six trauma patients were analyzed with 307 chest tubes and 189 pigtails. The choice of drainage was at the discretion of the surgeon at the time. Primary outcomes included initial drainage, complications, and failure rate which included further procedures to drain, which were similar in both tubes. Conclusion was that pigtail was not inferior to chest tubes.

5. Watkins JR, Farivar AS. Endoluminal therapies for esophageal perforations and leaks. *Thorac Surg Clin.* 2018;28:541–554.

   This review article summarizes esophageal perforations and the endoluminal therapies available. Complications and mortality rates are high, and diagnosis and time to treatment can improve outcomes. In those with early diagnosis and limited contamination, endoluminal therapies can be considered, including clips, stents, and wound vacuum systems, with effective outcomes to those of open surgery.

6. Dasari BV, Neely D, Kennedy A et al. The role of esophageal stents in the management of esophageal anastomotic leaks and benign esophageal perforations. *Ann Surg.* 2014;259:852–860.

   Review of safety and effectiveness of esophageal stents in benign esophageal perforation and anastomotic leaks. This is a systematic review of literature where the authors found a total of 27 case series with 340 patients. Technical and clinical success was 91% and 81%, respectively. Sub-analysis found plastic stents migrated more than metallic stents, which lead to more reinterventions. However, metallic stents had higher stricture rate. Overall, the article concluded that stenting is feasible and a viable option in early diagnosis with limited contamination.

7. Persson S, Rouvelas I, Irino T, Lundell L. Outcomes following the main treatment options in patients with a leaking esophagus: A systematic literature review. *Dis Esophagus.* 2017;30:1–10.

   This was a systematic literature review comparing metallic stent versus operative repair for esophageal leak. After applying their inclusion criteria, 17 articles for stent and 17 articles for open repair were identified for analysis. Overall, 88% success rate for stent was found with an in-hospital mortality of 7.5%. For open repair, 83% success rate was found with an in-hospital mortality of 17%. Conclusion was that esophageal stent can be a successful alternative therapy to esophageal leak.

8. Tong BC, Hanna J, Toloza EM et al. Outcomes of video-assisted thoracoscopic decortication. *Ann Thorac Surg.* 2010;89:220–225.

   Retrospective single-center study identified adult patients with benign conditions who underwent open decortication or VATS in a 10-year period. One of the largest comparing VATS to open thoracotomy, 420 patients were identified, of which 289 were VATS. However, these patients included other diagnoses in addition to empyema, such as complex pleural effusion and hemothorax. Results found VATS with shorter operating time, shorter HLOS, fewer postop complications, and lower 30-day mortality. Conversion rate to open decortication was 11.4%. However, the retrospective nature of the study and multiple diagnosis may have a selection bias to those who underwent VATS versus open decortication. Conclusion is that VATS show at least an equivalent outcome to open decortication and may be a good first option for patients so a larger operation is not necessary.

9. Reichert M, Pösentrup B, Hecker A et al. Thoracotomy versus video-assisted thoracoscopic surgery (VATS) in stage III empyema—An analysis of 217 consecutive patients. *Surg Endosc.* 2018;32:2664–2675.

   Retrospective paper looking specifically at stage 3 empyema treatment of thoracotomy versus VATS. The single-institution paper notes that prior to 2011, only open thoracotomy was performed, while VATS was performed after with the same group of surgeons. These two cohorts were compared to HLOS. Aside from longer operation time with the open technique, LOS, recurrence, complications, and air leaks were no different. However, after adjusting for relevant confounders, there was a statistically significant decrease in HLOS in VATS patients. Conclusion was that VATS is feasible in stage III empyema.

10. Pan H, He J, Shen J, Jiang L, Liang W, He J. A meta-analysis of video-assisted thoracoscopic decortication versus open thoracotomy decortication for patients with empyema. *J Thorac Dis.* 2017;9(7):2006–2014.

    Meta-analysis of VATS versus open decortication for only patients with empyema. Inclusion criteria included original publications with >20 patients, VATS or open decortication for empyema or pleural infection, and reported in the English language. Five total publications were used for analysis. Despite that, conclusions from this meta-analysis found VATS to have shorter operative time, hospital length of stay (HLOS), decreased air leak and chest tube need, and decreased morbidity and mortality. Unfortunately, the authors acknowledge that each paper may have reported outcomes differently, and the patients in each arm are likely different populations, and they hope to repeat the meta-analysis when better designed studies are published.

RANDOMIZED CLINICAL TRIAL OF PIGTAIL CATHETER VERSUS CHEST TUBE IN INJURED PATIENTS WITH UNCOMPLICATED TRAUMATIC PNEUMOTHORAX

Kulvatunyou N, Erickson L, Vijayasekaran A, Gries L, Joseph B, Friese RF, O'Keeffe T, Tang AL, Wynne JL, and Rhee P, *BJS.* 2014;101:17–22

ABSTRACT

Background   Small pigtail catheters appear to work as well as the traditional large-bore chest tubes in patients with traumatic pneumothorax, but it is not known whether the smaller pigtail catheters are associated with less tube-site pain. This study was conducted to compare tube-site pain following pigtail catheter or chest tube insertion in patients with uncomplicated traumatic pneumothorax.

Methods   This prospective randomized trial compared 14-Fr pigtail catheters and 28-Fr chest tubes in patients with traumatic pneumothorax presenting to a level I trauma center from July 2010 to February 2012. Patients who required emergency tube placement, those who refused, and those who could not respond to pain assessment were excluded. Primary outcomes were tube-site pain, as assessed by a numerical rating scale, and total pain medication use. Secondary outcomes included the success rate of pneumothorax resolution and insertion-related complications.

Results   Forty patients were enrolled. Baseline characteristics of 20 patients in the pigtail catheter group were similar to those of 20 patients in the chest tube group. No patient had a flail chest or hemothorax. Pain scores related to chest wall trauma were similar in the two groups. Patients with a pigtail catheter had significantly lower mean (s.d.) tube-site pain scores than those with a chest tube, at baseline after tube insertion (3.2(0.6) vs. 7.7(0.6); P < 0.001), on day 1 (1.9(0.5) vs. 6.2(0.7); P < 0.001), and day 2 (2.1(1.1) vs. 5.5(1.0); P = 0.040). The decreased use of pain medication associated with pigtail catheter was not significantly different. The duration of tube insertion, success rate, and insertion-related complications were all similar in the two groups.

Conclusion   For patients with a simple, uncomplicated traumatic pneumothorax, use of a 14-Fr pigtail catheter is associated with reduced pain at the site of insertion, with no other clinically important differences noted compared with chest tubes.

Editor Notes

Assessment: What is most important about this paper is that it tries to brings some scientific rigor to challenge the dogma that a large chest tube is superior to a small pigtail catheter in the management of pneumothorax. This work clearly demonstrated, using a randomized clinical trial, the feasibility of this technique during emergency care, the benefits of this technique in regard to resolution of pneumothorax, and the advantages of the pigtail catheter over chest tubes in regard to minimizing pain.

Limitations: The study did not assess the benefits of this technique in the patient with hemothorax or flail chest. In addition, tube site pain may have been substantially eclipsed by the chest wall pain related to rib fractures and associated injuries. This may account for the lack of differences in pain medications administered. Certainly, narcotics given for chest wall pain may have obscured differences in pain from the tubes. Also, the larger chest tubes often employed (36-Fr) were not utilized in this study. This makes the noted reduction in tube-site pain with small pigtail tubes even more impressive. It is true that the assessors of pain were not blinded as to group, so bias may have occurred.

Conclusions: The superiority of large-bore chest tube over smaller pigtail-type catheters for management of pneumothorax was clearly refuted in this randomized clinical trial.

CHAPTER 30

Complications of Bariatric Surgery

Review by Contributors: Jazmín M. Cole, Vishwanath Chegireddy,
Nabil Tariq, and Daniel J. Bonville

Obesity and its associated comorbidities affect over one-third of the US population (Sanni et al., 2014). There has been a significant rise in the number of bariatric surgery procedures performed over the past few decades, which directly correlates with the escalating rate of obesity in the population and the rising number of those seeking treatment. In 1967, Mason and Ito were the first to perform open Roux-en-Y gastric bypass (RYGB) for weight loss, which is now regarded as the gold standard by most bariatric surgeons (Tucker et al., 2007). Currently, approximately 270,000 bariatric surgeries were performed in 2015–2016 in the United States, about a third of which were RYGBs (Sebastian, 2018).

Due to bariatric surgery's popularity in combatting the obesity epidemic and laparo-scopic RYGB being the most commonly performed bariatric procedure worldwide (Husain et al., 2007), surgeons are encountering an increasing frequency of postop-erative complications, including marginal ulceration with perforation, bleeding, and bowel obstruction. Marginal ulcerations occur at a rate of 4%, are associated with tobacco and NSAID use, and can lead to perforation at the gastrojejunostomy site (Ma and Madura, 2015). Perforations are often closed over an endoscope and buttressed with omentum with care taken to avoid narrowing the gastrojejunostomy. A gastros-tomy tube may be placed in the remnant stomach should the repair fail.

Intestinal obstruction can also be caused by endoluminal bariatric devices, such as intragastric balloons. Balloons left in place longer than the 4–6 months indicated to induce weight loss are at risk of rupturing and migrating distally. Instead of adhesive disease or internal hernias causing bowel obstruction from extrinsic compression of the bowel in post-surgical bariatric patients, intragastric balloons can cause intralumi-nal intestinal obstruction.

Bleeding is another complication that can be associated with marginal ulceration late after surgery and is primarily managed endoscopically, as the most common site is the gastrojejunostomy. Rarely, patients may develop bleeding ulcers in the gas-tric remnant requiring interventional radiology or open gastrotomy for endoscopic evaluation of the gastric remnant. Operative intervention for bleeding is rare. The reported overall incidence of small intestinal obstruction (SBO) following RYGB varies between 0.8% and 5% (Paroz et al., 2006) and appears to be more common following laparoscopic compared to open procedures, particularly within the first few weeks to months following surgery (Paroz et al., 2006; Tucker et al., 2007). There are now hundreds of thousands of patients in the United States who have undergone RYGB and it is therefore more likely that the acute care surgeon may encounter these complications.

Intestinal obstructions following gastric bypass can often present a diagnostic challenge to even an experienced bariatric surgeon, and it is a vital part of the acute care surgeon's repertoire to be familiar with these patients and their unique surgical needs. The onset of SBO after RYGB can vary; it may occur early acute, which is less than 30 days postop, early late, which is between 30 days to 12 months postop, and chronic, which is greater than 12 months postop (Tucker et al., 2007). The clinical presentation of patients presenting with SBO after gastric bypass varies depending on the onset of SBO. Chronically obstructed patients most frequently present with recurrent episodes of colicky abdominal pain (Paroz et al., 2006). Due to the small gastric pouch created during RYGB, patients with intestinal obstructions may not complain of nausea or report voluminous emesis as may be anticipated with intestinal obstruction (Husain et al., 2007). Instead, dry heaving or clear emesis may be reported. Upper gastrointestinal intestinal (GI) contrast studies and computerized tomography (CT) scans are both used regularly in the evaluation of post-bypass patients presenting with abdominal pain; however, their effectiveness in diagnosing intestinal obstructions, and particularly obstructions due to internal hernias, can vary. Husain et al. reported the overall sensitivity in diagnosing small bowel obstructions due to internal hernias with CT scan was 51.1%, while the diagnostic sensitivity using upper GI studies was 56.6%. In this series of patients, CT scans seemed to be more effective in diagnosing obstructions due to adhesive disease rather than internal hernias. Also, there must be a high degree of suspicion for closed-loop obstruction if the imaging reveals a dilated biliopancreatic limb with the gastric remnant, as this can lead to peritonitis, intestinal ischemia, and eventual death if it is unrecognized.

Other etiologies for SBOs in post-gastric bypass patients include roux limb strictures, anastomotic stricture, jejunojejunostomy stenosis, intussusception of jejunojejunostomy, adhesions, port-site hernias, and angulation or obstruction at the jejunojejunostomy which may be difficult to discern on imaging studies. Regardless of the presumed etiology, approaching the diagnosis of a bowel obstruction following gastric bypass should follow a systematic thought process represented by the "ABC's" of bowel obstruction locations described by Tucker et al. "A" stands for the alimentary limb or roux limb, "B" stands for the biliopancreatic limb, and "C" stands for the common channel distal to the jejunojejunostomy. In regard to location of the obstruction, various symptoms and laboratory values can guide the surgeon. Patients with obstruction of the alimentary limb or common channel can present with gastroesophageal reflux and significant vomiting. In addition, elevation of liver function tests and hyperamylasemia can suggest obstruction of the biliopancreatic limb or the common channel (Tucker et al., 2007). When the "B" limb is obstructed it can act like a closed-loop obstruction and thus require surgical correction and remnant gastrostomy tube decompression of the "B" limb.

SBO due to internal hernia has proven to be a diagnostic challenge due to the patients' altered anatomy, uncharacteristic presenting symptoms, imaging findings that can be difficult to interpret, and intermittent nature of the obstruction that may not be captured on imaging studies. As a result, a high index of suspicion must be maintained when post-gastric bypass patients present with abdominal pain, as a delayed diagnosis often results in longer segments of bowel requiring resection and a higher rate of conversion from laparoscopic to open exploratory procedures (Paroz et al., 2006). Of particular importance, patients with several emergency department visits for abdominal pain and a series of negative imaging studies should be strongly considered for diagnostic laparoscopy. In regard to operative approach, imaging studies can be used to guide safe entry into the patient's abdomen using either open Hassan or Optiview technique. During exploration, running the small bowel in retrograde fashion starting from the terminal ileum to the roux limb will help guide the surgeon to find the point of obstruction in regard to the complex anatomy. In evaluation of tissue integrity and perfusion, attention must also be paid to therapeutic reduction of any identified hernias and repair of mesenteric defects to prevent future obstructive episodes. The most common locations for mesenteric defects include the jejuno-jejunal anastomosis defect, Petersen's space (behind the Roux limb, whether retrocolic or antecolic), and transverse mesocolic window (if retrocolic), with some patients having multiple defects.

Except in acute obstructions, radiological findings often cannot confirm the diagnosis of intestinal obstruction due to an internal hernia. Therefore, it is paramount to maintain a high index of suspicion, particularly in post-gastric bypass patients with recurrent colicky abdominal pain. A low threshold for offering patients a diagnostic laparoscopy with repair of all mesenteric defects is the best way to prevent future obstructive episodes, avoid the need for bowel resection, and reduce mortality overall.

ANNOTATED REFERENCES FOR COMPLICATIONS OF BARIATRIC SURGERY

1. Tucker ON, Escalante-Tattersfield T, Szomstein S, Rosenthal RJ. The ABC system: A simplified classification system for small bowel obstruction after laparoscopic Roux-en-Y gastric bypass. *Obes Surg.* 2007;17:1549–1554.

   Electronic literature review of Embase, Cochrane, and Medline databases was performed between January 1999 and October 2006 to examine the history, presentation, diagnostic workup, and management of small bowel obstruction after laparoscopic Roux-en-Y gastric bypass. The ABC classification system is based on the site of anatomic obstruction after gastric bypass: A for alimentary limb, B biliopancreatic limb, C common channel.

2. O'Brien PE. Bariatric surgery: Mechanisms, indications and outcomes. *J Gastroenterol Hepatol.* 2010;25:1358–1365.

   A review of the evolution of bariatric surgery, a comparison of the efficacy of surgery versus nonsurgical therapies as well as various surgical options available.

3. Sanni A, Perez S, Medbery R et al. Postoperative complications in bariatric surgery using age and BMI stratification: A study using ACS-NSQIP data. *Surg Endosc.* 2014;28:3302–3309.

   Authors searched the ACS-NSQIP 2010–2011 Public Use File for patients who underwent elective laparoscopic adjustable gastric band, sleeve gastrectomy, and gastric bypass in an effort to identify trends in morbidity and mortality as it relates to age and body mass index (BMI). The odds of postoperative complications increased by 2% for every additional year of age or point increase in BMI.

4. Paroz A, Calmes JM, Giusti V, Suter M. Internal hernia after laparoscopic Roux-en-Y gastric bypass for morbid obesity: A continuous challenge in bariatric surgery. *Obes Surg.* 2006;16:1482–1487.

   The authors performed a retrospective review of 607 patients at two institutions who underwent Roux-en-Y gastric bypass with the goal of characterizing the incidence and presentation of internal hernias postoperatively. They concluded that radiographic studies were of little diagnostic use and recommended prevention by closing all mesenteric defects during initial operation.

5. Husain S, Ahmed AR, Johnson J, Boss T, O'Malley W. Small-bowel obstruction after laparoscopic Roux-en-Y gastric bypass: Etiology, diagnosis, and management. *Arch Surg.* 2007;142(10):988–993.

   The authors performed a single-institution retrospective review of 105 patients who underwent surgery for small bowel obstruction after laparoscopic Roux-en-Y gastric bypass to summarize common presenting symptoms, causes, and yield of radiographic studies. The authors concluded that the diagnosis of bowel obstruction in these patients was difficult due to altered gastrointestinal anatomy, vague complaints, and poor yield of imaging studies. Therefore, a solid understanding of the surgical anatomy and low level of suspicion are key in diagnosing bowel obstruction promptly.

6. Sebastian R, Howell MH, Chang KH et al. Robot-assisted versus laparoscopic Roux-en-Y gastric bypass and sleeve gastrectomy: A propensity score-matched comparative analysis using the 2015–2016 MBSAQIP database. *Surg Endosc* 2019;33(5):1600–1612.

   The authors used the 2015–2016 Metabolic and Bariatric Surgery Accreditation and Quality Improvement Program database to identify 269,923 patients who underwent sleeve gastrectomy or Roux-en-Y gastric bypass surgery and compared 30-day outcomes between robotic-assisted and laparoscopic procedures. They concluded that robotic-assisted approaches were associated with better postoperative outcomes overall, particularly with Roux-en-Y gastric bypass.

7. Ma IT, Madura JA II. Gastrointestinal complications after bariatric surgery. *Gastroenterol Hepatol.* 2015;11(8):526–535.

   The authors reviewed the short- and long-term complications associated with four bariatric procedures: adjustable gastric banding, sleeve gastrectomy, gastric bypass, and biliopancreatic diversion with duodenal switch. Complication rates have decreased overall and metabolic issues specific to each procedure must be considered when counseling patients prior to bariatric surgery.

SMALL-BOWEL OBSTRUCTION AFTER LAPAROSCOPIC Roux-en-Y GASTRIC BYPASS: ETIOLOGY, DIAGNOSIS, AND MANAGEMENT

Husain S, Ahmed AR, Johnson J, Boss T, and O'Malley W, *Arch Surg.* 2007;142(10):988–993

ABSTRACT

Objective To summarize our experience with small-bowel obstructions after laparoscopic Roux-en-Y gastric bypass.

Design Retrospective record review.

Setting University-affiliated hospital.

Patients One hundred five consecutive patients undergoing surgery for intestinal obstruction after laparoscopic Roux-en-Y gastric bypass between May 24, 2001 and December 1, 2006.

Main Outcome Measures Common presenting symptoms, causes, yield of radiological studies, and types of surgical procedures performed for post-gastric bypass bowel obstruction.

Results A total of 2325 laparoscopic Roux-en-Y gastric bypass procedures were performed during the study period. A total of 105 patients underwent 111 procedures. Bowel obstruction was confirmed in 102 patients, yielding an overall incidence of 4.4%. The most common presenting symptom was abdominal pain (82.0%), followed by nausea (48.6%) and vomiting (46.8%). Thirty-one patients (27.9%) presented with all of the three mentioned symptoms. The mean time to presentation was 313 days after bypass (range, 3–1215 days). Among the studies, results in 48.0% of computed tomographic scans, 55.4% of upper gastrointestinal studies, and 34.8% of plain abdominal radiography studies were positive for intestinal obstruction. In 15 patients (13.5%), all of the radiological study results were negative. The most common causes were internal hernias (53.9%), Roux compression due to mesocolon scarring (20.5%), and adhesions (13.7%). Laparoscopic explorations were carried out in 92 cases (82.9%). The incidences of bowel obstructions were 4.8% with retrocolic Roux placement and 1.8% with antecolic Roux placement.

Conclusions Altered gastrointestinal tract anatomy results in vague symptoms and a poor yield with imaging studies. A sound knowledge of altered anatomy is the key to correct interpretation of imaging studies and prompt diagnosis.

Editor Notes

Assessment: This was a single-institutional review of 105 patients who underwent surgery for small bowel obstruction after laparoscopic Roux-en-Y gastric bypass. The authors concluded that the diagnosis of bowel obstruction in these patients is complex due to altered gastrointestinal anatomy, vague complaints, and poor yield of imaging studies. Abdominal pain was the most common symptom associated with intestinal obstruction post-gastric bypass and was found in more than 80% of patients. Unfortunately, less than half of these patients had diagnostic confirmation on abdominal CT scan.

As nearly 300,000 bariatric procedures are performed yearly in the United States and as many as 5% develop intestinal obstruction, this complication looms large for clinicians in North America. It should be noted that complications of bariatric surgery are often evaluated initially by primary care providers and emergency room personnel and are operated upon by non-bariatric general surgeons.

Limitations: Small sample size limits our ability to generalize conclusions.

Conclusions: A solid understanding of the surgical anatomy and a low level of suspicion after bariatric surgical procedures are key in diagnosing bowel obstruction promptly. The authors recommended an early aggressive surgical approach to post-gastric bypass abdominal pain.

CHAPTER 31

Burns

Review by Contributor: Laura Johnson

Since the beginning of recorded history, burn wounds have been recognized and managed by physicians of all disciplines. Many of the preeminent surgeons of the twentieth century spent time studying wound healing, fluid resuscitation, and nutrition in the setting of burn injury, including G. Tom Shires, Joseph E. Murray, and Francis D. Moore, with significant resultant contributions to surgical practice. Management of burn patients engenders the development of a robust and engaging multidisciplinary team, as surgeons, therapists, nurses, scientists, pharmacists, nutritionists, and other allied health professionals have dedicated their careers to the care of these complex patients.

Today, burn injury results in approximately half a million emergency room visits per year in the United States, with approximately 10% of those requiring hospitalization and 1% dying from either fire or smoke inhalation injuries. Globally, 180,000 deaths occur per year from burn injury, and nonfatal burns are among the leading cause of disability-adjusted life-years lost in low- and middle-income countries.

Burn wounds are typically classified by the mechanism of injury (flame, scald, contact, chemical, electrical, and radiation), the depth of injury (superficial thickness, partial thickness [either superficial or deep], and full thickness), and the surface area involved. The Rule of Nines provides a rough estimation for calculating the total burn surface area (TBSA) involved, which is important for delineating patients at risk for the development of burn shock (TBSA >20%). The classic Parkland resuscitation described by Baxter and Shires in 1968 has been modified in the last decade to account for significant "fluid creep." The administration of excess fluid volumes (above 4 mL/kg/%TBSA) during resuscitations has been well documented, resulting in issues ranging from acute respiratory failure and compartment syndromes to multiple organ dysfunction. Calculations should begin with 2–4 mL/kg/%TBSA depending on the type of burn and age of the patient, with consideration for use of colloid and other adjuncts depending on patient response (Pham et al., 2008).

While the early burn wound is sparsely populated by bacteria, most being destroyed in the injury, Gram-positive species predominate. This gives way over the first week to the colonization of burn eschar with Gram-negative organisms. If left unchecked, burn wound sepsis can develop, with mortality over 50% in patients who go on to develop multiorgan system failure. The development of Sulfamylon and silver sulfadiazine in the mid-nineteenth century significantly decreased mortality from burn wound sepsis. (Pruitt and Curreri, 1971) To this day, despite some controversy over the impact of silver on wound healing, silver-containing wound products remain the mainstay of therapy for burn wounds. Nutritional supplementation is another component of successful burn infection control. Energy expenditure in patients after burn injury can be as high as 100% above normal, and catabolism of protein stores is profound. Enteral feeding started early (within 2–4 h of injury) can attenuate the hypermetabolic response to injury and potentially preserve mucosal gut integrity, thereby decreasing infection risk (Mochizuki et al., 1984). Surgical removal of burn wounds is also a critical component of infection control; colony counts in burn wounds can drop by as much as a factor of 10^2 after a correctly performed excision (Barett and Herndon, 2003).

Early excision of burn wounds has a myriad of positive effects on patient outcomes. Long waits for autolysis and eschar separation followed by grafting of the resulting granulation plate was coupled with significant mortality and extensive development of hypertrophic, functionally limiting scar. While the potential benefit of full thickness burn excision was recognized in the 1940s, the ability to manage the physiologic response to such surgery was not possible at that time. Jackson and colleagues were the first to suggest the safety of early fascial excision and grafting in the setting of large burns, but it was not until Zora Janzekovic in the 1960s that the idea of early tangential excision for deep second-degree burns became a staple of burn surgery (Janzekovic, 1970). Prevention of infection and burn wound sepsis as noted earlier, early return to work, and improvement in hypertrophic scar development and cosmesis have all been shown to be benefits (Burke et al., 1974).

While autograft has always been the gold standard in skin replacement, renewed interest in skin replacement and tissue engineering has led to a number of new options for how to approach post-excision autografting. In evaluating these products, it is important to understand the balance of requirements for skin replacement after burn injury. Optimally, replacement tissue should have the same cellular components as the uninjured skin, should minimize the donor site necessary to obtain the replacement, and be as simple to manipulate surgically and manage postoperatively as classically harvested split-thickness skin grafts. Both epidermal and dermal substitutes exist, but no current product provides the full spectrum of function encompassed by combined healthy epidermis and dermis. Most recently, the use of a noncultured autologous skin suspension has shown great promise in reducing donor site morbidity, as it requires approximately 1/40th the donor skin of a standard split thickness graft (Holmes et al., 2018).

Concurrent with acute surgical management of burn wounds is the consideration of patient rehabilitation. Occupational and physical therapy specialists in burn care are integral members of the team, and patients are started on active rehabilitation regimens as soon as they are admitted. Burn scar maturation is a process that evolves over at least a year after the last wound is closed. Targeted compression on a burn scar during the first year after injury can modulate scar fibroblast deposition and collagen rearrangement, resulting in more pliable, flexible scars (Tejiram et al., 2016). Another novel intervention that is increasingly demonstrating benefit for both scar pliability and issues related to neuropathy and pruritus is laser modulation of hypertrophic scar. Use of fractional lasers allows for the creation of small thermal injuries in the skin, prompting rapid healing between islands of uninjured tissue that promote more organized tissue remodeling (Issler-Fisher et al., 2017). While a relatively new tool in the burn surgeon's kit, laser scar revision is able to address the spectrum of issues associated with hypertrophic scar, and is complementary to the traditional scar release approaches.

ANNOTATED REFERENCES FOR BURNS FOR THE GENERAL SURGEON

1. Pham TN, Cancio LC, Gibran NS; American Burn Association. American Burn Association practice guidelines burn shock resuscitation. *J Burn Care Res.* 2008;29(1):257–266.

   The authors summarize the incidence and pathophysiology of burn shock, and discuss the issues with the classic formulas for burn shock resuscitation. They then describe the available literature on resuscitation practices, and how those have evolved to create the current American Burn Association guidelines for burn shock resuscitation.

2. Pruitt BA Jr, Curreri PW. The burn wound and its care. *Arch Surg.* 1971;103(4):461–468.

   In this paper, the authors specifically describe the impact of mafenide acetate (Sulfamylon) on the development of Pseudomonas burn wound infection and subsequent sepsis, and compares it to silver sulfadiazine, at that time still an "investigational" product (Table 2). Much of the wound care approaches discussed are additionally relevant in today's resource-strapped environment.

3. Mochizuki H, Trocki O, Dominioni L, Brackett KA, Joffe SN, Alexander JW. Mechanism of prevention of postburn hypermetabolism and catabolism by early enteral feeding. *Ann Surg.* 1984;200(3):297–310.

   In a guinea pig model of thermal injury, the authors sought to address the question of timing of enteral feeding initiation after injury with the goal of attenuating hypercatabolism and hypermetabolism. Timing was set at 2 hrs post-injury vs. 3 days post-injury; today's readers should not be surprised that early feeding resulted in maintenance of initial weight (less than 5% loss over 2-week period), early preservation of gut thickness, and lower resting energy expenditures at 2 weeks. This study prompted additional work in early enteral support across surgical specialties, with nearly all report improvement in infection rates, decreased ileus and overall decreased length of stay.

4. Barret JP, Herndon DN. Effects of burn wound excision on bacterial colonization and invasion. *Plast Reconstr Surg.* 2003;111(2):744–750; discussion 751–2.

   The authors of this study demonstrate that excision and grafting can decrease burn wound organism counts by a factor of 10^2, with anticipated improvement in postoperative outcomes when this operation is performed early after a burn injury. It is worth noting that even after technically complete excisions, no wounds were ever completely sterile at the time of grafting; despite this, none of the patients in the early excision group had evidence of graft loss.

5. Janzekovic Z. A new concept in the early excision and immediate grafting of burns. *J Trauma.* 1970;10(12):1103–1108.

   Both technical aspects of tangential excision and outcomes related to the utilization of this technique in thermally injured patients is described for the first time by the author. This author single-handedly changed the surgical approach to the management of burn patients.

6. Burke JF, Bondoc CC, Quinby WC. Primary burn excision and immediate grafting: A method shortening illness. *J Trauma*. 1974;14(5):389–395.

The authors present their work using the combination of early tangential excision for smaller, deep second-degree burns coupled with facial excision for large burns; this is the first time the combination of early excision at multiple levels (fascial and tangential) was demonstrated to improve both mortality and hospital length of stay.

7. Tejiram S, Zhang J, Travis TE et al. Compression therapy affects collagen type balance in hypertrophic scar. *J Surg Res*. 2016;201(2):299–305.

While pressure therapy had been used for scar modulation in burn patients prior to this study, the understanding of its impact on gene expression and collagen content of scar was limited prior to this study. The authors were able to successfully demonstrate both an animal model with consistent application of pressure over times comparable with those used in patients, and demonstrable difference in collagen deposition in scars treated with pressure over time, paving the way for more complex experimentation into post-burn scar modulation.

8. Issler-Fisher AC, Waibel JS, Donelan MB. Laser modulation of hypertrophic scars: Technique and practice. *Clin Plast Surg*. 2017;44(4):757–766.

These authors, leaders in the field of laser surgery, have written a review paper on the technical aspects of laser scar revision for hypertrophic burn scar. Covering the physics of lasers in medicine, the basic science of laser scar modulation, current clinical results with pictorial examples, and perioperative management, this paper is a great reference for surgeons starting to incorporate laser surgery into their practice.

Landmark Article of the 21st Century

A COMPARATIVE STUDY OF THE RECELL® DEVICE AND AUTOLOGOUS SPLIT-THICKNESS MESHED SKIN GRAFT IN THE TREATMENT OF ACUTE BURN INJURIES

Holmes JH IV, Molnar JA, Carter JE, Hwang J, Cairns BA, King BT, Smith DJ, Cruse CW, Foster KN, Peck MD, Sood R, Feldman MJ, Jordan MH, Mozingo DW, Greenhalgh DG, Palmieri TL, Griswold JA, Dissanaike S, and Hickerson WL, *J Burn Care Res*. 2018;39(5):694–702

ABSTRACT

Early excision and autografting are standard care for deeper burns. However, donor sites are a source of significant morbidity. To address this, the ReCell® Autologous Cell Harvesting Device (ReCell) was designed for use at the point of care to prepare a noncultured, autologous skin cell suspension (ASCS) capable of epidermal regeneration using minimal donor skin. A prospective study was conducted to evaluate the clinical performance of ReCell versus meshed split-thickness skin grafts (STSG, Control) for the treatment of deep partial-thickness burns. Effectiveness measures were assessed to 1 year for both ASCS and Control treatment sites and donor sites, including the incidence of healing, scarring, and pain. At 4 weeks, 98% of the ASCS-treated sites were healed compared with 100% of the Controls. Pain and assessments of scarring at the treatment sites were reported to be similar between groups. Significant differences were observed between ReCell and Control donor sites. The mean ReCell donor area was approximately 40 times smaller than that of the Control (P < .0001), and after 1 week, significantly more ReCell donor sites were healed than Controls (P = .04). Over the first 16 weeks, patients reported significantly less pain at the ReCell donor sites compared with Controls (P ≤ .05 at each time point). Long-term patients reported higher satisfaction with ReCell donor site outcomes compared with the Controls. This study provides evidence that the treatment of deep partial-thickness burns with ASCS results in comparable healing, with significantly reduced donor site size and pain and improved appearance relative to STSG.

Original Author Commentary: James Holmes

Most of the major advancements in skin grafting have occurred within the last 200 years. These include identification of free epidermal grafts as an option for wound coverage, the development of tools to improve quality and consistency of harvests, and the evolution of expansion techniques to increase the wound area covered. This last is of particular interest as donor sites carry significant morbidity, and in patients with large burns, a limited amount of uninjured skin is available for harvest. With the optimization of mechanical expansion reached in the 1950s, the laboratory approach to further expansion initially resulted in cultured epithelial autografts. However, the multi-week time frame required to harvest, grow, and apply these can be prohibitive on multiple levels. ReCell is an autologous skin harvesting device that allows for intraoperative cellular harvest and immediate grafting of patients at an expansion ratio of 1:80. With the safety studies completed previously, the effectiveness of this approach in achieving wound closure can now be discussed. Our multidisciplinary group has shown that wound closure rates are equivalent to the gold standard with a substantially smaller, less morbid donor site, leaving the door wide open for a radical change in the approach to the treatment of thermal injury. Large areas of thermal injury can now potentially be removed and wounds definitively closed without substantially increasing a patient's wound burden; this has significant implications for shutting down the inflammatory response to thermal injury. In addition, with smaller donor sites, significant patient morbidity can be eliminated even in smaller burns, which has the potential to improve both the physical and mental recovery of patients after this traumatic injury.

CHAPTER 32

Urologic or Gynecologic Surgery

Review by Contributors: Vasiliy Sim and Samuel Hawkins

UROLOGIC SURGERY

General surgeons frequently encounter management issues related to the urinary tract while taking care of surgical patients, most often related to perioperative management of urinary catheters and of postoperative urinary retention. While the general approach to the use of urinary catheters has changed over the past two decades, little controversy remains. It has become standard to use urinary catheters as little and for as short a time as possible, as their contribution to iatrogenic infection has been firmly established. The first large study of perioperative catheter placement found that risk of infection increases significantly at 48 h (Wald et al., 2008), but is likely increased with any exposure. Catheters that are placed for surgery should be removed immediately after in the absence of persistent bladder dysfunction. While rectal surgeons may remain reluctant to embrace early catheter removal due to proximity of their dissection to the bladder, the literature firmly supports early catheter removal even in this patient group. Practices regarding catheter placement and removal are now largely driven by institutional protocol and require little clinician input or judgment.

The most common indication for maintaining urinary catheters in the postoperative period is postoperative urinary retention (POUR). Estimates of the incidence of POUR range widely, from 4%–13% in the general surgical population, and vary based on the type of surgery performed. While POUR has a clear impact on catheter use and other metrics of quality related to catheters, it remains poorly defined. In general, excluding the diagnosis requires both voiding and a post-void residual (PVR) volume of less than 1/3 the starting volume, or less than 200 mL. The most common method of defining POUR utilizes a spontaneous voiding trial, where the catheter is removed and the patient is given a set time in which to void, at which time the PVR is determined using a bladder scanner. A more precise method is the retrograde voiding trial, where a set volume of sterile saline (300 mL) is instilled in the decompressed bladder followed by immediate catheter removal. After 15 minutes, the volume voided can be compared directly to the expected volume. A full review of POUR diagnosis and treatment is not possible here, but it is worth noting that the general surgeon can impact the prevention of POUR. Any use of urinary catheters is a risk factor for POUR, another reason to limit their use. There is also evidence that perioperative prophylactic administration of alpha-1 adrenergic blocking agents can significantly reduce POUR, with a meta-analysis of RCTs finding an absolute reduction of over 15%, though the studies had significant heterogeneity (Ghuman et al., 2018).

Another topic of great interest to general surgeons is whether the use of ureteral stents will help prevent ureteral injury during retroperitoneal dissection. The incidence of ureteral injury during colorectal surgery has been reported as 0.15% to just over 1% (Palaniappa et al., 2012; Beraldo et al., 2013; Andersen et al., 2015). While some studies show increase in ureteral injuries with laparoscopic procedures, others do not (Beraldo et al., 2013; Andersen et al., 2015; Llarena et al., 2015). Patterns in the use of prophylactic preoperative ureteral stenting vary by surgeon. Some place prophylactic stents for all their colorectal cases, while others place stents selectively for those with expected difficult retroperitoneal dissection, such as patients with radiation exposure, previous surgery, and invasive cancer. There is a lack of Grade A evidence to support adoption of prophylactic stenting. The majority of studies used historic comparisons after switching to universal prophylactic stenting, while in other studies the practice of stenting was left to the surgeon's discretion. There are also no studies that actually show a decrease in ureteric injury. Ureteral stenting has its own set of complications such as hematuria, urinary tract infection, and although very rare, ureteric perforation. It adds operating room utilization time and requires coordination with a urologist. With these considerations and the paucity of benefit found in the literature, there is little to support routine use of these stents.

The landmark paper looked at a cohort of 374 open colectomies performed over 5 years in a tertiary level center (Andersen et al., 2015). The baseline characteristics were mildly different, with the most important ones being malignancy (38% vs. 30%) and elective status (75% vs. 35%) in the prophylactic ureteral stent group. There were no statistically significant differences in either primary outcome (ureteral injury) or most of the secondary outcomes. The only significant difference was a higher rate of urinary complications in the stented group. The only ureteral injury occurred in a stented group, and what is more interesting is that it was not identified intraoperatively. While having all the weaknesses of a cohort study, it does show no difference in ureteral injury whether patients receive a stent or not.

GYNECOLOGIC SURGERY

The general surgeon most commonly interacts with the gynecologic surgeon when that service causes an iatrogenic injury to a non-gynecologic structure. A recent systematic review looked at 474,063 gynecologic laparoscopies performed between 1972 and 2014 to identify the incidence of iatrogenic bowel injury (Llarena et al., 2015). The rate of bowel injury was 1 in 769 cases (0.13%) and varied by procedure: 1 in 3333 (0.03%) for sterilization and 1 in 256 for hysterectomy. The small bowel was the most frequently damaged region, with 166 of 354 (47%), followed by colon (30%), rectum (18%), and stomach (6%). These injuries mainly occurred during access and insufflation with a Veress needle or trocar (55%), followed by electrocautery (29%) and lysis of adhesions (11%). Missed injuries were primarily managed with laparotomy (80%) and have a mortality rate of 3.2%. This study's biggest weakness was the lack of a strict definition of bowel injury. Most studies did not differentiate between serosal and full thickness injury, while others did not report injuries that were diagnosed intraoperatively.

Another consideration for general surgeons is how to manage iatrogenic injury to intra-abdominal gynecologic structures caused during non-gynecologic surgery. Such injuries are infrequent, and our insight into their management relies on literature from gynecological studies and trauma. A few principles when encountering injuries to these structures should be observed. It is of course a first principle that the main priority when addressing any accidental injury is bleeding control, and this applies to injury of gynecological organs, which are highly vascular. The uterus and adnexa are not life-sustaining and can be resected if the need arises to save a patient's life. For women of childbearing age or who are premenopausal, once hemostasis is achieved one can consider preservation of organ function. For the adnexa, the consequences to consider are straightforward. Bilateral oophorectomy will lead to immediate menopause and should be avoided, and repair of a fallopian tube should be avoided as the resultant scar increases the risk of ectopic pregnancy.

Approach to the repair of uterine injury is well studied, taking into account the literature on cesarean incisions. Uterine scarring has been thought to carry the risk of uterine rupture during a future pregnancy and delivery; however, despite the theoretical risk, the actual incidence of uterine rupture appears to be low. One systematic review found that the actual incidence of uterine rupture from a cesarean scar in the setting of a trial of labor was about 0.5%, which dropped to less than 0.03% when delivery was by planned cesarean (Guise et al., 2010). Notably, for the general surgeon who may encounter uterine lacerations of variable depths, these numbers are in a population where every person suffered a large full-thickness laceration to the uterine wall. Nonetheless, it has been a consideration whether the risk of uterine rupture may be impacted by the closure technique. There has been no standard closure technique for cesarean incisions, with published practices including single- and two-layer closure and the use of a variety of closure devices. A Cochrane review of closure techniques published in 2008 and updated in 2014 concluded that the optimal technique for hemostasis was a single-layer closure but could not assess the impact on closure technique on risk of rupture (Dodd et al., 2014). In radiologic studies and in studies of gross uterine specimens, there is significant variability in thickness of the scar, but there is no good association between this outcome and the closure technique. In fact, when this is examined it appears to make no difference (Hamaret al., 2007). One may conclude from the current state of the literature that a standard single-layer closure is acceptable and non-inferior in closing uterine lacerations of any depth.

ANNOTATED REFERENCES FOR GENERAL SURGICAL ISSUES SPECIFIC TO UROLOGIC OR GYNECOLOGIC SURGERY

1. Wald HL, Ma A, Bratzler DW, Kramer AM. Indwelling urinary catheter use in the postoperative period: Analysis of the National Surgical Infection Prevention Project data. *Arch Surg.* 2008;143(6):551–557.

   This retrospective cohort study included data from 35,904 patients in 2001 who underwent non-gynecologic surgery at one of 2965 US hospitals and had a catheter placed during their admission, a subset of the National Surgical Infection Prevention Project dataset. The main outcome measure was UTI, with findings of a 1.21 hazard ratio for developing UTI if the catheter was in place longer than 48 h. The 48-h time point was significant at the time the study was published because despite there being several smaller studies suggesting that UTIs increased after 48 h it was still common practice, in the absence of evidence-based recommendations, for surgeons to leave in catheters longer than 48 h.

2. Ghuman A, de Jonge SW, Dryden SD, Feeney T, Buitrago DH, Phang PT. Prophylactic use of alpha-1 adrenergic blocking agents for prevention of postoperative urinary retention: A review and meta-analysis of randomized clinical trials. *Am J Surg.* 2018;215(5):973–979.

   This meta-analysis of randomized trials included 15 studies with a total of 1732 patients. The primary outcome was urinary retention, with an overall relative risk of 0.48 in the group that received alpha-1 adrenergic blocking agents. Notably, the definition of retention used in each study was not explicit, and the studies had overall high heterogeneity. The strongest effect in subgroup analysis was for men (no effect was found for women in subgroup analysis) and those undergoing spinal anesthesia.

3. Halabi WJ, Jafari MD, Nguyen VQ et al. Ureteral injuries in colorectal surgery: An analysis of trends, outcomes, and risk factors over a 10-year period in the United States. *Dis Colon Rectum.* 2014;57(2):179–186.

   This is a retrospective database study of ureteric injuries during colorectal procedures from 2001–2010 in the United States. They noted an increase in ureteric injuries during the latter half of the decade, but surprisingly the laparoscopic approach was protective.

4. Beraldo S, Neubeck K, Von Friderici E, Steinmüller L. The prophylactic use of a ureteral stent in laparoscopic colorectal surgery. *Scand J Surg.* 2013;102(2):87–89.

   The authors performed a retrospective review of prophylactic stent placement in their hospital. Their incidence of ureteral injury was 1.1% over a 3-year period after switching to prophylactic stenting for all laparoscopic colorectal surgeries. While the authors argue that the cost of prophylactic stenting is minimal in comparison to even one lawsuit for injured ureter, their study was not designed to compare prophylactic placement versus no ureteric stent placement.

5. Palaniappa NC, Telem DA, Ranasinghe NE, Divino CM. Incidence of iatrogenic ureteral injury after laparoscopic colectomy. *Arch Surg.* 2012;147(3):267–271.

   This was another retrospective review of database over a 5-year period. The authors noted an increase in ureteric injuries with laparoscopic colorectal surgeries. More so, they did not see any difference in the rate of intraoperative identification of injuries (50% in both prophylactic and no stenting groups).

6. Andersen P, Andersen LM, Iversen LH. Iatrogenic ureteral injury in colorectal cancer surgery: A nationwide study comparing laparoscopic and open approaches. *Surg Endosc.* 2015;29(6):1406–1412.

Authors of this study reviewed 18,474 patients in the Danish National Colorectal Cancer database. The study showed a twofold increase in ureteral injury in laparoscopic surgery for the rectal cancer group and no difference in the colon cancer group.

7. Llarena NC, Shah AB, Milad MP. Bowel injury in gynecologic laparoscopy: A systematic review. *Obstet Gynecol.* 2015;125(6):1407–1417.

This review pooled data from 90 studies representing both retrospective and prospective studies (with the vast majority being cohort studies) and 474,063 laparoscopic surgeries. Despite significant flaws stemming from the heterogeneity of the source data it represents one of the largest datasets used to answer questions about bowel injury in gynecological surgery. Notably, the vast majority, almost 55% of injuries, are made by Veress or trocar insertion.

8. Guise J-M, Denman MA, Emeis C et al. Vaginal birth after cesarean: New insights on maternal and neonatal outcomes. *Obstet Gynecol.* 2010;115(6):1267–1278.

This systematic review included qualitative descriptions of 28 studies that reported outcome on uterine rupture; however, only 8 in a total of 63,499 patients were deemed of acceptable quality to include in analysis. The difference in rupture rates between those who underwent a trial of labor (0.47%) and those who had a planned cesarean section (0.026%) are hard to interpret when considering an injury less extensive than a cesarean incision, but suggest that it is safe to quote rupture risk after iatrogenic injury as very low.

9. Dodd JM, Anderson ER, Gates S, Grivell RM. Surgical techniques for uterine incision and uterine closure at the time of caesarean section. *Cochrane Database Syst Rev.* 2014;(7):CD004732.

This Cochrane Review is notable for the sheer number and variety of techniques that have been studied in the closure of cesarean incisions, and considering that there appears to be equivalence between them it permits the general surgeon to use whatever technique is available in the circumstances to achieve hemostasis and gross closure without fear of closure-related complications.

10. Hamar BD, Saber SB, Cackovic M et al. Ultrasound evaluation of the uterine scar after cesarean delivery: A randomized controlled trial of one- and two-layer closure. *Obstet Gynecol.* 2007;110(4):808–813.

This randomized trial enrolled 30 women and randomized them to either single- or double-layer closure of the uterine incision. Their uterine thickness was measured by ultrasound preoperatively and then at 48 h, 2 weeks, and 6 weeks postoperatively. The ultrasound examiner was blinded to the closure technique. There was no difference between the two techniques in cesarean scar thickness.

Landmark Article of 21st Century

PROPHYLACTIC URETERAL STENT PLACEMENT VS. NO URETERAL STENT PLACEMENT DURING OPEN COLECTOMY

Merola J, Arnold B, Luks V, Ibarra C, Resio B, Davis KA, and Pei KY, *JAMA Surg.* 2018;153(1):87–90

ABSTRACT

The prophylactic placement of ureteral stents during colorectal surgery may facilitate ureteral identification and/or recognition of injury. However, reports have cautioned against routine use of ureteral stents owing to the potential of iatrogenic injury during insertion and postoperative complications, including stenosis and infection. At present, no evidence-based guidelines exist regarding indications for ureteral stenting during colorectal surgery. This cohort study compares the outcomes of open colectomy with ureteral stenting with the outcomes of open colectomy without ureteral stenting.

Editor Notes

Assessment: Prophylactic placement of ureteral stents is often employed during colorectal surgery purportedly to facilitate identification of the ureter to prevent injury or possibly to help recognize injury during operation. There remains considerable controversy related to the concern that the placement of ureteral stents is not without risks or cost. This was a cohort study of 374 consecutive patients who underwent open colectomy. Stent placement was associated with increased operative times and increased rates of postoperative urinary complications. Patients who received the stents also had higher rates of new-onset urinary complications (OR 4.3, $p < 0.001$).

Limitations: Although this was a retrospective review, it did support several observations. First is that ureteral injury is quite rare. In fact, there was only one ureteral injury encountered, and it was in a patient who had received a prophylactic ureteral stent. The study is obviously underpowered to answer the question of whether the use of prophylactic stent is valuable or not. Prophylactic stent placement was done in 86% of the patients, suggesting a selection bias. The rate of injury in the stent group is 1/322 and we currently do not know what the rate of injury would be if they had performed similar number of cases without the stent. None of the 54 patients experienced ureteral injuries when stents were not placed.

Conclusions: This study showed that the surgery takes longer if a prophylactic stent is placed, and may be associated with a higher rate of urinary complications. Since the rate of ureteral injury was very low, it is difficult to say if the use of the ureteral stent aids in preventing or recognizing ureteral injuries. How many ureteral injuries would have occurred if it the number of patients in the non-stented group was over 300?

CHAPTER 33

Pregnancy

Review by Contributors: Manuel Castillo-Angeles and Ali Salim

More than 8000 urgent non-obstetrical surgical procedures are performed each year, impacting up to 2% of all pregnancies. The evaluation of the pregnant patient must weigh the risks and benefits of diagnostic methodology and therapy not only on the mother, but the fetus as well. Complicating care is the fact that the normal physiologic and anatomic changes that occur in pregnancy may make it difficult to interpret signs usually used in early diagnosis of emergency conditions. The delay in diagnosis and treatment of the surgical abdomen in the pregnant patient because of fear of unnecessary procedures and tests contributes to the high complication rate in this patient population (McGory et al., 2007).

The physiologic changes that comprise maternal adaptation to pregnancy involve almost every organ system. The plasma volume in pregnancy increases by almost 50%, whereas the red cell mass increases by only 20%, resulting in the "physiologic anemia of pregnancy." Maternal hypovolemia may be marked by fetal distress before any evidence of maternal tachycardia or hypotension is present. Gastrointestinal motility is decreased, and pregnant patients have an increased risk of aspiration with general anesthesia. Hematologically, there is a relative leukocytosis (white cell count can reach as high as 25,000/mm^3) often complicating the diagnosis of infection. The state of relative hypercoagulability in pregnant patients is well known to increase the risk for thromboembolic complications. Anatomically, the uterus becomes an intra-abdominal organ at approximately 12 weeks of gestation, and it can complicate invasive procedures such as port placement in laparoscopic surgery.

Laparoscopy has emerged as a diagnostic and therapeutic tool in the care of the pregnant patient with abdominal pain. Laparoscopy is well tolerated by both mother and fetus with minimal adverse effects in all trimesters. Although a 2012 meta-analysis of 11 studies found low-grade evidence that laparoscopic compared to open appendectomy was associated with a higher rate of fetal loss (Wilasrumee et al., 2012), a more recent Nationwide Inpatient Sample study of 20,000 patients found a three times higher risk of an adverse obstetrical outcome associated with open surgery (Sachs et al., 2017). In the late second trimester and beyond, laparoscopy becomes technically difficult and an open incision (vertical or over the point of maximal tenderness) can be utilized.

Making the diagnosis is often problematic for the following reasons: the expanding uterus, which displaces other intra-abdominal organs and thus makes physical exam difficult; the high prevalence of nausea, vomiting, and abdominal pain routinely encountered in the normal obstetric patient; and the general reluctance to operate unnecessarily on a gravid patient.

Acute appendicitis is the most common non-obstetric surgical emergency during pregnancy. The diagnosis is more frequently missed in pregnant than in non-pregnant patients, because signs and symptoms of appendicitis, such as leukocytosis, nausea, and vomiting, are also commonly seen during pregnancy. Maternal morbidity is usually the result of a delay in diagnosis. Fetal loss occurs in 3%–5% of pregnant patients without perforation but can be as high as 36% with perforation. This high risk of fetal loss with perforation explains the high rate (50% in many series) of normal appendices found at operation (McGory et al., 2007). Ultrasound, helical CT, MRI, or diagnostic laparoscopy can confirm the diagnosis. Appendectomy can be performed open or laparoscopically with equal safety to mother and fetus, although the laparoscopic approach has advanced to become the standard of care at many centers (Walsh et al., 2008). Interestingly, despite the upward displacement of intra-abdominal organs as the uterus enlarges, data suggest that the McBurney incision remains adequate, since the distance from the base of the appendix to the McBurney point changes by only 1.2 cm over the course of gestation (de Moya et al., 2015).

Biliary tract disease is the second most common non-obstetric surgical problem. Weight gain and hormonal changes predispose pregnant women to biliary sludge and gallstone formation. Surgical intervention is indicated for obstructive jaundice, acute cholecystitis failing medical management, and gallstone pancreatitis. Where once the nonoperative management with delayed cholecystectomy of symptomatic cholelithiasis was encouraged, data now suggests that pregnant patients with symptomatic cholelithiasis should undergo cholecystectomy early due to the increase in the rate of recurrent hospitalizations, preterm deliveries, spontaneous abortions, and fetal morbidity associated with nonoperative management (Dhupar et al., 2010). In addition, nonoperative management of symptomatic cholelithiasis increases the risk of gallstone pancreatitis up to 15%. Whereas once it was thought that the second trimester was the optimal time for cholecystectomy due to decreased spontaneous abortions and preterm labor, there is a growing body of evidence that suggests laparoscopy can be performed in all trimesters with equal safety (Gilo et al., 2009).

Choledocholithiasis in pregnancy is infrequent and is estimated to be around 1 in 1200 deliveries; however, therapeutic intervention is almost always required. The diagnosis of choledocholithiasis is similar in both pregnant and non-pregnant patients. Endoscopic treatment of choledocholithiasis is presently the treatment of choice in pregnant patients, especially in the presence of cholangitis.

Acute pancreatitis complicates approximately 1 in 1000–5000 pregnancies, usually occurring late in the third trimester or in the early postpartum period. Cholelithiasis is the most common cause and accounts for 67%–100% of cases, followed by ethanol use and hyperlipidemia. The medical management is the same as in pancreatitis in non-pregnant women and consists of bowel rest, fluid and electrolyte resuscitation, and the use of analgesics (Hernandez et al., 2007).

Pregnant patients are a specific population, where worry about the risk of harm to the fetus often overshadows clinical decision making when presented with a possible surgical diagnosis. While it is important to limit duration of exposure to radiation and unnecessary surgery in this population, delays in diagnosis and treatment can also harm both fetus and mother. Obtaining the correct diagnosis in the pregnant patient can be challenging because of the normal physiologic and anatomic changes that occur with pregnancy. Minimally invasive surgery may be performed safely depending on the surgeon's comfort level with the duration of pregnancy. In the case of an acute abdomen, a diagnosis should be rapidly sought and treatment offered, lest we should ever penalize a patient for being pregnant.

ANNOTATED REFERENCES FOR EGS IN PREGNANCY

1. McGory ML, Zingmond DS, Tillou A, Hiatt JR, Ko CY, Cryer HM. Negative appendectomy in pregnant women is associated with a substantial risk of fetal loss. *J Am Coll Surg*. 2007;205(4):534–540.

   The authors retrospectively analyzed all female patients undergoing appendectomy. They found that the rate of negative appendectomy was considerably higher in pregnant compared with non-pregnant women (23% vs. 18%). Rates of fetal loss and early delivery were considerably higher in women with complex appendicitis in comparison with negative and simple appendicitis. Complicated and negative appendicitis were major positive predictors of fetal loss.

2. Sachs A, Guglielminotti J, Miller R, Landau R, Smiley R, Guohua L. Risk factors and risk stratification for adverse obstetrical outcomes after appendectomy or cholecystectomy during pregnancy. *JAMA Surg*. 2017:E1–E6.

   The authors performed a cohort study using the Nationwide Inpatient Sample to identify maternal risk factors for adverse outcomes after appendectomy and cholecystectomy during pregnancy. They found that approximately 5% of women experience adverse obstetrical outcomes and major risk factors for such outcomes include preterm labor, cervical incompetence, vaginitis or vulvovaginitis, and sepsis.

3. Walsh CA, Tang T, Walsh SR. Laparoscopic versus open appendicectomy in pregnancy: A systematic review. *Int J Surg*. 2008;6(4):339–344.

   The authors performed a systematic review of reported cases of laparoscopic appendicectomy (LA) in pregnancy for a total of 637 cases. They found that LA in pregnancy is associated with a low rate of intraoperative complications in all trimesters. However, LA in pregnancy is associated with a significantly higher rate of fetal loss compared to open appendicectomy. Rates of preterm delivery appear similar or slightly better following a laparoscopic approach.

4. de Moya MA, Sideris AC, Choy G et al. Appendectomy and pregnancy: Gestational age does not affect the position of the incision. *Am Surg*. 2015;81(3):282–288.

   The authors reviewed abdominal or pelvic MRIs of 114 pregnant women to investigate the location of the appendix during pregnancy. They found that the distance from the base of the appendix to McBurney's point changed over the course of the gestation by only

1.2 cm, which did not amount to a clinically or statistically significant change in position. The authors concluded that the use of a McBurney's incision was justified regardless of the trimester.

5. Dhupar R, Smaldone GM, Hamad GG. Is there a benefit to delaying cholecystectomy for symptomatic gallbladder disease during pregnancy? *Surg Endosc.* 2010;24(1):108–112.

   The authors retrospectively examined all pregnant patients with the diagnosis of symptomatic cholelithiasis, choledocholithiasis, gallstone pancreatitis, biliary dyskinesia, or chronic cholecystitis. A total of 58 patients over a 3-year period were analyzed, of which 19 had an operation. Patients who were observed had a higher rate of pregnancy-related complications of 36%. The authors concluded that delaying cholecystectomy for hospitalized pregnant patients with gallbladder disease was associated with increased short- and long-term complications.

6. Gilo NB, Amini D, Landy HJ. Appendicitis and cholecystitis in pregnancy. *Clin Obstet Gynecol.* 2009;52(4):586–596.

   The authors provide a contemporary synopsis regarding the diagnosis and management of appendicitis and cholecystitis during pregnancy. They concluded that for these common concerns for the pregnant patient, diagnosis may be confounded by physiologic and anatomic changes during pregnancy. The safety and efficacy of the laparoscopic approach during pregnancy has been well established. Pregnancy outcomes are unlikely to be affected except in instances in which maternal morbidity and diagnostic delay are significant.

7. Hernandez A, Petrov MS, Brooks DC, Banks PA, Ashley SW, Tavakkolizadeh A. Acute pancreatitis and pregnancy: A 10-year single center experience. *J Gastrointest Surg.* 2007;11(12):1623–1627.

   The authors retrospectively analyzed 21 pregnant women presenting with 34 episodes of acute pancreatitis. They concluded that if treated conservatively, pregnant patients with biliary pancreatitis appear to have a high recurrence rate. Moreover, early surgical intervention is appropriate, safe, and does not increase the length of hospital stay.

Landmark Article of 21st Century

SYSTEMATIC REVIEW AND META-ANALYSIS OF SAFETY OF LAPAROSCOPIC VERSUS OPEN APPENDICECTOMY FOR SUSPECTED APPENDICITIS IN PREGNANCY

Wilasrusmee C, Sukrat B, McEvoy M, Attia J, and Thakkinstian A, *Br J Surg.* 2012;99(11):1470–1478

ABSTRACT

Background   Laparoscopic appendicectomy has gained wide acceptance as an alternative to open appendicectomy during pregnancy. However, data regarding the safety and optimal surgical approach to appendicitis in pregnancy are still controversial.

Methods   This was a systematic review and meta-analysis of studies comparing laparoscopic and open appendicectomy in pregnancy identified using PubMed and Scopus search engines from January 1990 to July 2011. Two reviewers independently extracted data on fetal loss, preterm delivery, wound infection, duration of operation, hospital stay, Apgar score, and birth weight between laparoscopic and open appendicectomy groups.

Results Eleven studies with a total of 3415 women (599 in laparoscopic and 2816 in open group) were included in the analysis. Fetal loss was statistically significantly worse in those who underwent laparoscopy compared with open appendicectomy; the pooled relative risk (RR) was 1.91 (95% confidence interval [CI] 1.31–2.77) without heterogeneity. The pooled RR for preterm labor was 1.44 (0.68–3.06), but this risk was not statistically significant. The mean difference in length of hospital stay was −0.49 (−1.76 to −0.78) days, but this was not clinically significant. No significant difference was found for wound infection, birth weight, duration of operation, or Apgar score.

Conclusion The available low-grade evidence suggests that laparoscopic appendicectomy in pregnant women might be associated with a greater risk of fetal loss.

Editor Notes

Assessment: This report addresses management of a difficult problem, appendectomy during pregnancy. With no available prospective data, the authors' pooled information was provided in 11 studies over a 20-year time period where both open and laparoscopic appendectomies were performed in 3415 pregnant women. Fetal loss was nearly twice as likely to occur with the laparoscopic approach. There were no other outcome differences noted with the two operative interventions, specifically in wound infection or hospital length of stay.

Limitations: The data reviewed fail to account for the severity of appendicitis and its impact upon fetal loss, irrespective of operative technique. Perforated appendicitis is known to dramatically increase the likelihood of fetal loss when compared to suppurative appendicitis. The findings of this meta-analysis are surprising, as this is a compilation of exclusively retrospective studies where selection bias should have led to more complicated patients undergoing open procedures, and therefore one would have expected the open group to be associated with more preterm labor and higher fetal loss.

Conclusions: This study is very important because it supports the idea that open appendiceal surgery may be preferred over the laparoscopic approach during pregnancy in regard to fetal health.

CHAPTER 34

Cellulitis and Superficial Abscess

Review by Contributor: Addison K. May

Whether adjunctive antibiotic therapy after incision and drainage of uncomplicated, superficial cutaneous abscesses improves outcome or simply increases cost, risk of adverse event, and unnecessary antibiotic exposure has been unanswered for some time. The recent report in January 2017 of the first death in the United States from a pan-resistant pathogen secondary to a postoperative skin and soft tissue infection highlights the importance of limiting unnecessary antibiotic exposure, as antibiotic exposure is strongly associated with infection with resistant pathogens (Chen et al., 2017). A recent randomized, placebo-controlled trial provides significant evidence that, in the era of highly prevalent MRSA skin and soft tissue infections, antibiotic therapy leads to higher cure rates, lower rates of subsequent surgical drainage, and fewer new infections (Talan et al., 2016).

Skin and soft tissue infections (SSTIs) are a common cause for antibiotic administration, hospitalization, and disability in the United States (May et al., 2009). The frequency of soft tissue infections has increased significantly in the last two and a half decades, with the annual number of emergency department visits expanding from 1.2 million to 3.4 million between 1993 and 2005 (Pallin et al., 2008). Most SSTIs are mild to moderate in severity and classified as uncomplicated cellulitis or superficial abscesses. Most do not require the involvement of a surgeon. Uncomplicated cellulitis can be treated with antibiotics alone. The majority of cases of uncomplicated cellulitis are caused Gram-positive organisms, mostly by streptococci, and respond to Gram-positive antibiotic therapy. However, bacteria are infrequently isolated in uncomplicated cellulitis, limiting access to data to assess the actual proportion. Determining whether cellulitis is, in fact, an uncomplicated superficial infection versus a manifestation of a deeper, more severe infection can be difficult and may require consultation of an acute care surgeon. This difficulty is highlighted by the fact that most patients who present with a necrotizing soft tissue infection have an original admitting diagnosis of cellulitis (May et al., 2009).

The increase in SSTIs presenting to emergency departments that has occurred over the past two and a half decades is primarily related to an increase in skin abscesses and is associated with a shift in SSTI epidemiology (Qualls et al., 2012). Over the same period, a dramatic rise in community-associated methicillin resistant *S. aureus* (CA-MRSA) infections in the United States and worldwide has resulted in this organism becoming the most common cause of SSTI (Moran et al., 2006). Due to the pathogenicity of CA-MRSA in SSTIs, this shift in the epidemiology has potential implications for the therapeutic approach to simple abscesses. CA-MRSA strains associated with SSTIs most commonly carry genes for several toxins, including the Panton-Valentin leucocidin (PVL) toxin, that increase the virulence of this organism within skin and skin structures (Deresinski et al., 2005). Undertreated CA-MRSA abscesses can produce severe, complicated abscesses, necrotizing SSTIs, and sepsis. Thus, while the need for antibiotic therapy following adequate drainage of a cutaneous abscess has been inadequately studied in the past, the epidemiologic shift to CA-MRSA likely alters the calculous for the benefit antibiotic therapy. Talan's study of antibiotic therapy versus placebo as adjunctive therapy following abscess drainage is the first of two adequately powered studies to demonstrate the benefit of antibiotic therapy, particularly in the era of CA-MRSA SSTIs (Talan et al., 2016).

Published at the end of 2016, the Talan paper presents the results of a multicenter, double-blind, randomized trial of trimethoprim-sulfamethoxazole (TMP-SMX) for 7 days versus placebo in over 1200 patients. Abscesses had to be present for less than 1 week, be greater than 2 centimeters in diameter, and be appropriate for outpatient treatment. Treatment with antibiotics resulted in an increased rate of clinical cures and lower rates of subsequent surgical drainage procedures, infections at new sites, and infections in other household members 7–14 days after the treatment period. MRSA was isolated in 45% of the patients, a rate that likely reflects the general frequency seen in emergency departments within the United States. Adverse events were similar except for a slight increase in mild gastrointestinal side effects in the TMP-SMX group. A second, adequately powered, though smaller study that compared antibiotics versus placebo in skin abscesses has been subsequently published with similar findings (Daum et al., 2017). Differing from the Talan study, this trial allowed treatment with either TMP-SMX or clindamycin in the treatment group. S. aureus was isolated in 67% of enrolled patients and MRSA in 49%. Of note in this study, the benefit of adjuvant antibiotics appeared to be limited to those infections where S. aureus was present. The use of TMP-SMX and clindamycin appears to be equally efficacious as adjuvant therapy following drainage of abscesses, with similar outcomes between the two agents in one randomized, controlled trial (Miller et al., 2015).

A subtle but important detail of the Talan study is that all trial personnel underwent standardized training on the appropriate technique for incision and drainage of cutaneous abscesses. Inadequate drainage, with or without antibiotic therapy, is a significant risk factor for progression of S. aureus cutaneous abscess progression to more severe disease, including necrotizing infections. Extension of incision to the margin of induration with adequate exploration of the abscess cavity is required to ensure proper drainage. There is limited efficacy of antibiotic therapy in the face of inadequate drainage.

In an era when antibiotic resistance threatens to limit our therapeutic options, all antibiotic indications should be scrutinized. Therapy should only be provided in settings with proven efficacy. Talan's study provides class I data for the use of adjuvant antibiotics when S. aureus or MRSA is a likely pathogen in cutaneous abscesses.

ANNOTATED REFERENCES FOR CELLULITIS AND SUPERFICIAL ABSCESS

1. Chen L, Todd R, Kiehlbauch J, Walters M, Kallen A. Notes from the field: Pan-resistant New Delhi metallo-beta-lactamase-producing *Klebsiella pneumoniae*—Washoe County, Nevada, 2016. *MMWR Morb Mortal Wkly Rep.* 2017;66(1):33.

   Brief clinical report of the first case in the United States of a fatality from a pan-resistant organism. The patient died of a postoperative skin and soft tissue infection from sepsis due to carbapenemase-resistant K. pneumonia *resistant to all 26 antibiotics available to treat Gram-negative bacteria.*

2. May AK, Stafford RE, Bulger EM et al. Treatment of complicated skin and soft tissue infections. *Surg Infect (Larchmt).* 2009;10(5):467–499.

   Extensive evidence-based management guideline for the treatment of complicated skin and soft tissue infections. Discusses the diagnosis and treatment of complicated cellulitis, abscesses, and necrotizing soft tissue infections.

3. Pallin DJ, Egan DJ, Pelletier AJ, Espinola JA, Hooper DC, Camargo CA Jr. Increased US emergency department visits for skin and soft tissue infections, and changes in antibiotic choices, during the emergence of community-associated methicillin-resistant *Staphylococcus aureus. Ann Emerg Med.* 2008;51(3):291–298.

   Epidemiologic study of the rates of skin and soft tissue infections treated in US emergency departments. Demonstrates the correlation of increased CA-MRSA with SSTIs.

4. Qualls ML, Mooney MM, Camargo CA Jr, Zucconi T, Hopper DC, Pallin DJ. Emergency department visit rates for abscess versus other skin infections during the emergence of community-associated methicillin-resistant *Staphylococcus aureus*, 1997-2007. *Clin Infect Dis.* 2012;55(1):103–105.

   Epidemiologic study that demonstrates that the increase in SSTIs treated in emergency rooms is primarily associated with an increase in CA-MRSA abscesses.

5. Moran GJ, Krishnadasan A, Gorwitz RJ et al. Methicillin-resistant *S. aureus* infections among patients in the emergency department. *N Engl J Med.* 2006;355(7):666–674.

   One of the first and most extensive epidemiologic studies that highlighted the dramatic increase in MRSA SSTIs treated in the US emergency departments.

6. Deresinski S. Methicillin-resistant *Staphylococcus aureus*: An evolutionary, epidemiologic, and therapeutic odyssey. *Clin Infect Dis.* 2005;40(4):562–573.

   Extensive review of the epidemiologic shift, pathogenicity, and therapeutic implications of CA-MRSA.

7. Daum RS, Miller RG, Immergluck L et al. A placebo-controlled trial of antibiotics for smaller skin abscesses. *N Engl J Med.* 2017;376(26):2545–2555.

   A randomized, double-blinded, placebo-controlled trial of antibiotic therapy in cutaneous abscesses. Smaller than the Talan study and provided an option of clindamycin or trimethoprim-sulfamethoxazole for treatment. Findings support the original findings of the Talan study.

8. Miller LG, Daum RS, Creech CB et al. Clindamycin versus trimethoprim-sulfamethoxazole for uncomplicated skin infections. *N Engl J Med.* 2015;372(12):1093–1103.

   A randomized, double-blinded, placebo-controlled trial comparing clindamycin with trimethoprim-sulfamethoxazole for the treatment of SSTIs. The study demonstrated equivalence of outcome for the two agents.

Landmark Article of 21st Century

TRIMETHOPRIM-SULFAMETHOXAZOLE VERSUS PLACEBO FOR UNCOMPLICATED SKIN ABSCESS

Talan DA, Mower WR, Krishnadasan A, Abrahamian FM, Lovecchio F, Karras DJ, Steele MT, Rothman RE, Hoagland R, and Moran GJ, *N Engl J Med.* 2016;374(9):823–832

ABSTRACT

Background   US emergency department visits for cutaneous abscess have increased with the emergence of methicillin-resistant *Staphylococcus aureus* (MRSA). The role of antibiotics for patients with a drained abscess is unclear.

Methods   We conducted a randomized trial at five US emergency departments to determine whether trimethoprim-sulfamethoxazole (at doses of 320 mg and 1600 mg, respectively, twice daily, for 7 days) would be superior to placebo in outpatients older than 12 years of age who had an uncomplicated abscess that was being treated with drainage. The primary outcome was clinical cure of the abscess, assessed 7–14 days after the end of the treatment period.

Results   The median age of the participants was 35 years (range, 14–73); 45.3% of the participants had wound cultures that were positive for MRSA. In the modified intention-to-treat population, clinical cure of the abscess occurred in 507 of 630 participants (80.5%) in the trimethoprim–sulfamethoxazole group versus 454 of 617 participants (73.6%) in the placebo group (difference, 6.9 percentage points; 95% confidence interval [CI], 2.1 to 11.7; $P = 0.005$). In the per-protocol population, clinical cure occurred in 487 of 524 participants (92.9%) in the trimethoprim-sulfamethoxazole group versus 457 of 533 participants (85.7%) in the placebo group (difference, 7.2 percentage points; 95% CI, 3.2–11.2; $P < 0.001$). Trimethoprim-sulfamethoxazole was superior to placebo with respect to most secondary outcomes in the per-protocol population, resulting in lower rates of subsequent surgical drainage procedures (3.4% vs. 8.6%; difference, −5.2 percentage points; 95% CI, −8.2 to −2.2), skin infections at new sites (3.1% vs. 10.3%; difference, −7.2 percentage points; 95% CI, −10.4 to −4.1), and infections in household members (1.7% vs. 4.1%; difference, −2.4 percentage points; 95% CI, −4.6 to −0.2) 7 to 14 days after the treatment period. Trimethoprim-sulfamethoxazole was associated with slightly more gastrointestinal side effects (mostly mild) than placebo. At 7–14 days after the treatment period, invasive infections had developed in 2 of 524 participants (0.4%) in the trimethoprim-sulfamethoxazole group and in 2 of 533 participants (0.4%) in the placebo group; at 42–56 days after the treatment period, an invasive infection had developed in one participant (0.2%) in the trimethoprim-sulfamethoxazole group.

Conclusions In settings in which MRSA was prevalent, trimethoprim-sulfamethoxazole treatment resulted in a higher cure rate among patients with a drained cutaneous abscess than placebo. (Funded by the National Institute of Allergy and Infectious Diseases; ClinicalTrials.gov Number, NCT00729937.)

Original Author Commentary: David A. Talan

Primary treatment of a skin abscess is drainage. Past studies of adjunctive antibiotics conducted before and after the emergence of community-associated methicillin-resistant *Staphylococcus aureus* (MRSA) in the United States and other regions were small and did not demonstrate benefit. In 2016, we reported a US randomized placebo-controlled trial (RCT) among 1265 mostly adults with a drained skin abscess ≥ 2 cm that demonstrated antibiotic treatment possessing in vitro activity against MRSA, TMP-SMX was associated with a significantly higher cure rate and fewer additional surgeries and new-site skin infections. Overall adverse event rates were similar, with only slightly more mostly mild gastrointestinal side effects in the TMP-SMX group, but no serious reactions. Subsequently, these findings were validated by another US RCT by Daum et al. (2017) in which 786 patients over 6 months of age with a small abscess receiving drainage were assigned to clindamycin, TMP-SMX, or placebo. In neither trial were there complications of *Clostridium difficile* reported. We later conducted a subgroup analysis and found that the TMP-SMX treatment effect existed regardless of abscess size or presence or absence of diabetes, other comorbidities, past MRSA infection, or fever. Both investigations found the antibiotic benefit only among patients with an abscess from which *S. aureus* was isolated, suggesting that antibiotics would also be effective in other parts of the world where MRSA predominates. Since drainage alone has a high cure rate, the benefits, costs, and risks associated with antibiotic treatment can be discussed as part of shared patient decision making.

CHAPTER 35

Necrotizing Soft Tissue Infection (NSTI)

Review by Contributor: Rondi B. Gelbard

Necrotizing soft tissue infections (NSTIs) encompass a wide a range of soft tissue infections that can arise in skin, adipose tissue, fascia, or muscle involving any part of the body. NSTIs can manifest as mild pyoderma, necrotizing cellulitis, myositis, or severe, rapidly progressing necrotizing fasciitis. Infection typically spreads along the tissue planes causing microvascular thrombosis and ischemia, followed by further microbial invasion and tissue necrosis. This in turn promotes further bacterial growth and dissemination of infection. The diagnosis of NSTI can be difficult, as cutaneous manifestations vary widely and may not be present at all. Once the infection has progressed, pain and signs of systemic toxicity may be out of proportion to physical findings. Unfortunately, NSTI is typically rapidly progressive, causing significant morbidity and mortality (20%–30% in recent literature) and by the time NSTI is suspected, extensive local tissue destruction has already occurred.

Descriptions of NSTI date back to the fifth century BC when Hippocrates first described complications of Streptococcal infection. In 1871, the Confederate Army surgeon Joseph Jones reported on "hospital gangrene" among 2642 patients, and in 1883, Fournier referred to an abrupt, rapidly progressive necrotizing infection of the genitalia affecting previously healthy young men. However, it was not until 1951 that Wilson used the term "necrotizing fasciitis" to describe the characteristic findings of fascial and subcutaneous tissue necrosis with sparing of the underlying muscle.

The incidence of NSTI varies widely depending on the season, patient population, and geographic location, but is estimated to be around 0.4 per 100,000 for group A streptococcal infections in the United States alone. The true incidence of all-cause NSTI is unknown due to inconsistency in the reporting and classification schemes for this disease. NSTIs are usually classified based on the infecting organism, with polymicrobial infections (Type 1) being most common (~80%). Polymicrobial infections typically involve a combination of aerobic and anaerobic organisms such as *Staphylococcal* and *Streptococcal* species, *Escherichia coli*, *Bacteroides fragilis*, or *Clostridium* species. Monomicrobial infections (Type II) account for approximately 10% of NSTI and usually involve Group A β-hemolytic streptococci or *Staphylococcus aureus*. Type III NSTIs are associated with *Vibrio vulnificans* (from exposure to contaminated seawater or consumption of raw seafood) while Type IV NSTIs are seen with fungal infections (*Candida* spp.) in the setting of trauma or an immunocompromised state.

Early diagnosis and treatment is essential to the management of NSTI but can be challenging due to a paucity of clinical exam findings. While bullae, ecchymosis, erythema, and crepitus are helpful for diagnosis, they are often late findings and are only present in a small number of patients. Laboratory values and imaging may be useful adjuncts in equivocal cases, but they have low positive predictive value and may delay definitive management. Various scoring systems have also been developed to facilitate diagnosis. The Laboratory Risk Indicator for Necrotizing Fasciitis (LRINEC) score, developed by Wong et al. in 2004, has been used to distinguish NSTI from other soft tissue infections, with a score ≥6 having a 92% positive predictive value for NSTI (Wong et al., 2004). However, more recent studies of the LRINEC score failed to demonstrate its utility for changing outcomes, and it should not be used in isolation to guide treatment decisions. Similarly, the Fournier's Gangrene Risk index has not been found to be superior to the Charlson Comorbidity Index for predicting outcomes in NSTI.

Early, radical surgical debridement of all infected and necrotic tissue is fundamental to the treatment of NSTI and is associated with improved survival compared to delayed intervention (Kobayashi et al., 2011; Gelbard et al., 2018). Margins of debridement should extend to healthy bleeding tissue and may require extensive resection of adjacent organs, or amputation when extremities are involved. Repeated debridement may be required, and surgical re-exploration should be carried out within 24 hours. Some suggest a skin-sparing approach to facilitate future wound coverage, minimize restricted movement from scarring, and improve quality of life. At Harborview Medical Center, various incision patterns are used to preserve critical perforators that perfuse spared skin. With these techniques, they have achieved a delayed primary wound closure rate as high as 87%. Broad-spectrum empiric antibiotics may vary by institution (and local incidence of methicillin-resistant *Staphylococcus aureus* [MRSA] infection), but should include adequate Gram-negative, Gram-positive, and anaerobic coverage. Antibiotics should be narrowed based on cultures and continued until adequate source control is achieved.

In terms of adjunctive therapies, the role of intravenous immunoglobulin (IVIG) for neutralizing Streptococcal and Clostridial exotoxins remains unclear. Several small observational studies found improved survival with IVIG, but randomized controlled trials are lacking. The use of hyperbaric oxygen therapy (HBOT) for the management of NSTI is also somewhat controversial. HBOT is thought to promote wound healing by increasing oxygen delivery and the generation of reactive oxygen species that have antimicrobial effects. While some larger studies have found the use of HBOT to be associated with a lower mortality, it is costly, can increase hospital lengths of stay, and not all NSTI patients are stable enough for transport to a hyperbaric chamber. Again, the quality of the evidence is limited by the small number of trials, small sample sizes, and the risks of bias in existing studies (Jallali et al., 2005).

Newer pharmacologic therapies for NSTI are now being developed. Reltecimod (AB103) was recently found to be a safe, new agent for modulation of inflammation in NSTI. In the first randomized placebo-controlled trial of AB103, Bulger et al. found improvements in the SOFA scores at 14 days among patients receiving the study drug (Bulger et al., 2014). Her group subsequently found that organ dysfunction on admission was associated with worse outcomes, and they developed and validated a necrotizing infection clinical composite endpoint (NICCE) for patients with NSTI that incorporated local tissue injury, systemic organ dysfunction, and mortality. A Phase III study of AB103 utilizing this composite endpoint is currently underway.

The management of NSTI is extremely complex and does not end with the final operative debridement. NSTI patients should be treated at tertiary care centers that are equipped to perform the necessary debridements as well as provide long-term multidisciplinary care. These patients may be best served on burn, emergency general surgery (EGS), or trauma services capable of performing radical debridement, optimal wound care, and definitive closure of these wounds, which can sometimes require more complex reconstruction (Gunter et al., 2008).

ANNOTATED REFERENCES FOR NECROTIZING SOFT TISSUE INFECTION (NSTI)

1. Wong C, Khin L, Heng K, Tan K, Low C. The LRINEC (Laboratory Risk Indicator for Necrotizing Fasciitis) score: A tool for distinguishing necrotizing fasciitis from other soft-tissue infections. *Crit Care Med.* 2004;32(7):1535–1541.

   This well-cited study discusses one of the most widely used scoring systems to assist with early diagnosis of NSTI. This validated scoring system is based on laboratory values found to be independent predictors of disease but should not be used in isolation to guide management.

2. Kobayashi L, Konstantinidis A, Shackelford S et al. Necrotizing soft tissue infections: Delayed surgical treatment is associated with increased number of surgical debridements and morbidity. *J Trauma.* 2011;71(5):1400–1405.

   This retrospective review of 47 patients with NSTI found that a delay in surgical intervention >12 hours contributes to higher mortality, septic shock, and renal failure, and is associated with an increased number of debridements than patients whose initial debridement is <12 hours after admission. This confirms that early initial debridement leads to improved outcomes in NSTI.

3. Gelbard RB, Ferrada P, Yeh DD et al. Optimal timing of initial debridement for necrotizing soft tissue infection: A practice management guideline from the eastern association for the surgery of trauma. *J Trauma Acute Care Surg.* 2018;85(1):208–214.

   This practice management guideline using GRADE methodology provides evidence-based recommendations for the optimal timing of surgical management of NSTI. Despite the low quality of evidence, the authors recommend early operative debridement within 12 hours of suspected diagnosis to decrease mortality. Institutional and regional systems should be optimized to facilitate prompt surgical evaluation and debridement.

4. Jallali N, Withey S, Butler PE. Hyperbaric oxygen as adjuvant therapy in the management of necrotizing fasciitis. *Am J Surg.* 2005;189(4):462–466.

   This literature review does not find consistent evidence to support the routine use of HBO as an adjunctive therapy in the management of NSTI. These findings have since been corroborated in a recent Cochrane review that failed to locate relevant clinical evidence to support or refute the effectiveness of HBOT in the management of necrotizing fasciitis.

5. Bulger EM, Maier RV, Sperry J et al. A novel drug for treatment of necrotizing soft-tissue infections: A randomized clinical trial. *JAMA Surg.* 2014;149(6):528–536.

   This is the first interventional trial using an immunomodulatory agent to treat necrotizing soft tissue infections. In this multicenter study, 40 adult patients with NSTI were randomized to receive AB103 within 6 hours of diagnosis. AB103-treated patients had an improvement in SOFA score from baseline, although it did not appear to decrease the overall number of debridements.

6. Gunter OL, Guillamondegui OD, May AK, Diaz JJ. Outcome of necrotizing skin and soft tissue infections. *Surg Infect (Larchmt).* 2008;9(4):443–450.

   This study identifies risk factors for mortality, including APACHE II score and lactate levels. It also focuses on the benefit of primary management by an EGS service to facilitate prompt surgical intervention.

Landmark Article of 21st Century

IMPACT AND PROGRESSION OF ORGAN DYSFUNCTION IN PATIENTS WITH NECROTIZING SOFT TISSUE INFECTIONS: A MULTICENTER STUDY

Bulger EM, May A, Bernard A, Cohn S, Evans DC, Henry S, Quick J, Kobayashi L, Foster K, Duane TM, Sawyer RG, Kellum JA, Maung A, Maislin G, Smith DD, Segalovich I, Dankner W, and Shirvan A, *Surg Infect (Larchmt).* 2015;16(6):694–701

ABSTRACT

Background   Necrotizing soft tissue infections (NSTIs) represent a rare but devastating disease for which the systemic manifestations have been poorly characterized. In an effort to define an optimal endpoint for clinical trials in this condition, the objective of this study was to establish the pattern of organ dysfunction over time and determine the correlation between organ dysfunction and clinical outcome in patients with NSTI.

Methods   We conducted a multicenter, retrospective clinical study of patients with NSTI presenting to 12 academic medical centers in the United States during 2013. Patients with a diagnosis of NSTI confirmed by surgical findings were included. Organ dysfunction was assessed using a modified Sequential Organ Failure Assessment (mSOFA) score (excluding liver) on admission and on hospital days 1, 2, 3, 7, 10, and 14. The presence of organ dysfunction on admission and resolution of organ dysfunction were correlated with clinical parameters, including intensive care unit (ICU)-free days (of 28 d), ventilator-free days, number of debridements, and mortality rate. The incidence of acute kidney injury (AKI) and recovery also were assessed.

Results   There were 198 patients enrolled, of whom 62% were male, the mean age was 51 years, and 40% had monomicrobial infections. The mean mSOFA score on admission was 2.4 ± 3.0, with 49% of the patients having a score ≥ 2 and 35% a score of ≥ 3. Patients typically demonstrated worsening of the mSOFA score over the first 24 h followed by gradual resolution. An mSOFA $\geq$3 at admission was associated with a significant decrease in ventilator-free days (mean 20.1 vs. 25.6 days; $p < 0.001$); ICU-free days (15.2 vs. 23.1, $p < 0.001$); more debridements (mean 2.3 vs. 2.0; $p = 0.11$); a higher mortality rate (15.9% vs. 3.1%; $p = 0.003$); and a higher rate of AKI (59.4 vs. 35.9%; $p < 0.001$). The persistence of organ dysfunction (mSOFA >1) among survivors at day 14 was associated with fewer ICU-free days (17.8 vs. 23.6; $p < 0.001$) and ventilator-free days (23.6 vs. 27; $p = 0.001$) and a lower recovery rate from AKI (38.7% vs. 81.3%; $p < 0.001$).

Conclusion   Early development of systemic organ dysfunction in patients with NSTI is associated with higher morbidity and mortality rates. Failure of the resolution of organ dysfunction by day 14 forecasts a poor outcome. The mSOFA score may be a useful marker for patient selection for inclusion in interventional trials, and the resolution of organ dysfunction by day 14 may be an important clinical endpoint.

Original Author Commentary: Eileen M. Bulger

This paper was inspired by a patient I cared for as a surgery resident who died as a result of his rib fractures. The patient was an elderly gentleman who was living independently, and fell from a ladder at his home. He suffered four rib fractures on the right side with a pneumothorax which required a chest tube. He had no major medical comorbidities and was admitted to a thoracic surgeon in a non-trauma center. He was treated with IV narcotics for management of his pain. Over the next few days he became increasingly delirious and subsequently had an aspiration event requiring intubation and transfer to the ICU. He then developed a nosocomial pneumonia which progressed to septic shock resulting in his death. I was struck by the fact that this isolated injury had led to such a devastating outcome.

In this study, we sought to define the problem by exploring the impact of age on outcome after rib fractures, defining the relationship between number of rib fractures and outcome, and evaluating the influence of analgesic technique on outcome. This was a retrospective chart review over 10 years from Harborview Medical Center (Seattle, Washington). The results demonstrated significantly worse outcome for patients over age 65 and raised awareness that even a limited number of rib fractures was associated with an increased risk of pneumonia in this patient population. The limitations of retrospective data did not allow us to draw conclusions about the influence of analgesia approach and we suggested in the discussion that further prospective analysis was needed. This led us to conduct a subsequent randomized controlled trial of epidural analgesia versus intravenous narcotics, which demonstrated that the epidural approach was associated with a twofold reduction in the risk of pneumonia and two fewer days on the ventilator for ventilated patients (Bulger et al., 2004). We also explored the contraindications to epidural use in trauma patients (Bulger et al., 2008).

Over the last 17 years, our group has continued to explore the process of care to improve outcomes for all patients admitted with rib fractures and recently published a review of our comprehensive inpatient rib fracture protocol, which was developed as a quality improvement project at Harborview (Witt and Bulger, 2017). As the geriatric population in the United States continues to increase, our trauma centers are faced with the challenges of a growing number of elderly patients admitted with what may seem like minor injuries, but very poor outcome. It is our hope that this work will lead to increased awareness of the importance of a standardized, multidisciplinary approach to these patients to optimize outcomes.

References

Bulger EM, Edwards WT, de Pinto M, Klotz P, Jurkovich GJ. Indications and contraindications for thoracic epidural analgesia in multiply injured patients. *Acute Pain.* 2008;10(1):15–22.

Bulger EM, Edwards T, Klotz P, Jurkovich GJ. Epidural analgesia improves outcome after multiple rib fractures. *Surgery.* 2004;136(2):426–430.

Witt CE, Bulger EM. Comprehensive approach to the management of the patient with multiple rib fractures: A review and introduction of a bundled rib fracture management protocol. *Trauma Surg Acute Care Open.* 2017;2(1):e000064.

CHAPTER 36

Diabetic Foot Infection

Review by Contributors: Jaime Benarroch-Gampel and James Middleton Chang

Diabetic foot ulcers and associated infections are a major burden for diabetic patients. In the United States, the annual incidence of diabetic foot ulcers has been reported to be as high as 6% (Margolis et al., 2011). An estimated 19%–34% of diabetic patients will develop a foot ulcer during their lifetime; half of these ulcers become infected, with up to 20% of patients undergoing an amputation. The 5-year mortality is 2.5 times higher in diabetics with foot ulcers (Prompers et al., 2007; Armstrong et al., 2017). After an amputation, the 5-year mortality rate has been reported to be as high as 70% for all diabetics, and in diabetics on renal replacement therapy, 2-year mortality may be up to 74% (Armstrong et al., 2017). Diabetic foot ulcers and associated infections generate more emergency department visits and hospital admissions than heart failure or kidney disease (Armstrong et al., 2017).

Risk factors associated with development of foot infections include ulcers associated with trauma, exposed bone, ulcer duration longer than 30 days, recurrent ulcers, prior amputation, neuropathy, and presence of concomitant peripheral arterial disease (PAD) (Hobizal and Wukich, 2012). The diagnosis of a diabetic foot infection is based on clinical signs and symptoms ranging from local (foul-smelling purulent discharge, pain, swelling, and erythema) to systemic sepsis and even ultimately to shock. A detailed vascular examination is critical to determine the presence and severity of PAD, as this increases the risk of non-healing ulcers, recurrence, and amputations (Armstrong et al., 2017).

Plain radiographs are commonly used in the initial evaluation of patients with diabetic foot infections for the presence of subcutaneous emphysema or foreign bodies which may necessitate urgent or more rapid intervention. The presence of signs of osteomyelitis may also influence planning for surgical debridement. If plain radiographs are inconclusive, magnetic resonance imaging (MRI) is considered the most sensitive (90%) and specific (79%) test to diagnose osteomyelitis or the presence of a deep tissue abscess (Hingorani et al., 2016). In patients who do not require an emergency intervention, vascular evaluation is mandatory. The American Diabetes Association recommends vascular assessment consisting of ankle-brachial index (ABI), toe Dopplers and pressures, or transcutaneous percutaneous oximetry (TcPO2) in all patients with diabetic foot ulcers (American Diabetes Association, 2003). Although all these tests can predict wound healing and amputation risk with varying predictive value, TcPO2 has been shown to have the most predictive value (Mills et al., 2014). Diminishing degrees of perfusion increase amputation risk, especially when the ABI is less than 0.4 and toe systolic pressures are less than 30 mmHg (Mills et al., 2014). ABI measurements may be falsely elevated in diabetics due to medial calcinosis, and in these cases toe Dopplers and pressures are particularly helpful. Other available vascular studies, including pulse volume recordings, skin perfusion pressures, and quantitative indocyanine green angiography, can be used but have not been as extensively evaluated (Wang et al., 2016).

The traditional Rutherford and Fontaine classifications describe acutely threatened limbs; however, these classification systems do not account for the impact of diabetes and the major factors being evaluated to determine outcomes is the presence and severity of ischemia (Mills et al., 2014). Other important information such as the presence of active infection (common in diabetics) or the depth of tissue loss is not taken into consideration. In 2014, the Society for Vascular Surgery created a new classification for the threatened lower extremity known as the "WIfI" classification (Wound, Ischemia, and foot Infection), which reflects the impact of diabetes on limb complications (Mills et al., 2014). In the WIfI classification, the presence of a foot infection conferred at least a moderate risk of amputation independently of the other factors, highlighting the impact of diabetic foot ulcers and associated infections in limb outcomes.

Patients with clinical signs of infection should be started on empiric antibiotic therapy. Based on current guidelines from the Infectious Diseases Society of America (IDSA) (Lipsky et al., 2012), patients with mild to moderate infections should be treated empirically, targeting Gram-positive cocci. Broader-antibiotic coverage (including Gram-negative bacilli) should be reserved for severe infections. To guide antibiotic therapy, a bone sample should be obtained in open wounds during the initial intervention. In patients with systemic signs of sepsis as well as those with abscesses or necrotizing or gas-forming infections, emergent surgical intervention in the form of extensive debridement of devitalized tissue, drainage of an abscess, or amputation is mandatory and should be expedited. Patients with mild to moderate infections are treated in a less urgent manner. In these cases, early involvement of vascular surgery to evaluate the need for revascularization prior to or in addition to debridement is of utmost importance. Sharp debridement is aimed at the removal of debris, eschar, and callus. A number of patients may require minor amputations (usually toes) to obtain full control of infected or devitalized tissue. During the postoperative management, redistribution of pressure and the selection of dressings that allow for moist wound healing and control of excess exudates is indicated (Lipsky et al., 2012; Mills et al., 2014). Ulcer recurrence is common, estimated to be up to 65% at 5 years (Armstrong et al., 2017).

The impact of diabetic foot ulcers and associated infections continues to rise as the prevalence of diabetes increases. Management of the diabetic foot should consist of multidisciplinary teams aimed at prevention of the development of foot ulcers, early recognition including the presence of associated infections, and early management with the involvement of vascular surgery in patients with signs of PAD, to maximize the chances of limb salvage.

ANNOTATED REFERENCES FOR DIABETIC FOOT INFECTION

1. Margolis DJ, Malay DS, Hoffstad OJ et al. Incidence of diabetic foot ulcer and lower extremity amputation among Medicare beneficiaries, 2006 to 2008: Data Points #2. *Data Points Publication Series*. Rockville (MD): 2011.

   A report of the incidence and outcomes of Medicare beneficiaries from 2006–2008. The incidence of diabetic foot ulcer is about 6%, lower extremity amputation about 0.5%. Microvascular and macrovascular complications occurred in 46% and 65%, respectively. The annual mortality rate is about 11% overall, up to 22% who have a lower extremity amputation.

2. Armstrong DG, Boulton AJM, Bus SA. Diabetic foot ulcers and their recurrence. *N Engl J Med*. 2017;376(24):2367–2375.

   A study of diabetics in the northwestern United Kingdom; the prevalence of active foot ulcers identified in screening diabetics was 1.7% and the annual incidence was 2.2%. Higher incidence rates have been reported in Medicare beneficiaries (6%), US veterans with diabetes (5%), and globally (6.3%). The lifetime incidence of diabetic foot ulcers is likely between 19%–34%.

3. Prompers L, Huijberts M, Apelqvist J et al. High prevalence of ischaemia, infection and serious comorbidity in patients with diabetic foot disease in Europe. Baseline results from the Eurodiale study. *Diabetologia*. 2007;50(1):18–25.

   Trial conducted of 1229 diabetic patients from 14 European hospitals in 10 countries with a new foot ulcer. PAD was diagnosed in 49% of patients. Twenty-four percent of patients had no infection or PAD, 27% had infection without PAD, 18% had PAD without infection, 31% had both PAD and infection. Serious comorbidity increased with severity of foot disease.

4. Hobizal KB, Wukich DK. Diabetic foot infections: Current concept review. *Diabet Foot Ankle*. 2012;3.

   Current concept review on the diagnosis and management of diabetic foot infections, including a literature review on the pathophysiology, risk factors, and evaluation. Most infections begin with a wound, with subsequent onset of infection. Infection increases the risk of hospitalization and amputation.

5. Hingorani A, LaMuraglia GM, Henke P et al. The management of diabetic foot: A clinical practice guideline by the Society for Vascular Surgery in collaboration with the American Podiatric Medical Association and the Society for Vascular Medicine. *J Vasc Surg*. 2016;63(2 Suppl):3S–21S.

   The Society for Vascular Surgery, in collaboration with the American Podiatric Medical Association and the Society for Vascular Medicine, developed practice guidelines for the management of the diabetic foot. Recommendations include using custom therapeutic footwear in high-risk diabetic patients. In patients with a diabetic ulcer MRI is recommended when concerned about soft tissue infection. Foot wounds should be given 4 weeks of standard wound therapy, with adjunctive options being pursued afterward. In the presence of PAD and diabetic foot ulcer, revascularization is recommended.

6. American Diabetes Association. Peripheral arterial disease in people with diabetes. *Diabetes Care*. 2003;26(12):3333–3341.

   Consensus statement from the American Diabetes Association regarding peripheral arterial disease in people with diabetes.

7. Mills JL Sr, Conte MS, Armstrong DG et al.; Society for Vascular Surgery Lower Extremity Guidelines Committee. The Society for Vascular Surgery Lower Extremity Threatened Limb Classification System: Risk stratification based on wound, ischemia, and foot infection (WIfI). *J Vasc Surg.* 2014;59(1):220–234 e221–e222.

The WIfI classification system, as described by the Society for Vascular Surgery, classifies threatened lower extremities that reflect important risk factors influencing amputation risk and clinical management. This system takes into account more than just ischemia, such as in the Rutherford classification or fontaine classification. Limb threat from foot ulcers is of particular danger to patients with diabetes.

8. Wang Z, Hasan R, Firwana B et al. A systematic review and meta-analysis of tests to predict wound healing in diabetic foot. *J Vasc Surg.* 2016;63(2 Suppl):29S–36S e21–e22.

A meta-analysis to review eight tests to predict wound healing: ankle-brachial index (OR 2.89 for amputation), ankle peak systolic velocity, transcutaneous oxygen measurement (OR 15.81 for wound healing, OR 4.14 for amputation), toe-brachial index, toe systolic blood pressure, microvascular oxygen saturation, microvascular oxygen saturation, skin perfusion pressure, and hyperspectral imaging. Transcutaneous oxygen measurement and ankle-brachial index were the only tests with enough available evidence to perform meta-analysis.

9. Lipsky BA, Berendt AR, Cornia PB et al. 2012 Infectious Diseases Society of America clinical practice guideline for the diagnosis and treatment of diabetic foot infections. *Clin Infect Dis.* 2012;54(12):e132–e173.

The presence of infection is confirmed by the presence of >2 classic findings of inflammation or purulence. Most infections are polymicrobial with aerobic Gram-positive cocci. In chronic infections or previously treated infections, Gram-negative bacilli are frequent co-pathogens. Osteomyelitis may be difficult to diagnose and treat, usually requiring surgical debridement or resection. Ischemic feet or nonresponding infections may require revascularization.

THE SOCIETY FOR VASCULAR SURGERY LOWER EXTREMITY THREATENED LIMB CLASSIFICATION SYSTEM: RISK STRATIFICATION BASED ON WOUND, ISCHEMIA, AND FOOT INFECTION (WIfI)

Mills JL Sr, Conte MS, Armstrong DG, Pomposelli FB, Schanzer A, Sidawy AN, and Andros G; Society for Vascular Surgery Lower Extremity Guidelines Committee, *J Vasc Surg.* 2014;59(1):220–234

ABSTRACT

Critical limb ischemia, first defined in 1982, was intended to delineate a subgroup of patients with a threatened lower extremity primarily because of chronic ischemia. It was the intent of the original authors that patients with diabetes be excluded or analyzed separately. The Fontaine and Rutherford systems have been used to classify risk of amputation and likelihood of benefit from revascularization by subcategorizing patients into two groups: ischemic rest pain and tissue loss. Due to demographic shifts over the last 40 years, especially a dramatic rise in the incidence of diabetes mellitus and rapidly expanding techniques of revascularization, it has become increasingly difficult to perform meaningful outcomes analysis for patients with threatened limbs using these existing classification systems. Particularly in patients with diabetes, limb threat is part of a broad disease spectrum. Perfusion is only one determinant of outcome; wound extent and the presence and severity of infection also greatly impact the threat to a limb. Therefore, the Society for Vascular Surgery Lower Extremity Guidelines Committee undertook the task of creating a new classification of the threatened lower extremity that reflects these important considerations. We term this new framework the Society for Vascular Surgery Lower Extremity Threatened Limb Classification System. Risk stratification is based on three major factors that impact amputation risk and clinical management: Wound, Ischemia, and foot Infection (WIfI). The implementation of this classification system is intended to permit more meaningful analysis of outcomes for various forms of therapy in this challenging but heterogeneous population.

Original Author Commentary: Joseph L. Mills

For nearly 50 years, lower extremity PAD was classified based upon degree of ischemia and the concept of CLI (critical limb ischemia). Wound descriptions lacked detail, and infection was ignored in the Fontaine or Rutherford classifications. Due to the global epidemic of diabetes and the evolution of endovascular therapy, it became evident that these classifications, which were never intended to be applied to diabetics, were insufficiently granular to stratify the range of risk for amputation across a heterogeneous spectrum of disease. One in four diabetic foot ulcers (DFUs) leads to major limb amputation. To reduce unnecessary amputations, a better classification system was needed to stage the limb and direct therapy. The concept of a single hemodynamic cutoff point for ischemia was overly simplistic, as various degrees of ischemia might prove "critical" depending on the overall status of the limb. Chronic limb-threatening ischemia (CLTI) from PAD is a spectrum.

The SVS Lower Extremity Threatened Limb Classification System defines the limb disease burden analogous to the tumor, node, metastasis (TNM) system in use to stage cancer. Each of the three major factors (Wound, Ischemia, and foot Infection [WIfI]) is graded on a scale from 0 to 3; based on the combination of grades, the limb is placed into one of four clinical stages correlating with increasing amputation risk. WIfI has been widely adopted and validated globally (United States, Europe, Asia) in over 5000 patients from diverse centers. WIfI stratifies at-risk limbs into four clinical stages that correlate with the likelihood and time of wound healing, 1-year amputation risk, major adverse limb events (MALE), re-intervention and restenosis events (RAS), intensity and costs of care, hospital length of stay, and allows the comparison of alternate treatment methods (e.g., open bypass vs. endovascular therapy vs. best medical care). A classification system should predict the natural history of the condition, correlate with important clinical outcomes, allow comparison of alternate modes of therapy, and help direct therapy to reduce preventable amputations. WIfI satisfies these previously unmet needs, and its structure allows stages to be adjusted with further application and accumulation of data.

CHAPTER 37

Surgical-Site Infections

Review by Contributor: Mark Sawyer

The prevention of surgical-site infections (SSIs) is a battle that has been waged since the first procedures were performed; the practice of trepanation, practiced from prehistorical times, finally waned during the Renaissance because of the high infection rate. SSIs have not been able to be completely eliminated despite our best efforts—only minimized. The acute care surgical patient represents a special case scenario, as not all the available tools at our disposal to prevent SSIs in the elective patient may be utilized. However, in the interest of the fact that certain elective procedures may be within the purview of the acute care surgeon, this review covers the more pertinent preventative measures in the elective patient as well.

PRE-, INTRA-, AND POSTOPERATIVE INTRAVENOUS ANTIBIOTICS

Preoperative prophylactic antibiotics are given without a second thought today, but surgical luminaries were arguing against their "indiscriminate use" as recently as the 1950s. In 1961, John F. Burke's animal study demonstrating the efficacy of preexisting levels of antibiotics in the tissues prior to inoculation set the stage for widespread adoption of preincisional antibiotics. Following that was a tendency to a "more is better" philosophy, using antibiotics postoperatively as well. Over time, the lack of data for the use of postoperative antibiotic prophylaxis has largely led to the abandonment of this except in certain circumstances. Even in the case of trauma with breach of the colon, 12 hours of antibiotics postoperatively were found to be as efficacious as 5 days. The standard recommendation remains preoperative dosing so optimal levels are present within the tissues at the time of incision (30–120 minutes, depending upon the antibiotic), with repeated intraoperative dosing to maintain tissue levels based on the half-life of the agent used.

The selection of prophylactic intravenous antibiotics is fairly straightforward in most patients, logically aimed at likely organisms. In patients undergoing Class I wounds, coverage is aimed toward Gram-positive bacteria. In Class II and the above wounds where there is contamination with mucosal flora, agents are chosen which provide coverage of both Gram-negative and anaerobic bacteria as well. Most acute care surgery patients fit in the latter category, requiring broad coverage of skin and enteric flora both prophylactically and as initial empiric therapy for intra-abdominal contamination, hollow viscus infection, or frank peritonitis. For coverage of specific circumstances and procedures, there is thorough and detailed guidance available; recommendations are now usually consensus papers put forth by experts in the field under the auspices of the relevant societies.

In the mid-1990s, it was recognized that *Staphylococcus aureus* colonization of the nasal passages increased the risk of nosocomial infections. This was pursued by a study team which in 2002 reported that among elective surgical patients with positive cultures for *S. aureus*, there was a significant reduction in SSIs in patients treated preoperatively with intranasal mupirocin. Even a short course of mupirocin can eradicate nasal *S. aureus*, which begs the question as to whether or not it is effective in the acute care surgical patient. Certainly, some acute care surgical patients would have an interval in the hospital where the treatment could be done, but the perioperative data only showed a significant difference in patients with demonstrated intranasal *S. aureus*.

Mechanical bowel preparation and oral antibiotics in elective colon surgery were initially shown to decrease SSIs, but research in the ensuing years did not clearly show an increase in efficacy in patients receiving intravenous prophylactic antibiotics, and it was largely abandoned. More recently, studies have shown that the combination of oral antibiotics and mechanical bowel preparation decreases SSIs when used in conjunction with intravenous prophylactic antibiotics.

SKIN PREPARATION: ANTISEPSIS, HAIR REMOVAL, AND ADHESIVE SKIN DRAPES

Skin antiseptic solutions have been shown to decrease surgical-site infections, particularly of superficial wound infection. Ideally, a skin preparation solution will kill Gram-positive and Gram-negative bacteria, have rapid and persistent antibacterial activity, maintain activity in the presence of organic material, have minimal systemic absorption, minimal toxicity to contacted tissues, and be nonflammable. No one product has all the desirable and none of the negative traits. Chlorhexidine solutions have been recommended by consensus-type reviews, but the validity of that data has been questioned because of investigator conflicts of interest. Alcohol-based solutions with the addition of a longer-acting agent such as iodine or chlorhexidine provide a good combination of rapid bacterial lethality and a longer lasting effect.

Adherent drapes, especially those impregnated with iodine, are often used with the aim of preventing SSIs. While they have been shown to decrease bacterial skin counts, they have not been shown to decrease the rate of SSIs.

Hair removal has been shown to adversely affect SSI rates; no hair removal appears to be the best, followed by clipping close to the time of incision, with the worst rates in patients in whom the skin is shaved, especially with longer times before the skin incision. Hair should be therefore be removed only when necessary.

Antibacterial cleansing of those participating in operative cases has long been performed, although there is no clear evidence that such cleansing reduces SSIs in the era of surgical gloves. Therefore, it is no surprise that the type of antibacterial solution has not been shown to matter either.

OTHER FACTORS: OXYGEN, NORMOTHERMIA, GLUCOSE CONTROL, AND TOBACCO USE

Normothermia has been shown to lower the incidence of SSIs, as has postoperative administration of oxygen. Glucose control is recommended as a general health item prior to elective surgery, but Hgb A1C normalization has not been shown to improve the rate of SSIs. Tobacco use, on the other hand, has been definitively implicated in not only increasing the incidence of SSIs, but multiple other perioperative complications as well.

SURGICAL GARB: GOWNS, GLOVES, CAPS BOOTIES, AND "MYTHUNDERSTANDINGS"

Bacterial transmission from surgeon to patient was recognized during the era of Oliver Wendell Holmes Sr. and Ignaz Semmelweis, which prompted the transition from simple aprons to protect a surgeon's clothing from gouts of blood to gowns, gloves, caps, and shoe covers to form a two-way barrier protecting the patient from the surgeon and the surgeon from the patient. Most of these were adopted before the age of evidence-based medicine and as a result, the surgeon's garb has the weight of history and tradition behind it, but not necessarily that of solid evidence. Most of the attire recommendations are commonsensical, but there has been a disagreeable trend to enact and enforce ever more stringent garb rules and regulations without a shred of evidence in their support. Recommendations which have no demonstrable effect on SSI prevention, such as banning cloth caps in the operating room (an element of the attire which exists solely to prevent the fall of hair into the wound) or mandating paper booties (whose sole legitimate purpose is to protect footwear from blood and other bodily effluents) do little besides adding to the regulatory burden of performing surgery.

ASPECTS OF SSI PERTINENT TO ACUTE CARE SURGERY

Surgical-site infections are of course far more common in acute care surgery, which usually entails an intra-abdominal or soft tissue infectious process. A higher wound class means not only a higher SSI rate in closed incisions, but an increased incidence of deep SSIs as well. In general, there is a timeline that progresses from contamination to infection intra-abdominally. A prototypical "time zero" contamination might be exemplified by a Class 2 wound—spillage intraoperatively which is immediately tidied up. While it increases the risk of an SSI over a Class 1 wound, postoperative antibiotics will not be helpful. A bit further along the spectrum would be a penetrating injury of the colon, operated on within 6 hours of injury, which has been shown to do well with a duration of antimicrobials on the order of 12 hours. The next step along the timeline might be exemplified by gangrenous appendicitis or a perforated ulcer, which represents the bacterial contamination of the peritoneal cavity for about 24–48 hours, and usually responds well to a few days of antibiotics. Peritonitis due to conditions such as diverticulitis, either purulent of feculent, is often present as a well-established infection at the time of surgery and requires a longer duration of antibiotics and has a much higher attendant risk of a subsequent deep SSI. There is a simplification of the bacterial flora from contamination (hundreds of species) to early infection (6–10 species in carefully cultured gangrenous or ruptured appendicitis) to perhaps 2–3 pathogenic bacteria present in a well-established infection. However, the most common agents in peritonitis are *Escherichia coli* and *Bacteroides fragilis*, so broad-spectrum coverage is still required.

SUMMARY

SSIs represent a particularly difficult area for acute care surgeons, with more research needed to adapt existing modalities to the immediacy of the discipline as well as discover new treatments and preventative measures which do not depend on the time available in an elective setting. An understanding of the current underlying risks, principles, and known efficacious measures is necessary for the optimal prevention, recognition, and treatment of SSIs in the acute care patient.

ANNOTATED REFERENCES FOR SURGICAL-SITE INFECTIONS

1. Burke JF. The effective period of preventive antibiotic action in experimental incisions and dermal lesions. *Surgery.* 1961; 50:161–168.

   This paper is the genesis of the ubiquitous practice of preoperative intravenous antibiotic administration to prevent wound infections. Burke showed in a guinea pig model that maximal prevention of skin incision infections occurs when the antibiotics are circulating in the tissue at the time of bacterial inoculation, and that the longer after bacterial inoculation the antibiotics are administered, the less effective they are. Burke was also influential in the adoption of the wound contamination classification system still in use today, which enjoyed widespread adoption by 1964.

2. Nichols RL, Gorbach SL, Condon RE. Alteration of intestinal microflora following preoperative mechanical preparation of the colon. *Dis Colon Rectum.* 1971;14(2):123–127.

3. Hawn MT, Houston TK, Campagna EJ et al. The attributable risk of smoking on surgical complications. *Ann Surg.* 2011;254(6):914–920.

   This retrospective review of 393,794 patients looked at a number of postoperative complications, one of which was smoking, and is an excellent overview of the negative effects of smoking on surgical patients. The rate of SSIs in never-smokers was 2.4%, 3.2% in prior smokers, and 3.4% in current smokers. Odds ratios of developing an SSI were 1.0, 1.11, and 1.18, respectively. Cessation of smoking prior to surgery therefore had a benefit, but it could be surmised that there was a residual effect on the risk of SSI development in patients who had smoked previously but quit.

4. Bratzler DW, Dellinger EP, Olsen KM et al.; American Society of Health-System Pharmacists; Infectious Disease Society of America; Surgical Infection Society; Society for Healthcare Epidemiology of America. Clinical practice guidelines for antimicrobial prophylaxis in surgery. *Am J Health Syst Pharm*. 2013;70(3):195–283.

Weighing in at 89 pages, this is THE exhaustively researched, meticulous guide to antimicrobial prophylaxis in surgery covering the all facets of antimicrobial prophylaxis—drugs, dosages, procedures, and so on, with detailed, specific recommendations.

5. Oreskovich MR, Dellinger EP, Lennard ES, Wertz M, Carrico CJ, Minshew BH. Duration of preventive antibiotic administration for penetrating abdominal trauma. *Arch Surg*. 1982;117(2):200–205.

The authors demonstrated that a much shorter course of antibiotic therapy than was standard at the time (4–12 days) was just as efficacious in penetrating abdominal trauma. It helps demonstrate the continuum from contamination to infection in intra-abdominal processes, and the attendant change in antimicrobial duration necessary.

6. Berríos-Torres SI, Umscheid CA, Bratzler DW et al.; Healthcare Infection Control Practices Advisory Committee. Centers for Disease Control and Prevention Guideline for the prevention of surgical-site infection, 2017. *JAMA Surg*. 2017;152(8):784–791.

An evidence-based update to the first version of the recommendations published in 2000. The authors used the GRADE system, where recommendations are presented by strength, and the quality of the data is assessed and presented with the recommendation. The advantage of the GRADE approach is that evidence at times may be impractical or even impossible to rigorously test in a prospective, randomized fashion. An example given for both its logical impact and humor value is the use of parachutes: there exists no prospective randomized study of parachutes versus no parachutes, nor will there ever be. Having stated this, however, no one would suggest abandoning the use of parachutes for lack of evidence that they are necessary, and a very strong recommendation for their continued use can be given with confidence.

7. Greif R, Akça O, Horn EP, Kurz A, Sessler DI; Outcomes Research Group. Supplemental perioperative oxygen to reduce the incidence of surgical wound infection. *N Engl J Med*. 2000;342:161–167.

An elegantly done study which demonstrated a dramatic decrease in SSIs with the administration of 80% oxygen intraoperatively and postoperatively for 2 hours; the comparison group was given 30% oxygen and had double the infection rate of the first group. Like the Leuven study with glycemic control, however, it demonstrates the need for multiple confirmatory studies before even beautifully demonstrated hypotheses become the standard of care. Subsequent studies have demonstrated mixed results, with some showing a benefit, others no benefit or even a detrimental effect. With SSIs having so many factors influencing their occurrence, halving the wound infection rate by changing one variable should at least raise a questioning eyebrow, and the underlying hypothesis that the relatively small amount of additional oxygen solvent in the tissues may be helpful has not been supported by the extant experience with hyperbaric oxygen therapy.

INTRANASAL MUPIROCIN TO PREVENT POSTOPERATIVE *STAPHYLOCOCCUS AUREUS* INFECTIONS

Perl TM, Cullen JJ, Wenzel RP, Zimmerman MB, Pfaller MA, Sheppard D, Twombley J, French PP, and Herwaldt LA; Mupirocin and the Risk of *Staphylococcus aureus* Study Team, *N Engl J Med*. 2002;346(24):1871–1877

ABSTRACT

Background   Patients with nasal carriage of *Staphylococcus aureus* have an increased risk of surgical-site infections caused by that organism. Treatment with mupirocin ointment can reduce the rate of nasal carriage and may prevent postoperative *S. aureus* infections.

Methods   We conducted a randomized, double-blind, placebo-controlled trial to determine whether intranasal treatment with mupirocin reduces the rate of *S. aureus* infections at surgical sites and prevents other nosocomial infections.

Results   Of 4030 enrolled patients who underwent general, gynecologic, neurologic, or cardiothoracic surgery, 3864 were included in the intention-to-treat analysis. Overall, 2.3% of mupirocin recipients and 2.4% of placebo recipients had *S. aureus* infections at surgical sites. Of the 891 (23.1% of the 3864 who completed the study) who had *S. aureus* in their anterior nares, 444 received mupirocin and 447 received placebo. Among the patients with nasal carriage of *S. aureus*, 4.0% of those who received mupirocin had nosocomial *S. aureus* infections as compared with 7.7% of those who received placebo (odds ratio for infection, 0.49; 95% confidence interval, 0.25–0.92; P = 0.02).

Conclusions   Prophylactic intranasal application of mupirocin did not significantly reduce the rate of *S. aureus* surgical-site infections overall, but it did significantly decrease the rate of all nosocomial *S. aureus* infections among the patients who were *S. aureus* carriers.

Editor Notes

Assessment: This was a large randomized, double-blind, placebo-controlled trial to determine if mupirocin (2% topical antibiotic ointment that decolonizes the anterior nares) can reduce the rate of *S. aureus* infections at surgical sites and prevent other nosocomial infections. Patients (n = 3864) who underwent general, gynecologic, neurologic, or cardiothoracic surgery were included in the intention-to-treat analysis. In this population there was no difference in infection. However, 891 patients had *S. aureus* in their anterior nares, and in this subgroup of patients the nosocomial *S. aureus* infection rates were significantly lower (4.0% vs. 7.7%, p = 0.02).

Limitations: This rigorous, well-designed study demonstrated useful information. The limitations are that since we do not always know who is colonized with *S. aureus* in their anterior nares before surgery, we may have to apply the ointment on all elective surgery patients in order to have an effect on the patients who are colonized. Since there is minimal risk to the strategy and the study did not identify any complications, it may be prudent to adopt the policy at one's institution. Compared to placebo, mupirocin eliminated the carriage of *S. aureus* (83%–93%) depending on the number of dosages. Overall, there was no difference in nosocomial infection rates (11%) or SSI (8.2%). The concern is that the wide use of mupirocin might lead to widespread resistance.

Conclusions: The Mupirocin and the Risk of *Staphylococcus aureus* (MARS) study showed that the use of mupirocin significantly decreased nosocomial *S. aureus* infections in patients who were carriers of *S. aureus* but failed to impact on the incidence of surgical-site infection.

CHAPTER **38**

Snake Envenomation

Review by Contributors: Anne Rizzo and Peter Rhee

There are 8–10,000 reported emergency room visits for snakebites each year (Lavonas et al., 2009). Most snakebites are not venomous, and when bitten by a venomous snake, 25% are "dry," meaning that venom was not injected. Of the 120 known indigenous snake species in North America, approximately 20 are venomous to human beings, most belonging to the families Viperidae (vipers) and Elapidae (cobras) (Adukauskienė et al., 2011). Most envenomations in the United States are by vipers (rattlesnake, cottonmouth, copperhead) and occasionally by cobras (cobra, coral, mamba). Although cobras are not indigenous to the United States, cobra bites from imported pets have been reported and can be deadly. The vast majority of snake bites require only local wound care and approximately only 1–5 deaths are reported each year from snake bite envenomation in the United States, which is very low compared to worldwide figures. Serious snake-bite envenomations are still a public health issue but most are in tropical regions and especially in South Asia, Southeast Asia, and sub-Saharan Africa. India reports the most snakebite deaths of any country (Gold et al., 2002).

The care for the wounds is relatively simple and includes cleaning, delayed debride-ment, prevention of secondary infection, and hygienic conservative wound care. Occasionally the edema can cause compartment syndrome. The wounds should not be incised or sucked, and tourniquets are ill-advised. The majority of snakebites nation-wide occur in men on their lower and upper extremity. The threat of loss of tissue and limb function, and ambiguity over the type of snake that might have caused the envenomation, has resulted in a substantial demand for antivenom. The venom can cause local symptoms of pain, redness, and blistering. Systemic symptoms of feeling faint, fear, lightheadedness, tachycardia, nausea, and vomiting have all been reported. Systemic problems of anaphylaxis, coagulopathy, renal failure, respiratory failure, and death are uncommon but have occurred.

The controversy with snake envenomation is in regard to the use of antivenom, as many question whether they are needed (Gale et al., 2016). Although most snakebites are not venomous, antivenom is readily available and patients as well as health care providers often want it and even demand it. There are approximately 25 snake anti-venoms available worldwide, but the main antivenom used and studied in the United States is the sheep antivenom (ovine polyvalent crotalidae immunoglobulin [CroFab] which are antibodies harvested from a sheep injected with small amount of crotali-dae venom). Horse serum antivenom has been recently introduced as a competitor. The complications of CroFab antivenom have been well documented and are typical of injecting ovine antibodies. While severe reactions, including strokes and fatalities, have been reported, in general the CroFab antivenom has been reported to be relatively safe (Schaeffer et al., 2012; Kleinschmidt et al., 2018). Since CroFab antivenom is currently used so widely and is almost a standard, ethical concerns have minimized scientific rigors about formulating a recent study to determine the usefulness of CroFab antivenom. Since the earlier randomized multicenter study in 2001 on 31 patients, efficacy studies have been few.

A recent randomized, double-blind, placebo-controlled, multicenter study was reported in 2015. This study, done in 18 centers, showed that the new F(ab')2 immunoglobulin, which has a longer plasma half-life than the previous Fab, reduced the risk of subacute coagulopathy and bleeding following treatment of envenomation. While previous studies have shown a wide variation in the use of antivenom for copperhead bites (0%–70%), the most current literature notes no need for therapy other than local wound care. Gerardo and colleagues undertook the first-ever multicenter, randomized, double-blind, placebo-controlled study to evaluate the effects of antivenom versus placebo in copperhead snakebite victims. They quantitated the antivenom use as well as the injury and dysfunction of the effected limbs. This study showed improved functional limb function at 14 days after copperhead bites. The early improvement in limb function (at 14 days) was statistically significant but evaporated with additional time to recovery at 28 days. The study was underpowered due to the enormity of the undertaking of enrolling protocolized patients in the emergency room across several states.

Only mild to moderate envenomation was included in the Gerardo study. Severe envenomation was defined as systemic symptoms or advanced local effects due to delay in presentation. There was also an arm of the study for "rescue" if the patient was progressing on placebo but there was no crossover into this group. To the credit of the investigators, all bites were confirmed by photos of the offending snake or the actual snake before enrollment to ensure that only copperhead bites were being evaluated by the protocol. This did not delay treatment, as many snakebite victims take photographs or bring the offending snake to the hospital for identification.

Currently, no studies yet have shown survival difference or limb salvage effect with the Crotaline Fab antivenom. Case series have reported reduction in pain and opiate use. The severe cases of viper envenomation in the United States can cause acute or subacute subclinical coagulopathy. Currently, in addition to symptom relief, the Crotaline Fab antivenom is mostly used to treat coagulopathy. Although copperhead bites do not generally cause systemic problems, it can cause local pain and limb injury. Only 3 of the 24 reported deaths due to snake envenomation since 2010 are due to copperheads, whereas rattlesnakes account for 18 and cobra, mamba, and cottonmouth have reported 1 death each. Deaths are relatively uncommon after snake envenomation.

Financial consideration for the $2000 price tag of a single vial of CroFab antivenom was discussed in the paper. The protocol requires 4–6 vials being administered on admission of the patient and acknowledgement of a snakebite. The authors acknowledge the significant cost differential for minimal improvement with the placebo group averaging $12,000 to $20,000.00 less in charges. A strategy of delaying antivenom administration until there are signs of systemic symptoms or progression warrants investigation in the future. CroFab antivenom should be used with highly vetted protocols mainly because it can be very expensive and its benefits have not been rigorously demonstrated. Since the CroFab antivenom is relatively safe, the criticism for liberal use is due to the high costs. The same antivenom from the same manufacturer is significantly cheaper in Mexico ($100) compared to the United States ($7900–39,652) and the investigations have identified that hospital markup is the major reason for the higher charges (Boyer, 2015). As the high cost of medical care continues to be evaluated, costly resources such as CroFab antivenom should be reserved for severe copperhead bites as well as rattlesnake bites where systemic illness is much more prevalent. Treatment of pain and coagulopathy is an endpoint that most protocols use.

ANNOTATED REFERENCES FOR SNAKE ENVENOMATION

1. Lavonas EJ, Schaeffer TH, Kokko J, Mlynarchek SL, Bogdan GM. Crotaline Fab antivenom appears to be effective in cases of severe North American pit viper envenomation: An integrative review. *BMC Emerg Med.* 2009;9:13.

   Good review of the literature with the authors reviewing 147 unique publications regarding FabAV during the period of 1996 to 2008. Has good general information regarding the Ovine Crotalid Polyvalent Immune Fab antivenom.

2. Adukauskienė D, Varanauskienė E, Adukauskaitė A. Venomous snakebites. *Medicina (Kaunas).* 2011;47(8):461–467.

   Good review article with interesting information on pathology and simple rules to go by when treating wounds. Snake venom can be classified into hemotoxic, neurotoxic, necrotoxic, cardiotoxic, and nephrotoxic according to the different predominant effects depending on the family (i.e., venom of Crotalidae and Viperidae snakes is more hemotoxic and necrotoxic, whereas venom of Elapidae family is mainly neurotoxic). The intoxication degree is estimated according to the appearance of these symptoms: (1) no intoxication ("dry" bite); (2) mild intoxication (local edema and pain); (3) moderate intoxication (pain, edema spreading out of the bite zone, and systemic signs); (4) severe intoxication (shock, severe coagulopathy, and massive edemas).

3. Gold BS, Dart RC, Barish RA. Bites of venomous snakes. *N Engl J Med.* 2002; 375(5):347–356.

   Good general review article with facts and epidemiology.

4. Gale SC, Peters JA, Allen L, Creath R, Dombrovskiy VY. FabAV antivenin use after copperhead snakebite: Clinically indicated or a knee-jerk reaction? *J Venom Anim Toxins Incl Trop Dis.* 2016;22:2.

   Because copperhead envenomations are usually self-limited, some physicians are reluctant to use this costly treatment routinely, while others follow a more liberal approach. A single-center 11-year study showed that only 14% received antivenin. Median dose was four vials. There were no deaths. Use of FabAV appears poorly correlated with patients' symptoms. This practice may expose patients to the risks of antivenin and increasing costs of medical care without improving outcomes. Guidelines used for treating other pit viper strikes, such as rattlesnake or cottonmouth snakebite, may be too liberal for copperhead envenomations. Their data suggest that most patients with mild or moderate envenomation appear to do well independent of FabAV use.

5. Kleinschmidt K, Ruha AM, Campleman S, Brent J, Wax P; ToxIC North American Snakebite Registry Group. Acute adverse events associated with the administration of Crotalidae polyvalent immune Fab antivenom within the North American Snakebite Registry. *Clin Toxicol (Phila)*. 2018;56(11):1115–1120.

Crotalidae Polyvalent Immune Fab (Fab Antivenom) is the primary Viperid antivenom used in the United States since 2000. Adverse event data associated with its use are limited. The purpose of this study was to describe the prevalence of acute adverse events associated with the use of Fab antivenom. In this prospective case registry of poisoned and envenomated patients (a review of 438 cases), 85% received at least one vial of Fab Antivenom. Adverse events occurred in 10 patients (2.7%). Rash was the most common adverse event. More severe adverse events (hypotension, bronchospasm, and/or angio-edema) occurred in four (1.1%) patients.

6. Schaeffer TH, Khatri V, Reifler LM, Lavonas EJ. Incidence of immediate hypersensitivity reaction and serum sickness following administration of Crotalidae polyvalent immune Fab antivenom: A meta-analysis. *Acad Emerg Med*. 2012;19(3):368.

The literature search revealed 11 unique studies of patients who received FabAV that contained information on immediate hypersensitivity reactions and serum sickness. In this systematic literature review and meta-analysis, the combined estimates of the incidence of immediate hypersensitivity reactions and serum sickness from FabAV in the treatment of symptomatic North American crotaline envenomations appear to be lower than previously reported, at 0.08 and 0.13, respectively.

7. Bush SP, Ruha AM, Seifert SA et al. Comparison of F(ab')2 versus Fab antivenom for pit viper envenomation: A prospective, blinded, multicenter, randomized clinical trial. *Clin Toxicol (Phila)*. 2015;53(1):37–45.

F(ab')2 immunoglobulin derivatives have longer half-lives than do Fab. The authors hypothe-sized that F(ab')2 antivenom would be superior to Fab in the prevention of late coagulopathy following treatment of patients with Crotalinae envenomation. They conducted a prospective, double-blind, randomized, clinical trial, comparing late coagulopathy. The primary efficacy endpoint was coagulopathy. One hundred twenty-one patients were randomized at 18 clinical sites and received at least one dose of study drug. One hundred fourteen patients completed the study. In this study, management of coagulopathic Crotalinae envenomation with longer-half-life F(ab')2 antivenom, with or without maintenance dosing, reduced the risk of subacute coagulopathy and bleeding following treatment of envenomation.

8. Gerardo CJ, Quackenbus E, Lewis B et al. The efficacy of Crotalidae Polyvalent Immune Fab (Ovine) Antivenom versus placebo plus optional rescue therapy on recovery from copperhead snake envenomation: A randomized, double-blind, placebo-controlled, clinical trial. *Ann Emerg Med*. 2017;70:233–244.

Two-year multicenter, randomized, double-blind, placebo-controlled, clinical trial to evaluate the effect of ovine Crotalidae polyvalent immune Fab (ovine) (CroFab; FabAV) antivenom therapy on recovery of limb function in patients with copperhead snake envenomation at 14 days. The primary outcome was limb function 14 days after envenomation, measured by the Patient-Specific Functional Scale. Seventy-four patients received study drug (45 FabAV, 29 placebo). Treatment with FabAV reduced limb dis-ability measured by the Patient-Specific Functional Scale 14 days after copperhead envenomation P = 0.04.

9. Bush SP, Seifert SA, Oakes J et al. Continuous IV Crotalidae Polyvalent Immune Fab (Ovine) (FabAV) for selected North American rattlesnake bite patients. *Toxicon*. 2013;69:29–37.

   In patients bitten by North American rattlesnakes and treated with Crotalidae Polyvalent Immune Fab (Ovine) (FabAV), late hematologic abnormalities can be persistent or have late new onset with deleterious outcomes. This study is a case series of five patients at three medical centers that managed the patients with a continuous intravenous infusion of FabAV for late hematologic abnormalities and/or associated bleeding complications. Several patients had received repeat bolus infusions of FabAV, with either inadequate or only transient beneficial response. All patients were then managed with a continuous intravenous infusion of FabAV and all appeared to respond to the continuous intravenous infusion of FabAV, titrated to effect. A continuous intravenous infusion of FabAV between two and four vials per day, titrated to effect, and continued for 6–14 days post-envenomation appeared to be associated with reversal of late hematologic effects of rattlesnake envenomation and, when combined with indicated human blood products, control of significant bleeding. Continuous intravenous infusion of FabAV may be safer, more efficacious, and more cost effective than observation without FabAV treatment or as-needed bolus dosing in selected patients with late hematologic abnormalities.

10. Weant KA, Bowers RC, Reed J, Braum KA, Dodd DM, Baker SN. Safety and cost effectiveness of a clinical protocol implemented to standardize the use of Crotalidae Polyvalent Immune Fab antivenom at an academic medical center. *Pharmacotherapy*. 2012;32(5):433–440.

    Seventy-five adults treated with FabAV for snake envenomations in the emergency department at an academic medical center that serves as the regional level I trauma center. Use of a clinical protocol related to snake envenomations resulted in approximately two fewer vials of FabAV required for each patient. This decreased in usage correlated to a cost savings of approximately $2000/patient. In addition, the treatment group experienced a shorter hospital length of stay without a corresponding increase in adverse events or envenomation progression. Data show that use of the protocol was cost effective. The development of institution-specific multidisciplinary protocols regarding snakebite envenomations is recommended.

11. Boyer LV. On 1000-fold pharmaceutical price markups and why drugs cost more in the United States than in Mexico. *Am J Med*. 2015;128(12):1265–1267.

    Editorial on the cost of the CroFab in Mexico ($100) compared to the cost in the United States ($7900–39,652). The drug is from the same manufacturer, but the markup is due to hospital markup.

UNIFIED TREATMENT ALGORITHM FOR THE MANAGEMENT OF CROTALINE SNAKEBITE IN THE UNITED STATES: RESULTS OF AN EVIDENCE-INFORMED CONSENSUS WORKSHOP

Lavonas EJ, Ruha AM, Banner W, Bebarta V, Bernstein JN, Bush SP, Kerns WP 2nd, Richardson WH, Seifert SA, Tanen DA, Curry SC, and Dart RC; Rocky Mountain Poison and Drug Center, Denver Health and Hospital Authority, *BMC Emerg Med*. 2011;11:2

ABSTRACT

Background Envenomation by crotaline snakes (rattlesnake, cottonmouth, copperhead) is a complex, potentially lethal condition affecting thousands of people in the United States each year. Treatment of crotaline envenomation is not standardized, and significant variation in practice exists.

Methods   A geographically diverse panel of experts was convened for the purpose of deriving an evidence-informed unified treatment algorithm. Research staff analyzed the extant medical literature and performed targeted analyses of existing databases to inform specific clinical decisions. A trained external facilitator used modified Delphi and structured consensus methodology to achieve consensus on the final treatment algorithm.

Results   A unified treatment algorithm was produced and endorsed by all nine expert panel members. This algorithm provides guidance about clinical and laboratory observations, indications for and dosing of antivenom, adjunctive therapies, post-stabilization care, and management of complications from envenomation and therapy.

Conclusions   Clinical manifestations and ideal treatment of crotaline snakebite differ greatly and can result in severe complications. Using a modified Delphi method, we provide evidence-informed treatment guidelines in an attempt to reduce variation in care and possibly improve clinical outcomes.

Original Author Commentary: Eric J. Lavonas

Although 9000 patients are treated in the United States each year, few physicians see enough snakebite patients to become comfortable with this serious condition. Envenomation is a dynamic process, with signs and symptoms rapidly evolving in the patient. We assembled a group of 12 experienced clinicians from across the United States, representing diverse clinical experience and practice approaches. After systematically gathering the best evidence, we hammered out a single approach to therapy that works well for all of the pit viper (genus *Crotalus*: rattlesnake, cottonmouth/water moccasin, and copperhead) species native to North America.

With the introduction of highly purified Fab antivenom in 2000, antivenom therapy has become central to the management of all significant cases of pit viper envenomation. Treatment no longer needs to be withheld due to safety concerns. Fab antivenom can be used early, resulting in prompt stabilization and reduced tissue injury.

Of special concern to the surgeon, prophylactic fasciotomy and debridement are no longer appropriate, because studies show better outcomes with antivenom alone. Compartment syndrome is very rare, affecting less than 2% of snakebite victims, but inflammation and edema in the superficial tissue planes often mimics compartment syndrome. The approach to suspected compartment syndrome is to give Fab antivenom and assess further.

Seven years after its publication, we are pleased that surgeons and other physicians find the Unified Treatment Algorithm a helpful guide to this uncommon and serious condition.

CHAPTER 39

Ruptured Abdominal Aortic Aneurysms

Review by Contributors: Abdul Q. Alarhayem and Mark G. Davies

Abdominal aortic aneurysms (AAA) affect 7%–9% of the population over the age of 65 years, with a higher prevalence in smokers. The natural course of an unrepaired AAA is continued growth, and ultimately rupture and death. Aneurysm diameter, expansion rate, female gender, low FEV_1, current smoking, and hypertension have all been associated with an increased risk of rupture.

Over the last two decades, there has been a decline in the incidence and mortality of ruptured abdominal aortic aneurysms (rAAA), likely secondary to decreased smoking, regionalization of care, development of well-defined protocols, and increased elective treatment of AAA (Reimerink et al., 2013b).

Factors contributing to high morbidity and mortality include delays in establishing the diagnosis, intraoperative injuries (i.e., iatrogenic), and patient comorbidities such as age >75 years, preexisting renal insufficiency, severe hypotension (SBP < 70 mmHg), cardiac arrest, and anemia (Hb < 9 g/dL).

In about 20% of cases, AAAs rupture freely into the peritoneal cavity; this is usually fatal prior to reaching medical care. In the remaining 80%, AAAs rupture into the retroperitoneal space, usually posterolaterally, with a retroperitoneal hematoma that temporarily tamponades the hemorrhage.

A high index of suspicion and prompt surgical intervention is crucial to salvaging these patients. The classic triad of abdominal pain, hypotension, and pulsatile abdominal mass is present in less than 60% of patients. In the hemodynamically stable patient, a CT scan of the abdomen and pelvis is expedient and not only aids in diagnosis but allows determination of anatomic suitability for endovascular repair. While ultrasound is useful for screening, its utility in the setting of rupture is limited due to poor visibility of the retroperitoneum.

Patients have the highest chance of survival if prompt treatment is delivered by a specialized team with a high caseload of aortic surgery by board-certified vascular surgeons. Similarities can be drawn in the preoperative strategies employed in patients with rAAA and hemorrhaging trauma patients. Minimizing time from rupture to hemorrhage control, permissive hypotension, minimizing the administration of fluids (crystalloids and/or colloids), and balanced resuscitation are advocated (Wanhainen et al., 2019).

Endovascular aortic occlusion provides expeditious hemorrhage control in both open and endovascular repair of rAAA. This maneuver can be done under local anesthesia, avoiding hemodynamic collapse associated with general anesthesia; it enables rapid deployment at multiple levels in the aorta and is associated with reduced intraoperative mortality compared to open aortic cross-clamping (Raux et al., 2015).

Endovascular aortic repair (EVAR) is now performed for the majority of elective AAA cases in the United States. The adoption of EVAR in the setting of ruptured AAA, however, has been met with caution, due to concerns over anatomic suitability, expediency of repair, availability of dedicated staff and equipment, and insufficient data on its efficacy. The benefits of the endovascular approach include a less invasive approach that can eliminate the need for general anesthesia and aortic cross-clamping, and an association with a shorter hospital length of stay.

While retrospective and prospective studies have shown that EVAR is associated with lower mortality and perioperative morbidity compared to open repair, randomized trials have not shown a difference (Veith et al., 2009; Mehta et al., 2013). It is thought that these studies are flawed by selection bias, with better-risk patients undergoing EVAR and worse-risk patients (including those not anatomically suitable) undergoing open repair.

The AJAX trial from Amsterdam and the ECAR trial from France randomized patients who were eligible for both repair (physiologically capable of withstanding surgery) and EVAR (anatomically suitable, especially neck aneurysm). While both trials showed no difference in 30-day mortality between EVAR and open repair, sample sizes were small and many patients screened were excluded from randomization, including unstable patients, who were not offered EVAR (Reimerink et al., 2013a; Desgranges et al., 2015).

The IMPROVE trial randomized patients with an in-hospital clinical diagnosis of ruptured aneurysm. The overall 30-day mortality rate in the EVAR group was 35% versus 37% in the open repair group ($P = .67$). Upon closer inspection, this was an intention-to-treat analysis, and a number of patients breached the randomization protocol, undergoing open repair after being randomized to EVAR due to anatomic unsuitability (patients were randomized before knowledge of whether anatomy was suitable for EVAR), or undergoing EVAR after being randomized to open repair as general anesthesia was thought to be too risky. The 30-day mortality rate for rAAA patients actually treated with EVAR was 24.7% (46 of 186), versus 38.1% (128 of 336) for those actually treated by open repair ($P < .002$). These rates are still higher than the AJAX and ECAR trials, likely as IMPROVE included patients not morphologically suitable for EVAR as well as patients who did not reach the OR alive (IMPROVE Trial Investigators, 2014).

Unfavorable aneurysm neck anatomy (neck length <10 mm) is the most common reason for lack of suitability for EVAR; these patients are known to have a higher mortality rate even after open repair (IMPROVE Trial Investigators, 2015). When EVAR can be performed, it may be a better treatment option. It is likely that an increasing proportion of a rAAA will be amenable to endovascular treatment as the available technology evolves, with possibly improved patient outcomes (Hinchliffe et al., 2015; Starnes et al., 2015).

The immediate postoperative period is frequently marked by hemodynamic lability, coagulopathy, and an increased risk of complications. The ICU physician caring for these patients is to maintain a high index of suspicion for consumptive and dilutional coagulopathy; hypothermia and acidosis must be aggressively managed. Where available, thromboelastography (TEG) should be used for targeted transfusion therapy, with the hopes of reducing transfusion requirements, and the risk of transfusion-related acute lung injury (TRALI) and transfusion acute circulatory overload (TACO). In the absence of significant bleeding, judicious use of crystalloid using appropriate endpoints of resuscitation is indicated.

Postoperatively, myocardial infarction is the most common cause of death. Patients are also at increased risk of atrial fibrillation and should be monitored with continuous telemetry. Up to 75% develop varying degrees of AKI, with a culminant increased risk of death and prolonged hospitalization.

Regardless of the method of repair, all rAAA patients are at high risk for developing abdominal compartment syndrome (ACS). Decreasing urine output, pulmonary compliance, and mean arterial pressure, especially in the setting of increasing abdominal distension, should prompt immediate assessment. Mortality in patients who develop ACS after rAAA repair has been reported to be as high as 50%; decompressive laparotomy should thus be considered before the development of ACS (Rubenstein et al., 2015).

Ischemic colitis is another complication worth special mention. Worsening abdominal pain, distension, fever, unexplained leukocytosis, and bloody or frequent bowel movements should prompt immediate evaluation with a bedside flexible sigmoidoscopy/colonoscopy. In the absence of full-thickness involvement, patients frequently respond to bowel rest, intravascular volume repletion, IV antibiotics, and avoiding the use of vasopressors. Patients with full-thickness colonic involvement, peritonitis, or sepsis should undergo immediate laparotomy and segmental versus total colectomy. Patients should undergo a second-look operation in 24–48 hours to assess bowel viability.

While treatment of rAAA has improved over time, it continues to carry significant operative mortality. Ultimately, it is our duty as physicians to effectively communicate with patients and their families to help elucidate patient's goals of care and help guide decision making, especially when a favorable outcome is unlikely in spite of aggressive medical care.

ANNOTATED REFERENCES FOR RUPTURED
ABDOMINAL AORTIC ANEURYSMS

1. Desgranges P, Kobeiter H, Katsahian S et al. A French randomized controlled trial of endovascular versus open surgical repair of ruptured aorto-iliac aneurysms. *Eur J Vasc Endovasc Surg.* 2015;50(3):303–310.

   One hundred seven patients with ruptured aorto-iliac aneurysms were randomized to either endovascular (EVAR) or open surgical repair (OSR). Hemodynamically unstable patients were excluded from selection. Delay to treatment was higher in the EVAR group. Mortality at 30 days and 1 year was no different between the groups (18% in the EVAR group vs. 24% in the OSR group at 30 days, and 30% vs. 35%, respectively, at 1 year). EVAR was associated with shorter ICU and hospital length of stays, as well as lower pulmonary complications.

2. IMPROVE Trial Investigators; Powell JT, Sweeting MJ et al. Endovascular or open repair strategy for ruptured abdominal aortic aneurysm: 30 day outcomes from IMPROVE randomised trial. *BMJ.* 2014;348:f7661.

   Of the 316 patients who were initially randomized to the endovascular strategy group, only 154 were actually treated by EVAR while 112 underwent open repair. Of the 297 patients who were randomized to the open repair group, 220 underwent open repair.

3. IMPROVE Trial Investigators. The effect of aortic morphology on peri-operative mortality of ruptured abdominal aortic aneurysm. *Eur Heart J.* 2015;36(21):1328–1334.

   The IMPROVE Trial Investigators studied the impact of aortic morphology in rAAA patients on mortality and reinterventions within 30 days. Patients with shorter aneurysm neck lengths were more likely to undergo open repair. Aneurysm neck length was inversely associated with mortality for open repair and overall survival.

4. Mayer D, Rancic Z, Veith FJ, Pecoraro F, Pfammatter T, Lachat M. How to diagnose and treat abdominal compartment syndrome after endovascular and open repair of ruptured abdominal aortic aneurysms. *J Cardiovasc Surg (Torino).* 2014;55(2):179–192.

   A contemporary review of the clinical presentation and management strategies of intra-abdominal hypertension (IAH) and abdominal compartment syndrome (ACS) in patients with rAAA.

5. Mehta M, Byrne J, Darling RC 3rd et al. Endovascular repair of ruptured infrarenal abdominal aortic aneurysm is associated with lower 30-day mortality and better 5-year survival rates than open surgical repair. *J Vasc Surg.* 2013;57(2):368–375.

   A single-center retrospective review of 283 patients with rAAA treated with EVAR versus open surgical repair. EVAR was associated with a lower 30-day mortality (29/120 [24.2%] vs. 72/163 [44.2%]; P <.005) that was maintained at 5 years (37% vs. 26%; P <.005). 23% of EVAR patients required secondary interventions.

6. Raux M, Marzelle J, Kobeiter H et al. Endovascular balloon occlusion is associated with reduced intraoperative mortality of unstable patients with ruptured abdominal aortic aneurysm but fails to improve other outcomes. *J Vasc Surg.* 2015;61(2):304–308.

   In a retrospective review of 72 hemodynamically unstable rAAA patients, endovascular occlusion was associated with reduced intraoperative mortality compared to open aortic cross-clamping (19% vs. 3%, P =.031), but not in-hospital mortality.

7. Reimerink JJ, Hoornweg LL, Vahl AC et al. Endovascular repair versus open repair of ruptured abdominal aortic aneurysms: A multicenter randomized controlled trial. *Ann Surg.* 2013a;258(2):248–256.

One hundred sixteen (of 520 patients screened) with rAAA from three Dutch centers were randomized to EVAR versus open repair (OR). There was no significant difference in 30-day mortality or composite death and severe complications between EVAR and OR.

8. Reimerink JJ, van der Laan MJ, Koelemay MJ, Balm R, Legemate DA. Systematic review and meta-analysis of population-based mortality from ruptured abdominal aortic aneurysm. *Br J Surg.* 2013b;100(11):1405–1413.

A systematic review and meta-analysis of 24 retrospective population-based studies reporting both prehospital and in-hospital mortality in patients with rAAA published between 1977 and 2012. A decline in mortality was observed over time, 86% before 1990 versus 74% after 1990. Almost one-third of patients died before reaching hospital.

9. Hinchliffe RJ, Powell JT, Veith FJ, Rockman CB. What does the current evidence on EVAR for ruptured AAA tell us? *Endovascular Today.* 2015.

A contemporary review of the randomized trials in patients with ruptured AAAs, with authors discussing the pros and cons of EVAR versus open surgical repair.

10. Rubenstein C, Bietz G, Davenport DL, Winkler M, Endean ED. Abdominal compartment syndrome associated with endovascular and open repair of ruptured abdominal aortic aneurysms. *J Vasc Surg.* 2015;61(3):648–654.

A single-center retrospective review of 73 patients with rAAA treated with either open repair or EVAR. Mortality was 31% (9 of 29) in the EVAR group and 48% (21 of 44) in open repair. ACS developed in 21 patients (29%) and was associated with a higher mortality (13 of 21 [62%] vs. 17 of 52 [33%]; P = .022). Intraoperative fluid and blood product requirements were significantly higher in EVAR patients who developed ACS compared with those who did not.

11. Starnes BW et al. *Ruptured Abdominal Aortic Aneurysm.* Springer; 2015.

A comprehensive manual that covers pathogenesis, clinical presentation, diagnosis, management, and postoperative complications of patients with ruptured abdominal aortic aneurysm (AAA).

12. Veith FJ, Lachat M, Mayer D et al. Collected world and single-center experience with endovascular treatment of ruptured abdominal aortic aneurysms. *Ann Surg.* 2009;250(5): 818–824.

A retrospective multicenter study comparing EVAR and open repair (OR) of ruptured abdominal aortic aneurysms. In centers performing EVAR for RAAAs whenever possible, EVAR (n = 680) was associated with a significantly lower 30-day mortality compared to open repair (n = 763), 19.7% vs. 36.3%, P < 0.0001.

13. Wanhainen A, Verzini F, Van Herzeele I et al. European Society for Vascular Surgery (ESVS) 2019 clinical practice guidelines on the management of abdominal aorto-iliac artery aneurysms. *Eur J Vasc Endovasc Surg.* 2019;57.

Current clinical practice guidelines for the management of abdominal aortic aneurysms (AAAs) by the European Society for Vascular Surgery (ESVS).

ENDOVASCULAR OR OPEN REPAIR STRATEGY FOR RUPTURED ABDOMINAL AORTIC ANEURYSM: 30-DAY OUTCOMES FROM IMPROVE RANDOMISED TRIAL

IMPROVE Trial Investigators; Powell JT, Hinchliffe RJ, Thompson MM, Sweeting MJ, Ashleigh R, Bell R, Gomes M, Greenhalgh RM, Grieve RJ, Heatley F, Thompson SG, and Ulug P, *BMJ*. 2014;348:f7661

ABSTRACT

Objective   To assess whether a strategy of endovascular repair (if aortic morphology is suitable, open repair if not) versus open repair reduces early mortality for patients with suspected ruptured abdominal aortic aneurysm.

Design   Randomized controlled trial.

Setting   30 vascular centers (29 UK, 1 Canadian), 2009–2013.

Participants   613 eligible patients (480 men) with a clinical diagnosis of ruptured aneurysm.

Interventions   316 patients were randomized to the endovascular strategy (275 confirmed ruptures, 174 anatomically suitable for endovascular repair) and 297 to open repair (261 confirmed ruptures).

Main outcome measures   30-day mortality, with 24-hour and in-hospital mortality, costs, and time and place of discharge as secondary outcomes.

Results   30-day mortality was 35.4% (112/316) in the endovascular strategy group and 37.4% (111/297) in the open repair group: odds ratio 0.92 (95% confidence interval 0.66–1.28; P = 0.62); odds ratio after adjustment for age, sex, and Hardman index 0.94 (0.67–1.33). Women may benefit more than men (interaction test P = 0.02) from the endovascular strategy: odds ratio 0.44 (0.22–0.91) versus 1.18 (0.80–1.75). Thirty-day mortality for patients with confirmed rupture was 36.4% (100/275) in the endovascular strategy group and 40.6% (106/261) in the open repair group (P = 0.31). More patients in the endovascular strategy than in the open repair group were discharged directly to home (189/201 (94%) vs. 141/183 (77%); P < 0.001). Average 30-day costs were similar between the randomized groups, with an incremental cost saving for the endovascular strategy versus open repair of £1186 (€1420; $1939) (95% confidence interval −£625 to £2997).

Conclusions   A strategy of endovascular repair was not associated with significant reduction in either 30-day mortality or cost. Longer-term cost-effectiveness evaluations are needed to assess the full effects of the endovascular strategy in both men and women.

Original Author Commentary: Janet Powell

The IMPROVE Trial for the Management of Ruptured Abdominal Aortic Aneurysms

This pragmatic multicenter trial was designed to mimic the real-life situation and assess the benefits of having 24/7 access to emergency endovascular repair. Any trial in the emergency setting is challenging, including giving fully conscious patients a chance to give consent rapidly and using relative and other consents where this was not possible. A decade earlier, I had seen my father die of a more proximal aortic rupture after three hospital transfers over 2 days without any intervention, and I wanted current patients to fare better. Amazingly, we randomized about half of all eligible patients, with 613 randomized patients with an in-hospital diagnosis of ruptured abdominal aortic aneurysm (AAA) to either endovascular repair, if morphologically suitable, or open repair. In this emergency setting, unselective randomization was challenging and about 10% of each randomized group did not receive their allocated treatment (mainly operational or morbidity issues). At 30 days, mortality was similar (~35%) in each group, although women (22% of the cohort) had lower mortality in the endovascular strategy group (24% vs. 52%). Other analyses showed that aortic morphology affected survival, a long proximal aneurysm neck favoring survival irrespective of treatment modality. Patients had an input to trial design and running: their preferred outcomes relating to early discharge home and quality of life were significantly better in the endovascular strategy group and their most dreaded outcome (amputation) also was lower after endovascular repair. To provide full health economic outcomes, all patients were followed up for at least 3 years. Interestingly, after 3 years mortality was lower in the endovascular strategy group (48% vs. 56%), there was no excess of re-interventions, and this group had a net gain in quality-adjusted life years. Taken together, this meant that the endovascular strategy was likely to be very cost effective (an important driver of health care within the UK National Health Service). After 3 years, women continued to gain more survival benefit from the endovascular strategy than men. Pragmatic randomized trials can be conducted successfully in the emergency setting, but should not focus only on short-term outcomes.

CHAPTER 40

Global Surgery

Review by Contributor: Andrew J. Michaels

Acute care surgery is a discipline born of necessity and forms a core element of our health care safety net. Recognition that many surgical emergencies were not being managed in a timely fashion led to an evolution of trauma and critical care into a more encompassing specialty providing care to all forms of emergencies requiring surgical interventions. This evolution has been a natural extension of the training, experience, and temperament of trauma surgeons, and the application of a systems-based approach so characteristic of mature trauma programs has greatly benefited this essential component of health care (Institute of Medicine Committee, 2006; Kutcher and Peitzman, 2017). Understanding how the application of these skills—clinical, administrative, and academic—to the global burden of disease that is amenable to surgical intervention can provide many opportunities for a well-rounded acute care surgeon.

In 1980, the Director-General of the World Health Organization (WHO), Halfdan Mahler, identified surgery as an integral part of primary health care and appealed to the surgical community to address the global inequities in access to surgical care as a "social injustice" (Mahler, 1980). Global surgery is an area of study, research, practice, and advocacy that seeks to improve health outcomes and achieve health equity for all people who require surgical care, with a special emphasis on underserved populations and populations in crisis. It uses collaborative, cross-sectoral, and transnational approaches and is a synthesis of population-based strategies with individual surgical care (Dare et al., 2014). Surgery, because it is neither a disease entity nor does it target a specific demographic, has not been a priority for global health initiatives. The recognition of the enormous proportion of health problems requiring surgical intervention has begun to change that perception (Hedges et al., 2010). The Lancet Commission on Global Surgery convened in 2014 to outline the human and economic impact of surgical conditions in low- and middle-income countries (LMICs). The Commission was comprised of 25 commissioners and hundreds of collaborators from more than 110 countries and 6 continents. Their report, "Global Surgery 2030: Evidence and Solutions for Achieving Health, Welfare, and Economic Development" (Meara et al., 2015) is the topic of this review and a landmark paper in public health, social justice, and health economics as well as acute care surgery.

KEY MESSAGE 1

In 2010, it was estimated that 16.9 million lives were lost from conditions requiring surgical care. This figure represents one-third of all deaths worldwide and far eclipses the number of lives lost to HIV/AIDS, TB, and malaria combined (Shrime et al., 2015). In 2015, 5 billion people lacked access (in four dimensions: timeliness, surgical capacity, safety, and affordability) to safe, affordable surgical and anesthesia care when needed. This is most severe in LMICs where 9 out of 10 people cannot access basic surgical care. In 2012, of the more than 300 million surgical procedures performed worldwide, only 6.3% were done in countries comprising the poorest 37% of the world's population (Weiser et al., 2015).

KEY MESSAGE 2

Surgical care is needed in some way for all Global Health Estimate disease subcategories, and more than 300 million surgical procedures are necessary worldwide to meet this need. The distribution of unmet need is greatest in sub-Saharan Africa and south and southeast Asia, and a conservative estimate is that an additional 143 million surgical procedures are needed each year to save lives and prevent disabilities.

KEY MESSAGE 3

Currently, 33 million individuals face catastrophic health expenditure due to payment for surgery and anesthesia each year. In addition, when non-medical costs of illness and injury are considered, another 48 million cases of catastrophic expenditure occur annually. An estimated 3.7 billion people risk catastrophic expenditures because they lack financial risk protection. This burden and risk are distributed unequally, with the greatest risk being in the poorest countries and within the poorest segment of each country, a disparity that increases with national gross domestic product (GDP).

KEY MESSAGE 4

The value of lost productivity between 2015 and 2030, secondary to surgical conditions, is estimated to be responsible for a cumulative loss to the global economy of $20.7 trillion or 1.3% of projected economic output. More than half of these losses will occur in LMICs. The most conservative estimate of the cost for expanding surgical services in the 88 LMICs would be $550 billion, a fraction of anticipated cost. Investment in surgical and anesthesia services is affordable, saves lives, and promotes economic growth.

KEY MESSAGE 5

Surgery is an indivisible, indispensable part of health care. More than two-thirds of the world's population lack access to surgical care and 50% risk catastrophic expenditure should they require this care. The authors state: "broad scale-up of quality surgical services will prevent deaths, limit disability, palliate suffering, promote economic growth, and help achieve maximum gains in health, welfare, and development for all."

The Commission also recommended several metrics by which progress can be measured and compared. These indicators include access to timely essential surgery, surgical specialist workforce density, surgical volume, perioperative mortality rate, and protection against catastrophic expenditure. The Commission will continue to monitor and measure progress and demand accountability at national and international levels for surgical capacity and outcomes in LMICs. The Lancet Commission has made important observations, novel analyses, and issued a challenge as a moral imperative for social justice in the form of universal health coverage (UHC) with surgical and anesthesia services as a critical component.

Acute care surgeons have always served as the last line of defense and frequently the first point of contact with the health care system for the most physiologically and socially challenged. Trained in emergency surgery, critical care, trauma, and often systems development, administration, quality, and research, acute care surgeons have opportunities to contribute meaningfully, and these opportunities are becoming both more prevalent and more valid (Krishnaswami et al., 2018). There are significant considerations regarding equity, culture, context and sustainability of efforts from practitioners in high income countries, but the staggering needs outlined by the Lancet Commission provide many opportunities and new challenges for today's acute care surgeon from any type of practice and at any phase of their career (Mock et al., 2018).

ANNOTATED REFERENCES FOR GLOBAL SURGERY

1. Institute of Medicine Committee on the Future of Emergency Care in the US Health Care System. *Hospital-Based Emergency Care: At the Breaking Point.* Washington, DC: National Academy Press; 2006.

   This Institute of Medicine report outlines the challenges facing emergency care systems as they struggle to provide, in addition to hospital-based emergency and trauma care, safety net support for the uninsured, public health surveillance, disaster preparedness, and other essential functions.

2. Kutcher ME, Peitzman AB. A history of acute care surgery (emergency surgery). In: *Acute Care Surgery Handbook.* Di Saverio S, Catena F, Ansaloni L, Coccolini F, Velmahos G. (Eds). Cham: Springer; 2017.

   This chapter outlines the origins and evolution of acute care surgery as a specialty and advocates for the inclusion of elective general surgery into spectrum of care provided by surgeons typically experienced in trauma, critical care, and emergency surgery.

3. Mahler H. Surgery and Health for All. Address by Dr H. Mahler, Director-General of the World Health Organization. *XXII Biennial World Congress of the International College of Surgeons*, Mexico City, Sunday 29 June 1980.

   The quest for social justice in health formed the moral basis of that momentous decision of WHO's Health Assembly in 1977 that the main social health target of governments and WHO in the coming decades should be the attainment by all the people of the world year 2000 of a level of health that will permit them to lead a socially and economically productive life. Surgery has an important role to play in primary health care, and surgery will play its proper role in bringing the people of the world nearer to the goal of health for all by the turn of the century.

4. Dare AJ, Grimes CE, Gillies R et al. Global surgery: Defining an emerging global health field. *Lancet.* 2014;384(9961):2245–2247.

   This short viewpoint outlines the importance of a robust definition for the multidisci-plinary fields that constitute global surgery. The authors emphasize that global refers not only to geographical considerations but also to the holistic nature of surgical service development, practice, and evaluation.

5. Hedges JP, Mock CN, Cherian MN. The political economy of emergency and essential surgery in global health. *World J Surg.* 2010;34:2003–2006.

   Emergency and essential surgery (EES) remains a low priority on global health agendas even though a growing body of evidence demonstrates that EES is a cost-effective public health intervention and that it holds the potential to prevent a sizable number of deaths and disabilities. The inferior status of EES should be considered, in part, a political problem and subject to political analysis. This type of political economy examination has been used for other important global health issues but has not been applied to EES. By addressing political concerns and prospects, EES can be better positioned on interna-tional agendas, thus improving surgical care delivered to the poor.

6. Meara JG, Leather AJ, Hagander L et al. Global Surgery 2030: Evidence and solutions for achieving health, welfare, and economic development. *Lancet.* 2015;386(9993):569–624.

   Four-and-a-half billion people do not have access to safe, affordable surgical and anesthesia care. One hundred forty-three million additional surgical procedures are needed in LMICs each year to save lives and prevent disability. Thirty-three million individuals face catastrophic health expenditure due to payment for surgery and anesthesia care each year. An additional 48 million cases of catastrophic expenditure are attributable to the non-medical costs of accessing surgical care. Without an investment in basic surgical scale-up of approximately US$350–420 billion over 15 years, LMICs will incur cumulative losses estimated at US$12.3 trillion.

   The human and economic consequences of untreated surgical conditions in LMICs are large and for many years have gone unrecognized. Surgery is an "indivisible, indispens-able part of health care." Surgical and anesthesia care should be an integral component of a national health system in countries at all levels of development.

7. Shrime MG, Bickler SW, Alkire BC, Mock C. Global burden of surgical disease: An estimation from the provider perspective. *Lancet Glob Health.* 2015;3(Suppl 2):S8–9.

   More than 30% of the global burden of disease requires a surgical or anesthesia inter-vention. This estimation is robust to multiple estimation methods and avoids limiting the delineation of "surgical disease" only to patients who end up on an operating table. The scale-up of a functional surgical system could have a beneficial impact on a large portion of the global burden of disease.

8. Weiser TG, Haynes AB, Molina G et al. Estimate of the global volume of surgery in 2012: An assessment supporting improved health outcomes. *Lancet.* 2015;385(Suppl 2):S11.

   Surgical volume is large and continues to grow in all economic environments. A single-procedure cesarean delivery comprised almost a third of surgical volume in the most resource-limited settings. Surgical care is an essential part of health care and is associated with increased life expectancy, yet many low-income countries fail to achieve basic levels of service. Improvements in capacity and delivery of surgical services must be a major component of health system strengthening.

9. Krishnaswami S, Stephens CQ, Yang GP et al. An academic career in global surgery: A position paper from the Society of University Surgeons Committee on Academic Global Surgery. *Surgery.* 2018;163(4):954–960.

Academic global surgery creates avenues for interested surgeons to combine scholarship and education with their clinical global surgery passions through incorporation of basic/translational, education, clinical outcomes, or health services research with global surgery. This paper reviews the development of academic global surgery, delineates the framework and factors critical to training global surgeons, and proposes models for establishing an academic career in this field.

10. Mock C, Debas H, Balch CM et al. Global surgery: Effective involvement of US academic surgery: Report of the American Surgical Association Working Group on global surgery. *Ann Surg.* 2018 Oct;268(4):557–563.

US academic surgery can most effectively decrease the burden from surgically treatable conditions in LMICs. The task will be most successful (1) if the epidemiologic pattern in each country is taken into account by focusing on those surgically treatable conditions with the highest burdens; (2) if emphasis is placed on those surgical services that are most cost effective and most feasible to scale up; and (3) if efforts are harmonized with local priorities and with existing global initiatives. The ethical principles of maximally and transparently engaging with and deferring to the interests and needs of local surgeons and their patients are of paramount importance.

GLOBAL SURGERY 2030: EVIDENCE AND SOLUTIONS FOR ACHIEVING HEALTH, WELFARE, AND ECONOMIC DEVELOPMENT

Meara JG, Leather AJ, Hagander L, Alkire BC, Alonso N, Ameh EA, Bickler SW, Conteh L, Dare AJ, Davies J, Mérisier ED, El-Halabi S, Farmer PE, Gawande A, Gillies R, Greenberg SL, Grimes CE, Gruen RL, Ismail EA, Kamara TB, Lavy C, Lundeg G, Mkandawire NC, Raykar NP, Riesel JN, Rodas E, Rose J, Roy N, Shrime MG, Sullivan R, Verguet S, Watters D, Weiser TG, Wilson IH, Yamey G, and Yip W, *Lancet.* 2015;386(9993):569–624

Editor Notes

Assessment: This remarkable monograph was created by a large Lancet Commission to address the surgical needs globally. World leaders in the Commission gathered epidemiologic data from which they produced five key messages: (1) 5 billion people do not have access to safe affordable surgical and anesthesia care; (2) 143 million additional surgical procedures are needed in LMICs (low-income and middle-income countries) to save lives and prevent disability; (3) 33 million individuals face catastrophic health expenditures due to payment for surgery and anesthesia care each year; (4) investing in surgical services in LMICs is affordable, saves lives, and promotes economic growth; (5) surgery is an "indivisible, indispensable part of health care."

Limitations: The study presents epidemiological data from a variety of national and world organizations to support their conclusions. Databases are limited by the accuracy of the material included.

Conclusions: This paper highlights the immense need for surgical interventions in LMICs and supports the global perspective that investment in expansion of surgical resources is essential.

CHAPTER 41

Early versus Late Parenteral Nutrition in Critically Ill Adults

Review by Contributor: Mark L. Shapiro

Since Stanley Dudrick's (Dudrick et al., 1968) seminal work and publication of parenteral nutrition in the late 1960s, alternatives to delivering the maximum amount of micro- and macronutrients have been ferociously debated. No longer was there a singular method to deliver nutrition, and the benefits of supporting patient physiology through intravenous nutrition were about to flourish in the literature. Further advances came in the 1970s where specific lipid emulsions (macronutrient) were added to the complex carbohydrate, mineral, and salt formulations (Fell et al., 2015). This was a very important advancement. Though complex physiologic interactions are beyond the scope of this chapter, parenteral nutrition induced liver disease is less common and its safety has vastly improved. The recognition that the fat-free formula can sometimes leads to essential fatty acid deficiency (EFAD) has also been a recognized breakthrough. Research continues to improve parenteral nutrition (PN) formulae for in adults and children.

Among clinicians, patients, and even hospital administrators, few can deny the contributions of enteral and parenteral nutrition to the routine or critically ill patient (Herbert et al., 2018). Wounds began to heal, infections have decreased, and length of stay both in the hospital and the ICU have improved with the appropriate focus on nutritional support. Still, many questions remain as arguably two debates were borne from the adjunct of PN. The debates of enteral versus parenteral nutrition continue but they should be evidenced based (Sackett, 1997; Chang and Lee, 2018). Both references hold significant importance regardless of topic, and the subject of initiating early versus late parenteral nutrition in the intensive care unit should also be evidence based.

Enteral nutrition has been used in hospitalized patients with great success (Zhuang et al., 2013). It is easily delivered orally, directly into the stomach, the duodenum, or the jejunum (Gramlich et al., 2004). Critically ill patients have similar aspiration risks when fed into the stomach or duodenum. Jejunal feeds have some supportive literature demonstrating decreased aspiration risk, and some institutions will feed patients in the OR for non-visceral surgical cases. Enteral nutrition is cost effective, simple to prepare, and can be delivered in a variety of methods (Gabriel and Ackermann, 2004). One of the greatest risks of delivering enteral nutrition is aspiration, or intolerance. In addition, some institutional policies include checking gastric residuals. The thought process is that some predetermined volume increases aspiration risk. Contemporary studies are calling into question this practice as newer results contradict this practice (McClave et al., 2005).

Aspiration pneumonitis can lead to prolonged length of stay, ICU days, inappropriate or appropriate antibiotic usage, ventilator days, and death. These complications without a doubt are at the nidus of impassioned pleas for early PN. Another attempt at avoiding aspiration risk includes the practice of continuous feeds into the stomach rather than bolus feeds. Bolus feeds would be the more physiologic method of delivering nutrition, and is arguably more efficient for the caregiver. Continuous feeds, via an electronic pump device, would in theory deliver lower volumes over prolonged periods of time. Once again, the literature has been controversial. More recent studies have stronger evidence to support that bolus feeds are safe to administer (Ichimaru, 2018).

PN can be delivered in two forms, peripheral (delivered through a peripheral vein, should have a concentration of <900 mOsm/L, does not meet specific nutritional goals, and has a higher risk of thrombosis and phlebitis) and total forms. Although both have been demonstrated to be delivered safely in the critically ill patient, benefits of partial parenteral nutrition remain unclear when enteral and total parenteral nutrition (TPN) are available (Anderson et al., 2003). Multiple complex concerns must be addressed prior to prescribing TPN. These range from access and economic concerns to the ethical and social controversies.

Supportive evidence for TPN in patients who have the ability to tolerate enteral nutrition is sparse. The timing of TPN is also controversial. The ability of a surgeon at the time of an operation to predict gastroparesis or a postoperative ileus has yet to be investigated, and as such it proves challenging to determine which patient requires immediate postoperative nutritional support. In addition, the literature has mixed reviews which continue to weigh concerns for delays in nutritional delivery versus actual delivery and outcomes. From these concerns, a select number of high-quality investigations have delivered surprising results for those who have been taught and endorse early, calorie-dense supplementation, specifically when augmented parenterally (National Heart, Lung, and Blood Institute Acute Respiratory Distress Syndrome [ARDS] Clinical Trials Network, Rice et al., 2012; TARGET Investigators, 2018).

The Casaer Trial is one such study (Casaer and Van den Berghe, 2011). This multicenter, randomized, prospective trial addressed a European standard (early delivery of PN as defined as <48 hours) against the American and Canadian standard (late delivery of PN as defined as 8 days). Over 4500 patients were enrolled (8700 initially screened from 7 ICUs) and randomized to each group over a 40-month period. These patients were nutritionally at risk but were not chronically malnourished. The primary intent was to determine if the group could prevent caloric deficiencies during critical illness. Should the group be successful, potential complications may be prevented. This information was analyzed and reported as secondary outcomes for this trial. Euglycemia was maintained between 80 and 110 mg/dL via insulin infusion. Of the roughly 4000 patients, 3600 were deemed ineligible; most exclusions (1344) were <18 years old, 548 were taking oral nutrition, 458 did not give consent, and 328 did not have a catheter placed centrally. Those included in the study in both arms did not demonstrate any statistical differences and were well matched in their randomization, including APACHE II score

(23 ± 10–11, both arms). Initial nutrition included 20% dextrose for 2 days in the early TPN group and 5% dextrose for the late TPN group. The results demonstrated statistical significance in favor of those patients in the late TPN arm in the following categories: ICU length of stay, new infections (blood, pulmonary, and wound), duration of mechanical ventilation when >2 days as well as medial duration of renal replacement therapy, hospital length of stay, and mean total incremental health care cost (a difference of about USD $1600). There were twice as many (81 compared to 45) episodes of hypoglycemia in the late arm, and median peak C-reactive protein levels during the ICU stay was higher in the late group. Interestingly, the functional status (6-minute walk distance and activities of daily living) of patients from both arms were equivalent at discharge.

This investigation contradicts what many have reported and practiced for years, that early and dense nutrition is beneficial and improves outcomes. This study and subsequent other well-designed, prospective trials have contradicted previous studies and conventional practice. The tendency to "overtreat" rather than "undertreat" should not be taken lightly, as the results of these contemporary studies demonstrate higher risks or no difference in outcomes with increased costs and potential complications. The improvements in the quality of catheters, catheter care, insertion techniques, heightened awareness of central line–associated bloodstream infections (CLABSI), and data collection suggest a decreased risk of infectious and mechanical complications in the delivery of PN (Pittiruti et al., 2009). Similarly, thoughtful consideration must be exercised when deciding when to initiate nutritional therapy as well as the route and concentration (energy density). The critically ill patient appears to be at risk for the consequences of emergent deployment of TPN. The Casaer investigation strictly addresses the adult critically ill patient. Interestingly, some of the same authors (Fivez et al., 2016) found similar findings in the pediatric population in a subsequent investigation. Differences in outcomes of the routine (non-critically ill) patient are challenging to determine, as they may be more immunocompetent.

The embodiment of the nutrition literature has been low level (III/IV) and low grade (expert opinion). The American Society for Parenteral and Enteral Nutrition (ASPEN) Guidelines are no exception. The recent contributions of prospective, randomized, controlled studies introduced in this chapter remain the standard and give the necessary direction required for decision making regarding both evidence-based and interpersonal-based medicine.

ANNOTATED REFERENCES FOR EARLY VERSUS LATE PARENTERAL NUTRITION IN CRITICALLY ILL ADULTS

1. Dudrick SJ, Wilmore DW, Vars HM, Rhoads JE. Long-term total parenteral nutrition with growth, development and positive nitrogen balance. *Surgery*. 1968;64:134–142.

   One in a large series of landmark papers demonstrating the ability to treat malnutrition via the bloodstream. Dudrick and colleagues at UPENN under Dr. Rhoads in the field of parenteral nutrition have saved countless lives and will forever be discussed and challenged in the surgical literature.

2. Fell GL, Nandivada P, Gura KM, Puder M. Intravenous lipid emulsions in parenteral nutrition. *Adv Nutr*. 2015;6(5):600–610.

   Although largely pediatric based, this reference goes into detail to explain the importance and mechanism of lipid emulsions in PN. It further explains the potential pathology and complications associated with and without these formulations.

3. Zhuang CL, Ye XZ, Zhang CJ, Dong QT, Chen BC, Yu Z. Early versus traditional postoperative oral feeding in patients undergoing elective colorectal surgery: A meta-analysis of randomized clinical trials. *Dig Surg*. 2013;30(3):225–332.

   Interesting study examining early versus late oral feeding in colorectal patients. Primary outcomes included length of stay, anastomotic dehiscence, and infectious complications. Secondary outcomes included vomiting, 30-day mortality, and cost. Early postoperative feeding decreased length of stay and total postoperative complications. There was no difference in anastomotic leak, mortality, pneumonia, and wound infections.

4. Gramlich L, Kichian K, Pinilla J, Rodych NJ, Dhaliwal R, Heyland DK. Does enteral nutrition compared to parenteral nutrition result in better outcomes in critically ill adult patients? A systematic review of the literature. *Nutrition*. 2004;20(10):843–848.

   Meta-analysis of 13 studies that met inclusion criteria which demonstrated the benefits of enteral nutrition (EN) over PN in critically ill patients. Infectious complications were lowest in the EN group, and four studies had lower costs associated with EN. Ventilator days and length of stay were not significantly different. Intolerance to EN was inconclusive.

5. Sackett DL. Evidence based medicine. *Semin Perinatol*. 1997;21(1):3–5.

   One of the earliest and most cited papers on the call for the practice of evidence-based medicine (EBM). It nicely balances the idea of EBM, experience, and measured decision making as it applies to the individual patient.

6. Chang S, Lee T. Beyond evidence-based medicine. *N Engl J Med*. 2018;379:1983–1985.

   Introduction to a more contemporary paradigm of "interpersonal medicine." This looks at the gap between the strictly dogmatic practice of hard EBM and outcomes versus the practicality of the patient's ability to adhere to the rigorous plans clinicians set forth. The article examines the patient's circumstances, capabilities, and preferences.

7. Herbert G, Perry R, Andersen HK et al. Early enteral nutrition within 24 hours of lower gastrointestinal surgery versus later commencement for length of hospital stay and postoperative complications. *Cochrane Database Syst Rev*. 2018 Oct 24;10.

   Large Cochran database review. This large meta-analysis suggests improved length of stay. Key elements in outcomes (mortality, complications, etc.) were mixed and demonstrate the fallibility in these types of reviews and the equipoise of the authors who call for better designed, more conclusive investigations.

8. Gabriel SA, Ackermann RJ. Placement of nasoenteral feeding tubes using external magnetic guidance. *JPEN J Parenter Enteral Nutr*. 2004;28(2):119–122.

   One of the recent advances in enteral nutrition is the external magnetic guidance of a feeding tube. It can be placed at bedside with low cost and has been shown to be safe and effective. It is supported by an 80% success rate into the jejunum in recent studies. This adds to the literature safety profiles for decreased risk of aspiration compared to those placed in the stomach or "post-pyloric" (a more unfortunate and confusing term). Post-pyloric implies anywhere past the pylorus, making it difficult to decipher earlier works on burned children demonstrating equivalent aspiration risks when feeding tubes are placed in the stomach or duodenum. Jejunal placement had significantly lower aspiration events.

9. McClave SA, Lukan JK, Stefater JA et al. Poor validity of residual volumes as a marker for risk of aspiration in critically ill patients. *Crit Care Med.* 2005;33(2):324–330.

Frequently quoted study examining gastric residual volumes and their lack of utility and poor sensitivity in predicting aspiration when used routinely. It is a small (40 patients), randomized study with multiple samples (>1100 samples) comparing aspirates, residual volume, and patient management based on the residual volume of 200 mL versus 400 mL. It also addresses the lack of benefit in using adjuncts such as methylene blue. The importance of the physical exam, tube placement, and location remain important in preventing aspiration risk. Gastric residual volume is not recommended for routine management of tube-fed patients. Percutaneous gastric tubes may be more beneficial than nasoenteric tubes in decreasing the risk of aspiration.

10. Ichimaru S. Methods of enteral nutrition administration in critically ill patients: Continuous, cyclic, intermittent, and bolus feeding. *Nutr Clin Pract.* 2018;33(6):790–795.

From the ASPEN Society, a review article comparing intermittent versus bolus feeding. The existing studies remain low-level studies without a definitively superior method. Bolus feeds, however, appear to have advantages in muscle protein synthesis, gastrointestinal hormone secretion, and efficiency when the feeding tube is in the stomach. Higher-grade studies are required to determine a conclusive recommendation.

11. Anderson ADG, Palmer D, MacFie J. Peripheral parenteral nutrition. *BJS.* 2003;90(9):1048–1054.

Large meta-analysis performed addressing a lack of consensus guidelines. Results demonstrate that 50% of inpatients may benefit from PPN. This publication discusses best practices for delivery, formula, cannula, and infusion techniques. The advantage of PPN over TPN is unclear.

12. National Heart, Lung, and Blood Institute Acute Respiratory Distress Syndrome (ARDS) Clinical Trials Network, Rice TW, Wheeler AP, Thompson BT et al. Initial trophic vs. full enteral feeding in patients with acute lung injury: The EDEN randomized trial. *JAMA.* 2012;307(8):795–803.

Randomized, multicenter, open-label trial of 1000 critically ill adults with acute lung injury or ARDS supplemented with trophic (50%–65% of goal) or goal enteral feeds. Results demonstrated no differences in mortality at 60 days, infectious complications, or ventilator-free days. Patients fed with trophic level supplementation did significantly better, with less vomiting, gastric residual volumes, constipation, and fluid balance at 7 days.

13. TARGET Investigators, for the ANZICS Clinical Trials Group. Energy-dense versus routine enteral nutrition in the critically ill. *N Engl J Med.* 2018;379:1823–1834.

Large multicenter, randomized, double-blinded trial examining energy-dense (1.5 kcal/mL) versus routine (1 kcal/mL) enteral nutrition. Supplementation was delivered as 1 mL/Kg ideal body weight per hour. This was initiated within 12 hours of delivering nutritional support in ventilated patients. Results of this study demonstrated no difference between groups when it came to survival time, number of days alive out of the ICU, end organ support, or incidence of infectious complications or adverse events. This is an important contribution to the literature due to its design and message that more calories are not equivalent to improved outcomes. Requests for TPN in addition to enteral feeds to increase calories may not be beneficial and should be definitively studied.

14. Pittiruti M, Hamilton H, Biffi R, MacFie J, Pertkiewicz M. ESPEN Guidelines on Parenteral Nutrition: Central venous catheters (access, care, diagnosis and therapy of complications). *Clin Nutr.* 2009;28:365–377.

   This review is specifically directed toward TPN and commonly upheld concerns regarding complications. It elegantly highlights the concerns and points out the timeless concerns which are being addressed and practiced today. "Scrub the Hub" campaigns, timely removal, vigilance, and "champions" have contributed to improvements in line care and complications. Adding various anticoagulants has not improved thrombosis rates and is not recommended. Ultrasound guidance for placement of centrally placed lines has decreased some complications and is currently the standard of care. These European guidelines do not differ significantly from the American guidelines. With the exception of ultrasound guidance, the evidence in most of the literature thus far remains low (Grade B/C).

15. Fivez T, Kerklaan D, Mesotten D et al. Early versus late parenteral nutrition in critically ill children. *N Engl J Med.* 2016;374:1111–1122.

   Well designed multicenter, randomized, controlled trial of >1400 critically ill children. All children were started on enteral feeds and gradually increased to 80% goal. TPN was initiated either early (within 24 hours) or late (on the 8th day) to deliver a goal of 80% of their caloric targets. Results demonstrated were similar to the adult study in that late parenteral nutrition decreased length of hospital and ICU stay, decreased ventilator days, provided earlier live discharge, and decreased proportion of patients requiring renal replacement therapy.

16. Casaer MP and Van den Berghe G. Early versus late parenteral nutrition in critically ill adults. *N Engl J Med.* 2011;365:506–517.

EARLY VERSUS LATE PARENTERAL NUTRITION IN CRITICALLY ILL ADULTS

Casaer MP, Mesotten D, Hermans G, Wouters PJ, Schetz M, Meyfroidt G, Van Cromphaut S, Ingels C, Meersseman P, Muller J, Vlasselaers D, Debaveye Y, Desmet L, Dubois J, Van Assche A, Vanderheyden S, Wilmer A, and Van den Berghe G, *N Engl J Med.* 2011;365:506–517

ABSTRACT

Background   Controversy exists about the timing of the initiation of parenteral nutrition in critically ill adults in whom caloric targets cannot be met by enteral nutrition alone.

Methods   In this randomized, multicenter trial, we compared early initiation of parenteral nutrition (European guidelines) with late initiation (American and Canadian guidelines) in adults in the intensive care unit (ICU) to supplement insufficient enteral nutrition. In 2312 patients, parenteral nutrition was initiated within 48 hours after ICU admission (early-initiation group), whereas in 2328 patients, parenteral nutrition was not initiated before day 8 (late-initiation group). A protocol for the early initiation of enteral nutrition was applied to both groups, and insulin was infused to achieve normoglycemia.

Results   Patients in the late-initiation group had a relative increase of 6.3% in the likelihood of being discharged alive earlier from the ICU (hazard ratio, 1.06; 95%

confidence interval [CI], 1.00–1.13; P = 0.04) and from the hospital (hazard ratio, 1.06; 95% CI, 1.00–1.13; P = 0.04), without evidence of decreased functional status at hospital discharge. Rates of death in the ICU and in the hospital and rates of survival at 90 days were similar in the two groups. Patients in the late-initiation group, as compared with the early-initiation group, had fewer ICU infections (22.8% vs. 26.2%, P = 0.008) and a lower incidence of cholestasis (P < 0.001). The late-initiation group had a relative reduction of 9.7% in the proportion of patients requiring more than 2 days of mechanical ventilation (P = 0.006), a median reduction of 3 days in the duration of renal-replacement therapy (P = 0.008), and a mean reduction in health care costs of €1110 (about $1600) (P = 0.04).

Conclusions   Late initiation of parenteral nutrition was associated with faster recovery and fewer complications, as compared with early initiation. (Funded by the Methusalem Program of the Flemish Government and others; EPaNIC ClinicalTrials. gov Number, NCT00512122.)

Original Author Commentary: Michael P. Casaer and Greet Van den Berghe

For decades, nutrition therapy in intensive care units (ICUs) strived at attenuating the dramatic acute catabolism. For this purpose, early administration of preferentially enteral nutrition (EN) was advocated. If EN could not cover the estimated needs, guidelines recommended complementing EN with parenteral nutrition (PN) but disagreed on when to initiate PN.

This question was addressed by the EPaNIC Trial, the first large nutrition RCT in ICU, adhering to new standards of trial registration and conduct. Patients were randomized to receive either PN, targeting nutritional target, if EN was insufficient on ICU-day 2 (early-PN) or to receive no PN before day 8 (late-PN).

Late-PN—despite the resulting nutritional deficit—resulted in faster recovery, fewer infections and complications, better muscle force, and a shorter ICU and hospital stay. In 517 patients, admitted after complicated abdominal or esophageal surgery, late-PN resulted in 1 week of near-starvation, yet its beneficial effects were even more pronounced.

Thereafter, we conducted a similar RCT (PEPaNIC) in pediatric ICUs in Belgium, the Netherlands, and Canada. Despite their limited reserves and higher presumed metabolic needs, children—and particularly neonates—benefited even more from late-PN.

The deleterious effect of early-PN on muscle force was explained by inhibition of autophagy, an intracellular mechanism for damage clearing. These data and detailed analyses of the relation between macronutrient intake and outcome in EPaNIC and PEPaNIC revealed that not the parenteral route per se, but the early high dose of—particularly—amino acids may have hampered recovery.

EPaNIC showed that it is possible, ethical, and crucial to evaluate established therapies in adequately powered RCTs.

Funding: MPC holds a Post-Doctoral Research Grant (18322817N) by FWO Flanders and a Project Grant (C24/17/070) by the Catholic University Leuven. GVdB holds an ERC (ERC-AdvG-2017-785809) and Methusalem (Meth-14/06) Grant.

CHAPTER 42

Sepsis

Review by Contributor: Craig M. Coopersmith

Sepsis is life-threatening organ dysfunction caused by a dysregulated host response to infection (Singer et al., 2016). Research during the last 15 years has led to a tremendous increase in the understanding of sepsis on multiple scales, ranging from molecular to whole organ (Hotchkiss et al., 2016). Despite this, over 150 negative clinical trials have been performed in sepsis, demonstrating profound difficulty in translating preclinical studies to the bedside.

In the absence of our ability to manipulate the host response for therapeutic gain, the mainstays of sepsis therapy include antimicrobial therapy, fluid resuscitation, and supportive care. Despite this simple-sounding approach, care of the septic patient is complex, and the most recent Surviving Sepsis campaign guidelines for the management of sepsis include 93 statements on the early management and resuscitation of sepsis and septic shock (Rhodes et al., 2016). These include 32 strong recommendations, 39 weak recommendations, and 18 best practice statements.

While guidelines are vitally important for the management of septic patients, their length and depth represent a double-edged sword. Compliance with a vast literature of evidence-based recommendations associated with improved outcomes should lead to decreased mortality in a disease that still carries a mortality of 20%–40%. At the same time, the sheer volume of recommendations and evidence can be overwhelming for many bedside practitioners.

In contrast to guidelines, bundles represent a small number of easily followed actions that can be used by practitioners worldwide. The Surviving Sepsis campaign initially instituted the concept of sepsis bundles in 2004, containing a 6-hour resuscitation bundle with six elements and a 24-hour management bundle with four elements. Compliance with the bundles was associated with decreased mortality in multiple studies. The largest of these examined 29,740 patients in 218 hospitals over 7 years and demonstrated that for every quarter that a site participated in the Surviving Sepsis campaign, mortality went down by 0.7% (Levy et al., 2015, 2018). Notably, mortality varied greatly with bundle compliance, with a nearly 10% absolute difference in mortality between sites with low versus high compliance for the resuscitation bundle (38.6% vs. 29.0%).

Over the subsequent 8 years, studies supporting multiple elements in the management bundle previously shown to be beneficial in randomized controlled trials (including tight blood glucose control and activated protein C) were unable to be replicated. At the same time, increasing evidence was published on the importance of timely antibiotics. Specifically, Kumar and colleagues examined the impact of delays in initiation of antibiotics in nearly 3000 patients with septic shock in 14 ICUs (Kumar et al., 2006). They found that for every hour antibiotics were delayed, mortality increased by 7.6%, and an increase in mortality was detectable by the second hour. Further, they demonstrated that only 50% of patients with septic shock received appropriate antibiotics within 6 hours.

Based upon an evolving literature (both positive and negative), the Surviving Sepsis bundles were revised in 2012 to include a 3-hour severe sepsis bundle and a 6-hour septic shock bundle. The 3-hour bundle contained four elements: (a) drawing a lactate level, (b) obtaining blood cultures, (c) initiating broad-spectrum antibiotics, and (d) administering 30 mL/kg of crystalloid for patients who were hypotensive or had an elevated lactate. The 6-hour bundle also contained four elements, including applying vasopressors to maintain mean arterial pressure >65 mmHg for patients who were not responsive to fluid resuscitation.

Subsequent studies validated the importance of the bundles. A study of over 5000 septic patients enrolled over 4.5 years demonstrated that even short delays in the elements of the 3-hour bundle were associated with increased mortality (range 20 minutes to 125 minutes depending on bundle element) and concluded that there is no evidence that waiting 3 hours to complete the bundle is safe (Pruinelli et al., 2018). Further, a retrospective study of nearly 12,000 septic patients in nine hospitals demonstrated that initiation of fluid boluses in 2 hours or less was associated with lower hospital mortality, length of study, ICU days, and mechanical ventilation (Leisman et al., 2017).

Despite evidence of efficacy of sepsis bundles, compliance has historically been quite low, with the largest study demonstrating compliance at less than 30% (Levy et al., 2015, 2018). However, in 2013, New York State began requiring hospitals to follow protocols for early identification and treatment of septic shock. Hospitals were allowed to choose their protocol as long as it complied with the 3- and 6-hour bundles. This allowed for a real-world test of time to treatment and mortality in a large-scale program with mandated sepsis treatment (Seymour et al., 2017). A total of 49,331 patients at 149 hospitals were studied, of which 82.5% completed the 3-hour bundle within 3 hours, with a median time to completion of 1.3 hours. The study demonstrated that a longer time to completion of the bundle was associated with higher risk-adjusted mortality, which increased with each hour bundle completion was delayed. Similar results were demonstrated for antibiotics, where longer time to administration of antibiotics was associated with higher mortality. Interestingly, time to completion of fluid bolus was not associated with mortality, which differed from prior studies showing a benefit of more rapid fluid initiation as opposed to bolus completion (Leisman et al., 2017).

Significant evidence suggests that any delay in early treatment of sepsis is associated with higher mortality. While there have been historic concerns regarding the feasibility of rapid sepsis care, mandates in the management of myocardial infarction have been remarkably successful with 93% of patients meeting the goal of a 90-minute time window from ED presentation to percutaneous coronary intervention (Masoudi et al., 2017). Based upon this, the Surviving Sepsis campaign revised its recommendations again to include a single hour bundle containing elements of the prior 3- and 6-hour bundles (lactate, blood cultures, antibiotics, 30 mL/kg crystalloid, pressors) (Levy et al., 2015, 2018). The recognition that sepsis is a true immediate life-threatening emergency with a "golden hour" similar to other time-sensitive conditions is a paradigm shift and should avoid preventable deaths caused by treatment delay.

ANNOTATED REFERENCES FOR SEPSIS

1. Singer M, Deutschman CS, Seymour CW et al. The Third International Consensus Definitions for Sepsis and Septic Shock (Sepsis-3). *JAMA*. 2016;315(8):801–810.

   The updated definition of sepsis (Sepsis 3) defines the syndrome as life-threatening organ dysfunction caused by a dysregulated host response to infection. Septic shock is defined as a subset of sepsis in which profound circulatory, cellular, and metabolic abnormalities are associated with a greater risk of mortality than sepsis alone. The concept of systemic inflammatory response syndrome (SIRS) disappears from this new definition as does the term "severe sepsis" since sepsis is life-threatening by definition.

2. Hotchkiss RS, Moldawer LL, Opal SM, Reinhart K, Turnbull IR, Vincent JL. Sepsis and septic shock. *Nat Rev Dis Primers*. 2016;2:16045.

   This review of the pathophysiology of sepsis outlines the prolonged inflammation, immune suppression, organ injury, and lean tissue wasting associated with the disease. It also covers the generally unsuccessful attempts to date at immunomodulation and identification of a biomarker for sepsis and septic shock.

3. Rhodes A, Evans LE, Alhazzani W et al. Surviving sepsis campaign: International guidelines for management of sepsis and septic shock: 2016. *Crit Care Med*. 2016;45(3):486–552.

   The Surviving Sepsis campaign guidelines are the most recent compendium of evidence-based recommendations for the management of early sepsis. The guidelines are comprehensive in nature, covering a diverse range of treatment issues ranging from infection management to resuscitation to pressors to mechanical ventilation.

4. Levy MM, Rhodes A, Phillips GS et al. Surviving sepsis campaign: Association between performance metrics and outcomes in a 7.5-year study. *Crit Care Med*. 2015;43(1):3–12.

   This study examines 29,740 subjects in 218 hospitals enrolled in the Surviving Sepsis campaign from 2005–2012. The study demonstrated that the adjusted odds ratio for mortality decreased by 0.7% per quarter while a site participated. Additionally, compliance (which averaged less than 30%) directly impacted survival with 38.6% mortality with low resuscitation bundle compliance compared to 29.0% mortality with high compliance.

5. Kumar A, Roberts D, Wood KE et al. Duration of hypotension before initiation of effective antimicrobial therapy is the critical determinant of survival in human septic shock. *Crit Care Med*. 2006;34(6):1589–1596.

   This retrospective study of 2731 patients in 14 ICUs examines the prevalence and impact on mortality in delays on initiation of effective antibiotic therapy after the onset of septic shock. Mortality increased by 7.6% for each hour antibiotics were delayed, with increases in death detectable by the second hour. Remarkably, only 50% of patients received appropriate antibiotic therapy within 6 hours of the diagnosis of septic shock.

6. Pruinelli L, Westra BL, Yadav P et al. Delay within the 3-hour surviving sepsis campaign guideline on mortality for patients with severe sepsis and septic shock. *Crit Care Med.* 2018;46(4):500–505.

This retrospective cohort study of 5072 patients from six hospitals and 45 clinics examines whether delays of specific elements from the Surviving Sepsis campaign 3-hour bundles are associated with increased mortality from sepsis or septic shock. The authors found that even short delays in bundle compliance were associated with increased mortality and that there was no evidence that 3 hours is a safe time for bundle completion. Depending on which element of the bundle was assessed, delays ranging from 20 minutes to 125 minutes were associated with increased mortality.

7. Leisman DE, Goldman C, Doerfler ME et al. Patterns and outcomes associated with time-liness of initial crystalloid resuscitation in a prospective sepsis and septic shock cohort. *Crit Care Med.* 2017;45(10):1596–606.

This retrospective study of 11,000 patients in nine hospitals examined the impact of timeliness of initial fluid resuscitation on mortality in sepsis and septic shock. The authors found that initiation of fluid bolus in <120 minutes was associated with significantly lower hospital mortality, mechanical ventilation, ICU days, and hospital length of stay.

8. Masoudi FA, Ponirakis A, de Lemos JA et al. Trends in US Cardiovascular Care: 2016 Report from 4 ACC National Cardiovascular Data Registries. *J Am Coll Cardiol.* 2017;69(11):1427–1450.

This recent report on 667,424 percutaneous coronary interventions from 1612 hospitals using the National Cardiovascular Data Registry demonstrates that 93.5% of patients with ST elevation myocardial infarction are treated within the guideline standard of 90 minutes from presentation to intervention. The average time from "door to balloon" was 59 minutes. This large-scale registry accounts for over 90% of hospitals with the capac-ity to perform percutaneous coronary interventions and is a real-world example of how logistical concerns can be overcome, and a complex intervention can be performed in a time-sensitive manner nationally.

9. Levy MM, Evans LE, Rhodes A. The surviving sepsis campaign bundle: 2018 update. *Crit Care Med.* 2018;46(6):997–1000.

The 2018 Surviving Sepsis campaign hour-1 bundle contains five elements: (a) measure lactate levels, remeasure if >2 mmol/L; (b) obtain blood cultures prior to administration of antibiotics; (c) administer broad-spectrum antibiotics; (d) begin rapid administration of 30 mL/kg of crystalloids for hypotension or lactate >4 mmol/L; and (e) apply vasopressors if patient is hypotensive during or after fluid resuscita-tion to maintain mean arterial pressure >65 mmHg. The fact that the revised bundle has all elements in a single 1-hour time frame recognizes that sepsis is a time-sensitive emergency.

Landmark Article of 21st Century

TIME TO TREATMENT AND MORTALITY DURING MANDATED EMERGENCY CARE FOR SEPSIS

Seymour CW, Gesten F, Prescott HC, Friedrich ME, Iwashyna TJ, Phillips GS, Lemeshow S, Osborn T, Terry KM, and Levy MM, *N Engl J Med*. 2017; 376(23):2235–2244

ABSTRACT

Background In 2013, New York began requiring hospitals to follow protocols for the early identification and treatment of sepsis. However, there is controversy about whether more rapid treatment of sepsis improves outcomes in patients.

Methods We studied data from patients with sepsis and septic shock that were reported to the New York State Department of Health from April 1, 2014 to June 30, 2016. Patients had a sepsis protocol initiated within 6 hours after arrival in the emergency department and had all items in a 3-hour bundle of care for patients with sepsis (i.e., blood cultures, broad-spectrum antibiotic agents, and lactate measurement) completed within 12 hours. Multilevel models were used to assess the associations between the time until completion of the 3-hour bundle and risk-adjusted mortality. We also examined the times to the administration of antibiotics and to the completion of an initial bolus of intravenous fluid.

Results Among 49,331 patients at 149 hospitals, 40,696 (82.5%) had the 3-hour bundle completed within 3 hours. The median time to completion of the 3-hour bundle was 1.30 hours (interquartile range, 0.65–2.35), the median time to the administration of antibiotics was 0.95 hours (interquartile range, 0.35–1.95), and the median time to completion of the fluid bolus was 2.56 hours (interquartile range, 1.33–4.20). Among patients who had the 3-hour bundle completed within 12 hours, a longer time to the completion of the bundle was associated with higher risk-adjusted in-hospital mortality (odds ratio, 1.04 per hour; 95% confidence interval [CI], 1.02–1.05; P < 0.001), as was a longer time to the administration of antibiotics (odds ratio, 1.04 per hour; 95% CI, 1.03–1.06; P < 0.001) but not a longer time to the completion of a bolus of intravenous fluids (odds ratio, 1.01 per hour; 95% CI, 0.99–1.02; P = 0.21).

Conclusions More rapid completion of a 3-hour bundle of sepsis care and rapid administration of antibiotics, but not rapid completion of an initial bolus of intravenous fluids, were associated with lower risk-adjusted in-hospital mortality. (Funded by the National Institutes of Health and others.)

Editor Notes

This is an important study which analyzed 49,331 patients with sepsis and septic shock at 149 hospitals in New York State over a three year period, to understand the potential benefits of early completion of a 3-hour sepsis bundle. The primary interventions were administration of antibiotics and fluid boluses.

Assessment: This very large experience suggested that completion of the antibiotic administration within 3 hours of arrival, which was noted in 82.5%, resulted in a lower likelihood of death. The timing of the fluid bolus did not appear to influence mortality.

Limitations: As this bundle was to be employed in all of the patients in New York state, failure to achieve completion of the bundle (and expeditious administration of antibiotics in particular), may reflect either poor care by clinicians at those hospitals or a delay in diagnosis of sepsis in a more obscure or complicated patient population.

Conclusions: This study supports the prevailing opinion that timely administration of antibiotics in patients with sepsis results in better outcomes. The lack of mortality benefit of early fluid infusion was informative.

CHAPTER 43

Ventilator-Associated Pneumonia

Review by Contributors: Atif Jastaniah and Morad Hameed

Ventilator-associated pneumonia (VAP), which, by definition, has its onset at least 48 hours after intubation and the initiation of mechanical ventilation, is the most common nosocomial infection in ventilated patients. It develops in 8%–20% of intensive care unit (ICU) patients and in up to 65% of patients in high-risk populations (Ibrahim et al. 2001; Chastre and Fagon, 2002; Safdar et al., 2005; Canadian Critical Care Trials Group, 2006) and has a significant impact on clinical and economic outcomes (Safdar et al., 2005; Canadian Critical Care Trials Group, 2006). It is estimated that VAP is associated with an increase in ICU length of stay (LOS) of up to 6 days, with mortality ranging from 20% to 50%, and up to 76% if the infection is caused by high-risk pathogens (Ibrahim et al. 2001; Chastre and Fagon, 2002; Safdar et al., 2005). Reducing the enormous burden of VAP requires diagnostic vigilance, prompt therapeutic action, and systemwide, evidence-based prevention measures.

DIAGNOSIS

The presence of VAP is signaled by clinical observations including fever, tachypnea, increased purulent secretions, and changes in ventilator mechanics including reduced tidal volumes or increased pressures. Laboratory findings include hypoxemia on blood gases and leukocytosis (Kalil et al., 2016). The diagnosis is established more definitively with two other findings: new or worsening infiltrates on chest x-ray and microbiological evidence of infection (Chastre and Fagon, 2002). Because chest x-ray infiltrates can suggest a broad differential diagnosis (including aspiration pneumonitis, pulmonary contusion, pulmonary hemorrhage, vasculitis, infiltrating neoplasms, cryptogenic organizing pneumonia, and acute respiratory distress syndrome [ARDS]) microbiologic data is a mainstay of diagnosis and an important guide for therapy.

The method of obtaining bacterial evidence of infection has been debated in multiple studies. Bronchioalveolar lavage (BAL) offers the theoretical benefits of high sensitivity and specificity, high diagnostic accuracy, and reductions in unnecessary antibiotic exposure, but it can be more expensive and time consuming than obtaining samples from endotracheal tube aspirates. In a randomized trial done by the Canadian Critical Care Trials Group, there was no difference in 28-day mortality between patients in whom BAL was used to obtain the sample compared to those who underwent noninvasive procurement of endotracheal aspirates (adjusted relative risk of death was 1.01). Also, there was no difference in treatment effect, ICU LOS, or hospital stay between the two diagnostic methods (Canadian Critical Care Trials Group, 2006).

Although recent guidelines have suggested that noninvasive endotracheal aspiration is sufficient to obtain diagnostic samples (Kalil et al., 2016), BAL with quantitative analysis is still justifiable and is widely used based on the rationale that cultures of endotracheal aspirates lack specificity for invasive infection. An influential cadaver study of ICU patients who were considered to have VAP confirmed infection in only 67% of subjects and suggested that we may be treating many non-infectious conditions with antibiotics (Marquette et al., 1995). The choice of diagnostic methods for VAP holds significant consequences for the scope and duration of antibiotic therapy, the development of antimicrobial resistance and antibiotic-associated complications, and the costs of health care.

TREATMENT

With the high mortality rates associated with VAP, diagnostic measures (sputum and blood cultures), source control (with effective antimicrobial treatment), and resuscitation should be initiated promptly. A delay in the initiation of the appropriate antibiotics beyond 24 h has a significant impact on the risk of mortality (Iregui et al., 2002).

The antimicrobial strategy must be aggressive up front, even in the face of diagnostic uncertainty, accounting for the possibility of infection with resistant organisms and host vulnerabilities, while balancing the implications of overuse of antibiotics (including the promotion of antibiotic resistance and the risk of complications such as *Clostridioides difficile* colitis). The strategy is guided by well-established risk factors for the presence of multidrug resistance (MDR) (Kalil et al., 2016):

1. Prior intravenous antibiotic use within the past 90 days
2. Five or more days in hospital prior to the suspicion of VAP
3. Septic shock at the onset of VAP
4. ARDS prior to the onset of VAP
5. Need for renal replacement therapy prior to the onset of VAP
6. Being treated in units with >10% MDR among Gram-negative bacilli, or where the prevalence of MDR among Gram-negative organisms are unknown
7. Being treated in units where >10%–20% of *S. aureus* isolates are methicillin resistant, or in units where the prevalence of methicillin-resistant *S. aureus* (MRSA) is not known

The latter two points emphasize the need for intensivists to be familiar with local antibiograms and to adjust therapies based on local knowledge and probabilities.

In the absence of any of these risk factors for MDR, suspected VAP can initially be treated empirically with single agents with activity against *Pseudomonas* and methicillin sensitive *S. aureus* (two usual and dangerous suspects), such as piperacillin-tazobactam (Kalil et al., 2016). Patients with any of the aforementioned risks for infection with MDR organisms should receive coverage with two agents with activity against *Pseudomonas* and other Gram-negative bacilli (e.g., piperacillin-tazobactam with an aminoglycoside or an anti-Pseudomonal fluroquinolone) and MRSA (e.g., vancomycin or linezolid) (Kalil et al., 2016). In the case of high local resistance patterns (Risks 6 and 7, as previously mentioned) without other clinical risk factors for multidrug resistance, dual therapy against Gram-negative organisms (for Risk 6), or Gram-negative monotherapy with MRSA therapy (for Risk 7), may be sufficient empiric coverage.

Empiric regimens should be narrowed once culture results are available at 48–72 hours to avoid the development of resistance- and antibiotic-associated complications. If no pathogens are identified in a good sample from a patient who is improving on empiric treatment, dual coverage against MDR Gram-negative organisms and coverage against MRSA can be dropped for the duration of therapy, (i.e., the antimicrobial regimen can be narrowed to single agents with activity against *Pseudomonas* and methicillin-sensitive *S. aureus*, as described previously).

Multiple studies have investigated the optimal duration of antibiotic therapy. Chastre and colleagues found that an 8-day antibiotic regimen was non-inferior to a 15-day course (Chastre et al., 2003). The survival rates were similar between the two groups. In addition, there was no difference between them in the recurrence of pulmonary infection, relapse, or superinfections. The recent guidelines published by the Infectious Diseases Society of America and the American Thoracic Society recommended that a 7-day course of antibiotics is sufficient (Kalil et al., 2016). Therapy may be prolonged on an individual basis for patients developing non-fermenting Gram-negative bacillus infections (Chastre et al., 2003), or for patients who are severely ill or immunocompromised. A low or decreasing procalcitonin level in patients who have demonstrated good clinical response may support discontinuation of therapy. Failure to respond by 72 hours should prompt a thorough search for complications of VAP (such as abscess or empyema) and a comprehensive reassessment of the differential diagnosis (different pathogens, different septic foci, or non-infectious issues).

PREVENTION

Given the impact of VAP on individual patients and the health care systems, many studies have explored strategies to prevent VAP. It has been shown that ventilator-weaning protocols are an effective method in reducing the duration of mechanical ventilation and result a decrease in VAP incidence, especially in trauma patients (Marelich et al., 2000). In a study by Marelich and colleagues, introduction of a weaning protocol reduced the duration of mechanical ventilation by a median 154 hours compared to physician-directed weaning (Marelich et al., 2000). Other measures that have been used to reduce the risk of VAP include semi-recumbent positioning (up to 45° in patients without contraindications) and the usage of closed endotracheal suction systems (Dodek et al., 2004).

Many individual prevention strategies including the ones mentioned previously and others (e.g., minimizing sedation, spontaneous breathing trials, head of bed elevation, thromboprophylaxis, early mobilization, low tidal volume ventilation, judicious fluid management, stress ulcer prophylaxis, aspiration of subglottic secretions, and silver-coated endotracheal tubes) have been rigorously studied, and some have been found to reduce the risk of VAP. Interestingly, almost none of these strategies have been found to have beneficial effects beyond the reduction of VAP (e.g., LOS, survival). This may be because some interventions may modify superficial VAP diagnostic criteria (which are numerous and often subjective or ambiguous) without significantly altering underlying pathophysiology, while others, when tested individually, may not have enough efficacy to alter hard outcomes such as mortality (Marquette et al., 1995; Klompas, 2009). There is, however, promising evidence that combining VAP prevention strategies into bundles might have more measurable benefits in terms of important ICU outcomes, including mortality (Pileggi et al., 2018).

SUMMARY

VAP is a serious, time-dependent illness that, like many surgical illnesses, requires early diagnosis, aggressive but thoughtful source control and resuscitation that accounts for patient factors (often in the face of incomplete information), and close follow-up. It is becoming increasingly clear that comprehensive and systematic approaches to management and prevention of VAP can alter the trajectories of our most vulnerable patients and substantially affect the burden of critical illness on individuals and society.

ANNOTATED REFERENCES FOR VENTILATOR-ASSOCIATED PNEUMONIA

1. Canadian Critical Care Trials Group. A randomized trial of diagnostic techniques for ventilator-associated pneumonia. *N Engl J Med*. 2006;355(25):2619–2630.

   What is the best technique to diagnose VAP? A classic randomized trial examining established diagnostic strategies for VAP.

2. Safdar N, Dezfulian C, Collard HR, Saint S. Clinical and economic consequences of ventilator-associated pneumonia: A systematic review. *Crit Care Med*. 2005;33(10):2184–2193.

   A review showing the impact of VAP on clinical outcomes and health systems.

3. Ibrahim EH, Ward S, Sherman G, Schaiff R, Fraser VJ, Kollef MH. Experience with a clinical guideline for the treatment of ventilator-associated pneumonia. *Crit Care Med*. 2001;29(6):1109–1115.

   The importance of standardization of clinical guidelines in the treatment of VAP.

4. Chastre J, Fagon J. Ventilator-associated pneumonia. *Am J Respir Crit Care Med*. 2002;165(7):867–903.

   Highly cited state-of-the-art article that summarizes VAP epidemiology, diagnosis, and treatment.

5. Kalil AC, Metersky ML, Klompas M et al. Management of Adults with Hospital-acquired and Ventilator-associated Pneumonia: 2016 Clinical Practice Guidelines by the Infectious Diseases Society of America and the American Thoracic Society. *Clin Infect Dis*. 2016;63(5):e61–e111.

   The most recent guidelines regarding management of ventilator-associated pneumonia by the ATA and IDSA.

6. Marquette CH, Copin MC, Wallet F et al. Diagnostic tests for pneumonia in ventilated patients: Prospective evaluation of diagnostic accuracy using histology as a diagnostic gold standard. *Am J Respir Crit Care Med.* 1995;151(6):1878–1888.

    Does a patient diagnosed with VAP really have one? A cadaveric study evaluating the accuracy of diagnosis.

7. Iregui M, Ward S, Sherman G, Fraser VJ, Kollef MH. Clinical importance of delays in the initiation of appropriate antibiotic treatment for ventilator-associated pneumonia. The American College of Chest Physicians. *Chest.* 2002;122(1):262–268.

    A study showing the importance of early treatment of VAP and increased mortality with delayed initiation of antibiotics.

8. Chastre J, Wolff M, Fagon J-Y et al. Comparison of 8 vs. 15 days of antibiotic therapy for ventilator-associated pneumonia in adults: A randomized trial. *JAMA.* 2003;290(19):2588–2598.

    How long should I treat my patient? The classic article of the chapter answers this important clinical question.

9. Marelich GP, Murin S, Battistella F, Inciardi J, Vierra T, Roby M. Protocol weaning of mechanical ventilation in medical and surgical patients by respiratory care practitioners and nurses: Effect on weaning time and incidence of ventilator-associated pneumonia. The American College of Chest Physicians. *Chest.* 2000;118(2):459–467.

    An article showing the importance of developing and following protocols to reduce length of mechanical ventilation and risk of VAP in medical and surgical patients.

10. Dodek P, Keenan S, Cook D et al. Evidence-based clinical practice guideline for the prevention of ventilator-associated pneumonia. *Ann Intern Med.* 2004;141(4):305–313.

    Evidence-based recommendations to reduce and prevent VAP.

11. Pileggi C, Mascaro V, Bianco A et al. Ventilator bundle and its effects on mortality among ICU patients: A meta-analysis. *Crit Care Med.* 2018;46:1167–1174.

12. Klompas M. The paradox of ventilator-associated pneumonia prevention measures. *Crit Care.* 2009;13(5):315.

    An insight to why VAP prevention measures failed to reduce mortality and length of stay.

COMPARISON OF 8 VS. 15 DAYS OF ANTIBIOTIC THERAPY FOR VENTILATOR-ASSOCIATED PNEUMONIA IN ADULTS: A RANDOMIZED TRIAL

Chastre J, Wolff M, Fagon JY, Chevret S, Thomas F, Wermert D, Clementi E, Gonzalez J, Jusserand D, Asfar P, Perrin D, Fieux F, and Aubas S; PneumA Trial Group, *JAMA.* 2003;290(19):2588–2598

ABSTRACT

Context The optimal duration of antimicrobial treatment for ventilator-associated pneumonia (VAP) is unknown. Shortening the length of treatment may help to contain the emergence of multiresistant bacteria in the intensive care unit (ICU).

Objective   To determine whether 8 days is as effective as 15 days of antibiotic treatment of patients with microbiologically proven VAP.

Design, Setting, and Participants   Prospective, randomized, double-blind (until day 8) clinical trial conducted in 51 French ICUs. A total of 401 patients diagnosed as having developed VAP by quantitative culture results of bronchoscopic specimens and who had received initial appropriate empirical antimicrobial therapy were enrolled between May 1999 and June 2002.

Intervention   A total of 197 patients were randomly assigned to receive 8 days and 204 to receive 15 days of therapy with an antibiotic regimen selected by the treating physician.

Main Outcome Measures   Primary outcome measures—death from any cause, microbiologically documented pulmonary infection recurrence, and antibiotic-free days—were assessed 28 days after VAP onset and analyzed on an intent-to-treat basis.

Results   Compared with patients treated for 15 days, those treated for 8 days had neither excess mortality (18.8% vs. 17.2%; difference, 1.6%; 90% confidence interval [CI], −3.7% to 6.9%) nor more recurrent infections (28.9% vs. 26.0%; difference, 2.9%; 90% CI, −3.2% to 9.1%), but they had more mean (SD) antibiotic-free days (13.1 [7.4] vs. 8.7 [5.2] days, $P < 0.001$). The number of mechanical ventilation-free days, the number of organ failure—free days, the length of ICU stay, and mortality rates on day 60 for the two groups did not differ. Although patients with VAP caused by non-fermenting Gram-negative bacilli, including *Pseudomonas aeruginosa*, did not have more unfavorable outcomes when antimicrobial therapy lasted only 8 days, they did have a higher pulmonary infection recurrence rate compared with those receiving 15 days of treatment (40.6% vs. 25.4%; difference, 15.2%, 90% CI, 3.9%–26.6%). Among patients who developed recurrent infections, multiresistant pathogens emerged less frequently in those who had received 8 days of antibiotics (42.1% vs. 62.0% of pulmonary recurrences, $P = 0.04$).

Conclusions   Among patients who had received appropriate initial empirical therapy, with the possible exception of those developing non-fermenting Gram-negative bacillus infections, comparable clinical effectiveness against VAP was obtained with the 8- and 15-day treatment regimens. The 8-day group had less antibiotic use.

Original Author Commentary: Jean Chastre

Two decades ago, most experts were recommending that treatment of ventilator-associated pneumonia (VAP) last 14–21 days. This recommendation was largely empirical and only justified by a higher theoretical risk of infection relapse after a short duration of antibiotic administration. However, unduly prolonging the duration of therapy may not improve the outcome and lead to the emergence of multidrug-resistant microorganisms. This is why we undertook a randomized trial in 1999 to compare the outcomes of therapy with an 8-day or 15-day antibiotic regimen in ICU patients who had developed VAP. In this study, we observed no benefit in patients randomized to the 8-day regimen. The confidence intervals for the between-group differences in mortality and pulmonary infection recurrence rates exclude an absolute difference exceeding 10% in favor of the 15-day regimen. No differences in other outcome parameters could be established, including duration of mechanical ventilation, number of organ failure–free days, the evolution of signs and symptoms potentially linked to pulmonary infection, number of infection recurrences, or status at hospital discharge. Pertinently, multiresistant pathogens emerged more frequently for patients with pulmonary infection recurrence who had received 15 days of antibiotics. These results are consistent with those of other studies conducted after the publication of our trial that also clearly demonstrated the possibility of safely reducing antibiotic exposure in ICU patients by shortening duration of therapy. Thus, although appropriate antibiotics may improve the survival rate of patients with VAP, their indiscriminate use after 8 days of therapy should be strongly discouraged.

CHAPTER 44

Delirium

Review by Contributors: Anchit Mehrotra and Natasha Keric

"Sundowning" used to be a common description for a patient suffering from what we now describe medically as delirium. The definition of sundowning is that it is a symptom of "late-day confusion" associated with dementia. Sundowning is quite different from the definition of delirium, which is a DSM-5 criterion. Delirium is described as "a disturbance in attention and awareness, which develops acutely and tends to fluctuate in severity, causes a disturbance in cognition that cannot be better explained by preexisting dementia or does not occur in the context of severely reduced level of arousal or coma, with evidence of an underlying organic cause or causes."

Sundowning and delirium were used interchangeably and not much gravitas was given to a patient exhibiting cognitive dysfunction and agitation until Dr. Ely's groundbreaking landmark study described delirium as a form of organ dysfunction that was an independent predictor of mortality and longer hospital stays for patients on mechanical ventilation. This study has brought to light much of what we now understand and practice regarding delirium.

For many practicing intensive care medicine, this information was truly earthshattering. Yet even as the longstanding belief that delirium is an inevitable or a normal part of critical illness is slowly falling out of favor with those involved in critical care (Brummel et al., 2013). A decade later, delirium continues to be difficult to appreciate, diagnose, and manage among many medical providers.

Delirium in critically ill patients can affect up to 80% of mechanically ventilated adult intensive care unit (ICU) patients, is a manifestation of acute brain dysfunction, and is an important independent predictor of negative clinical outcomes in ICU patients, including increased mortality, hospital length of stay, cost of care, and long-term cognitive impairment consistent with a dementia-like state (Barr et al., 2013). Although the mechanically ventilated patient is at greatest risk, with the incidence being found at greater than 75%, delirium has also been reported to occur in 16%–89% of hospitalized patients and is seen in approximately a third of patients aged 70 years or older. Delirium can be considered the most common surgical complication in older adults, with increasing rates after high-risk procedures such as hip fracture repair and cardiac surgery (Marcantonio, 2017). The BRAIN-ICU Study investigators found that of the patients who developed delirium during their hospital stay, 40% had decreased global cognition and executive function at 3 months, and these deficits persisted at 12 months in both younger and older patients. These deficits were similar to patients with moderate traumatic brain injury and mild Alzheimer's disease and independently associated with longer duration of delirium.

Identification is the key to detecting and treating delirium sooner and possibly improving outcomes. Current guidelines endorse routine monitoring for all ICU patients with validated screening tools such as the Confusion Assessment Method for the ICU (CAM-ICU) and the Intensive Care Delirium Screening Checklist (ICDSC), both found to be sensitive and specific in the identification of critically ill patients suffering from delirium at the bedside in less than 2 minutes (Gusmao-Flores et al., 2012). Despite these valid and reliable assessment tools, providers continue to use their gestalt and miss the diagnosis in 75% of patients suffering from delirium.

Management of delirium is rooted in first identifying risk factors and physiologic causes (such as sepsis) and employing prevention strategies. In a landmark trial published in *Lancet*, early mobilization was shown to reduce the incidence of delirium in mechanically vented critically ill patients and is still considered one of the most important non-pharmacologic prevention practices utilized today. The Awakening and Breathing Coordination, Delirium Monitoring/Management, and Early Exercise/Mobility (ABCDE) bundle incorporates the best available evidence related to delirium prevention in ICU patients. Implementing the ABCDE bundle decreased the likelihood of patients experiencing delirium, spending 3 less days on mechanical ventilation, and increased their mobility during their ICU stay (Balas et al., 2014).

Currently, there is no large randomized controlled trial that supports the use of pharmacologic interventions to treat and prevent delirium, and despite popular belief that benzodiazepines cause delirium there has been no single trial that has validated or disproved this. Benefits related to dexmedetomidine use when compared to benzodiazepine and propofol infusions have shown ventilator-free time and faster resolution of delirium symptoms; however, the studies with dexmedetomidine have had small sample sizes, and its use as a first-line treatment modality is not clearly indicated at this time. Similarly, there has been no proven benefit of antipsychotics for the treatment or prevention of ICU delirium. A recent small sample size comparison trial of antipsychotics and melatonin showed no difference in delirium-free days, duration of delirium, mortality, or ICU length of stay (Hayhurst et al., 2016; Daniels et al., 2018). Regardless of what pharmacologic interventions are employed, implementing a daily target sedation goal, with analgesia first treatment and titrating sedatives to maintain light sedation, is the key to success when trying to manage delirium in the ICU. Either the Richmond Agitation-Sedation Scale (RASS) or Sedation-Agitation Scale (SAS) may be used as they have been found to be the most valid, reliable, and discriminatory sedation assessment tools for measuring quality and depth of sedation in adult ICU patients.

Even with all the current research and interest in delirium, there are continued barriers in implementing evidence-based guidelines into practice. Studies show that multidisciplinary involvement of support staff with continued emphasis on education coupled with buy-in at the physician level will help to promote the diagnosis, treatment, and resolution of delirium in critically ill patients (Aparanji et al., 2018).

ANNOTATED REFERENCES FOR DELIRIUM

1. Marcantonio E. Delirium in hospitalized older adults. *N Engl J Med*. 2017;377: 1456–1466.

   A case-based vignette of hypoactive delirium discussing the current recommendations using CAM-ICU for diagnosis, management of agitation first with non-pharmacological interventions, avoidance of restraints, and the use of antipsychotic agents for unremitting symptoms. Consider proactive geriatrics consult for patients at high risk for delirium, with emphasis on scheduled Tylenol, local pain management, and no scheduled insomnia medications; based on data focused on the older population undergoing hip fracture repair.

2. Hayhurst C, Pandharipande P, Hughes C. Intensive care unit delirium: A review of diagnosis, prevention, and treatment. *Anesthesiology*. 2016;125:1229–1241.

   A review article providing detailed analysis of the validation of delirium screening tools, analysis of recent studies on the use of pharmacologic prophylaxis in the prevention of delirium, impact of sedation (benzodiazepine, opiate only, propofol, dexmedetomidine) in ventilated patients, impact of early mobility, and concept of sleep hygiene. A review of current data on potential delirium treatment options including the use of antipsychotics, dexmedetomidine, and anticholinesterase inhibitors.

3. Trogrlic Z, van der Jagt M, Bakker J et al. A systematic review of implantation strategies for assessment, prevention, and management of ICU delirium, and their effect on clinical outcomes. *Crit Care*. 2015;19:157.

   A systematic review of 21 studies, of which 9 studies reported both process measures and clinical outcomes. In meta-analyses, reduced mortality and ICU LOS was statistically significant when six or more implementation programs were employed when coupled with either PAD or ABCDE strategies. In addition, implementation strategies aimed at organizational change and behavioral change were associated with reduced mortality.

4. Gusmao-Flores D, Salluh JI, Chalhub RÁ, Quarantini LC. The confusion assessment method for the intensive care unit (CAM-ICU) and intensive care delirium screening checklist (ICDSC) for the diagnosis of delirium: A systematic review and meta-analysis of clinical studies. *Crit Care*. 2012;16:R115.

   A systematic review and meta-analysis of nine studies evaluating CAM-ICU and four studies evaluating ICDSC. The pooled analysis of the CAM-ICU studies showed a sensitivity of 80% and specificity of 96% with a diagnostic odds ratio of 103, indicating that the CAM-ICU is an excellent diagnostic tool in critically ill ICU patients. The pooled analysis of ICDSC showed a sensitivity of 74% and specificity of 82% with an odds ratio of 21.5, indicating that this is also an acceptable screening tool. Both tools can be used for the diagnosis of delirium in critically ill ICU patients.

5. Brummel NE, Vasilevskis EE, Han JH, Boehm L, Pun BT, Ely EW. Implementing delirium screening in the intensive care unit: Secrets to success. *Crit Care Med*. 2013;41(9):2196–2208.

   A review of available delirium screening tools, screening implementation, and common pitfalls encountered during delirium screening in the ICU. Implementation is feasible;

however, ICU culture must change to understand that delirium is not an inevitable or normal part of critical illness and must be viewed as a dangerous syndrome that can lead to poor outcomes but may be modifiable depending on patient circumstances.

6. Balas M, Vasilevskis E, Olsen KM et al. Effectiveness and safety of the awakening and breathing coordination, delirium monitoring/management, and early exercise/mobility bundle. *Crit Care Med.* 2014;42(5):1024–1036.

A prospective, cohort, before-and-after study (n = 146 pre-bundle, n = 150 post-bundle) to evaluate the effectiveness and safety of implementing the ABCDE bundle into everyday practice. Post-bundle cohorts spent 3 less days on the ventilator, were half as likely to experience delirium, and were twice as likely to be mobilized out of the ICU bed during their ICU stay. No increase in self-extubation or re-intubation rates. ABCDE bundle can be implemented safely.

7. Brummel NE, Jackson JC, Pandharipande PP et al. Delirium in the ICU and subsequent long-term disability among survivors of mechanical ventilation. *Crit Care Med.* 2014; 42(2):369–377.

A prospective cohort study (n = 126) nested within an RCT to analyze the hypothesis that duration of delirium in the ICU would be associated with subsequent disability and worse physical health status following critical illness. Follow-up at 3 (n = 80) months and at 12 (n = 87) months showed duration of delirium was independently associated with disability in ADLs in the year following critical illness. The longer a patient was delirious in the ICU, the more likely they were to report worse motor-sensory function. Early mobility interventions (early PT/OT in mechanically ventilated patients) designed to prevent ICU-acquired weakness were shown to be associated with a reduction in delirium duration and a return to baseline functional status.

8. Aparanji K, Kulkarni S, Metzke M, Schmudde Y, White P, Jaeger C. Quality improvement of delirium status communication and documentation for intensive care unit patients during daily multidisciplinary rounds. *BMJ Open Quality.* 2018;7:e00239.

After implementation of simulation-based education and delirium screening videos for nursing staff, an urban tertiary care hospital found compliance with delirium screening rise from 40% to 69% on day shift and 27% to 61% on night shift. With the addition of standardizing the screening tool and critical care progress note with specific required documentation of delirium status and management strategy and discussion on rounds by physicians, screening increased to 91% and documentation by physicians was 95%.

9. Daniels LM, Nelson SB, Frank RD, Park JG. Pharmacologic treatment of intensive care unit delirium and the impact of on duration of delirium, length of intensive care unit stay, length of hospitalization, and 28-day mortality. *Mayo Clinic Proc.* 2018;93(12):1739–1748.

A retrospective cohort study (n = 449) with ICU delirium as defined by positive CAM-ICU. Patients stratified into four treatment groups: no pharmacologic treatment, melatonin only, antipsychotics only, and both melatonin and antipsychotics. Exposure to melatonin or antipsychotic agents did not reduce duration of ICU delirium, ICU/hospital LOS, or 28-day mortality. Antipsychotic use only was associated with longer hospitalization.

10. Fowler B. Clinical education to decrease perceived barriers to delirium screening in adult intensive care units. *Crit Care Nurse Q.* 2019;42(1):41–43.

Emphasis on the nursing perspective for the implementation of education to decrease barriers to delirium screening using validated screening tools, while emphasizing a need for buy-in at the physician level and understanding of delirium as a syndrome that is not a benign or inevitable part of an ICU admission.

11. Barr J, Fraser GL, Puntillo K et al. Clinical practice guidelines for the management of pain, agitation, and delirium in adult patients in the intensive care unit. *Crit Care Med.* 2013;41:263–306.

    The American College of Critical Care Medicine assembled a 20-person, multi-disciplinary, multi-institutional task force with expertise in guideline development, pain, agitation and sedation, delirium management, and associated outcomes in adult critically ill patients. The task force, divided into four subcommittees, collaborated over 6 years and developed relevant clinical questions, using the Grading of Recommendations Assessment, Development and Evaluation method (http://www.gradeworkinggroup.org) to review, evaluate, and summarize the literature, and to develop clinical statements (descriptive) and recommendations (actionable). These guidelines provide a roadmap for developing integrated, evidence-based, and patient-centered protocols for preventing and treating pain, agitation, and delirium in critically ill patients.

12. Pandharipande PP, Girard TD, Jackson JC et al. Long-term cognitive impairment after critical illness. *N Engl J Med.* 2013;369:1306–1316.

    Eight hundred twenty-one patients admitted to the MICU or SICU with respiratory failure or shock were assessed for in-hospital delirium and global cognition and executive function at 3 and 12 months post-hospital discharge. Of the enrolled patients, 74% developed delirium during their hospitalization. At 3-month follow-up, 40% of patients had global cognitional results similar to those of moderate traumatic brain injury (TBI) patients and 26% had results similar to those with mild Alzheimer's disease. At 12-month follow-up, 34% and 24% of patients had scores similar to moderate TBI and mild Alzheimer's disease, respectively. A longer duration of delirium was independently associated with worse global cognition and worse executive function at both 3 and 12 months. The use of sedatives was not found to be statistically significant in relation to cognitive impairment at both follow-up intervals. Patients admitted to the ICU are at risk for long-term cognitive impairment, and a longer duration of delirium is associated with worse global cognition and executive function scores at 3- and 12-month follow-ups.

13. Schweickert D, Pohlman M, Pohlman S et al. Early physical and occupational therapy in mechanically ventilated, critically ill patients: A randomized control trial. *Lancet.* 2009;373:1874–1882.

    A randomized control trial focusing on sedation interruption with early mobilization and exercise (intervention group) and with therapy as ordered by the primary team in mechanically ventilated patients. Measured endpoints included patients returning to independent functional status upon discharge—defined as the ability to perform six activities of daily living and the ability to walk independently. Secondary endpoints included duration of delirium and ventilator-free days. Return to independent functional status was found to be statistically significant in the intervention group. Decreased duration of delirium and increased ventilator-free days were also found to be statistically significant in the intervention group. This study showed that interruption of sedation coupled with early physical and occupation therapy in the earliest days of critical illness provided a significant benefit to the patient in returning to independent functional status, reducing delirium, and increasing ventilator-free days.

Landmark Article of 21st Century

DELIRIUM AS A PREDICTOR OF MORTALITY IN MECHANICALLY VENTILATED PATIENTS IN THE INTENSIVE CARE UNIT

Ely EW, Shintani A, Truman B, Speroff T, Gordon SM, Harrell FE Jr, Inouye SK, Bernard GR, and Dittus RS, *JAMA*. 2004;291(14):1753–1762

ABSTRACT

Context In the intensive care unit (ICU), delirium is a common yet underdiagnosed form of organ dysfunction, and its contribution to patient outcomes is unclear.

Objective To determine if delirium is an independent predictor of clinical outcomes, including 6-month mortality and length of stay among ICU patients receiving mechanical ventilation.

Design, Setting, and Participants Prospective cohort study enrolling 275 consecutive mechanically ventilated patients admitted to adult medical and coronary ICUs of a US university-based medical center between February 2000 and May 2001. Patients were followed up for development of delirium over 2158 ICU days using the Confusion Assessment Method for the ICU and the Richmond Agitation-Sedation Scale.

Main Outcome Measures Primary outcomes included 6-month mortality, overall hospital length of stay, and length of stay in the post-ICU period. Secondary outcomes were ventilator-free days and cognitive impairment at hospital discharge.

Results Of 275 patients, 51 (18.5%) had persistent coma and died in the hospital. Among the remaining 224 patients, 183 (81.7%) developed delirium at some point during the ICU stay. Baseline demographics including age, comorbidity scores, dementia scores, activities of daily living, severity of illness, and admission diagnoses were similar between those with and without delirium (P > 0.05 for all). Patients who developed delirium had higher 6-month mortality rates (34% vs. 15%, P = 0.03) and spent 10 days longer in the hospital than those who never developed delirium (P < 0.001). After adjusting for covariates (including age, severity of illness, comorbid conditions, coma, and use of sedatives or analgesic medications), delirium was independently associated with higher 6-month mortality (adjusted hazard ratio [HR], 3.2; 95% confidence interval [CI], 1.4–7.7; P = 0.008) and longer hospital stay (adjusted HR, 2.0; 95% CI, 1.4–3.0; P < 0.001). Delirium in the ICU was also independently associated with a longer post-ICU stay (adjusted HR, 1.6; 95% CI, 1.2–2.3; P = 0.009), fewer median days alive and without mechanical ventilation (19 [interquartile range, 4–23] vs. 24 [19–26]; adjusted P = 0.03), and a higher incidence of cognitive impairment at hospital discharge (adjusted HR, 9.1; 95% CI, 2.3–35.3; P = 0.002).

Conclusion Delirium was an independent predictor of higher 6-month mortality and longer hospital stay even after adjusting for relevant covariates including coma, sedatives, and analgesics in patients receiving mechanical ventilation.

Editor Notes

Assessment: This was a prospective cohort study of 224 mechanically ventilated patients in an adult medical and coronary ICU. Using the Confusion Assessment Method and the Richmond Agitation-Sedation Scale, they found an association between delirium and clinical outcomes. The vast majority of patients (82%) developed delirium at some point in their ICU stay. Compared to the small number of patients who did not develop delirium, those who did had higher mortality and a 10-day longer length of stay. The development of delirium in the mechanically ventilated patients was associated with a threefold increase in risk of death after controlling for preexisting comorbidities, severity of illness, coma, and use of sedative and analgesic medications. Concerning medication use, only lorazepam was significantly associated with delirium. Delirium was persistent in 11% of the patients at the time of discharge.

Limitations: The definition of delirium is confusing, and numerous terminology and scales were used. Although it verified that the development of delirium is associated with a worse outcome, the causes of delirium and the prevention were not addressed in this paper. This study did not include surgical patients or trauma patients.

Conclusions: Patients developing delirium are worse off than those patients who do not develop delirium.

CHAPTER 45

Prevention of Central Line–Associated Bloodstream Infections

Review by Contributor: Stephen O. Heard

Central venous catheters are essential for the care of the critically ill patient. Mechanical and infectious complications are the most common complications associated with central venous catheterization. Early efforts to reduce catheter infection included scheduled removal and reinsertion of the catheter at a different site and/or scheduled exchange of the catheter for a new one over a guidewire. Although initial reports touted the efficacy of these approaches, neither strategy was found to be helpful in reducing central line–associated bloodstream infections (CLABSIs).

Studies in the early to mid-1990s showed that experience and education of the proceduralist was important in reducing the risk of CLABSIs. A simple educational program provided to interns was found to be effective in reducing the incidence of these infections (Sherertz et al., 2000). Use of maximum barrier precautions, where the proceduralist wears a cap and mask and sterile gown and gloves, and the patient is covered with a drape that covers the entire body, reduced the incidence of CLABSIs in outpatient cancer patients (Raad et al., 1994). Alcoholic chlorhexidine was also found to be superior to 10% povidone-iodine in preparing the patient for catheterization (Maki et al., 1991). Advances in catheter manufacturing resulted in the development of antimicrobial and antiseptic catheters which were associated with fewer CLABSIs compared to control catheters (Maki et al., 1997; Raad et al., 1997). Antimicrobial catheters appear to be the most effective (Darouiche et al., 1999). Use of a chlorhexidine-impregnated dressing or sponge also reduced the incidence of high-level catheter colonization. Post-hoc analyses of prospective, randomized trials studying the utility of anti-infective catheters indicated the subclavian site of insertion was associated with the lowest risk of infection, followed by the internal jugular and femoral sites. A recent large, prospective, randomized study has confirmed these findings (Parienti et al., 2015).

Despite periodic publication by the CDC of evidence-based guidelines to prevent intravascular catheter infections that date back to at least 1983, the incidence of CLABSIs during the 1980s and 1990s remained stubbornly high. At the end of the 1990s, the number of CLABSIs per year in US ICUs was estimated to be 16,000, resulting in a rate of 5.3 CLABSIs per 1000 catheter-days (Mermel, 2000). However, it was not until 2004 that Berenholtz and co-workers developed a true team approach to eradicate CLABSIs. All clinicians who inserted CLABSIs had to complete an educational program. A central line cart was created where all supplies were readily available. During rounds, discussion had to occur as to whether the catheter was needed. During insertion, a checklist was utilized to ensure all evidence-based guidelines (hand hygiene, preparation of skin with chlorhexidine, use of cap, mask, sterile gloves and gown, and maximum barrier precautions) followed, and the nurse was empowered to stop the insertion if sterile technique was breached. The authors found that this intervention resulted in a significant and sustained reduction in CLABSIs (Berenholtz et al., 2004). Subsequently, larger multicenter studies have demonstrated the efficacy of this approach (Pronovost et al., 2006). Studies that have incorporated a "larger" bundle (use of antibiotic-impregnated catheters and chlorhexidine-impregnated dressings and tracking high-risk catheters [emergency insertion and femoral catheters]), have shown a reduction in CLABSI rates to 0.3–0.8 per 1000 catheter-days that has persisted for over 8 years (Walz et al., 2015).

Use of ultrasonography has been shown to improve time to vessel cannulation and reduce mechanical complications compared to insertion by using anatomic landmarks. It would seem logical that ultrasonography would also reduce the risk of CLABSI. However, in ICUs where there is already a low CLABSI rate, use of ultrasonography has not been shown to further reduce the infection rate (Cartier et al., 2014).

Catheter infection can occur by either bacterial spread via the subcutaneous wound or by the development of an intraluminal biofilm. Early infection tends to occur via the wound, and most strategies of prevention focus on this route. However, several techniques have been developed to prevent infection via the catheter lumen. A meta-analysis of various lock solutions (e.g., ethanol, citrate, minocycline, EDTA, aminoglycoside, and heparin) have been shown to be helpful in preventing CLABSIs even in units that have a low baseline rate of infection. However, most patients in this analysis were receiving hemodialysis through a catheter. The findings may not be germane to the standard ICU patient (Zacharioudakis et al., 2014). Hubs represent another means by which bacteria can reach the catheter lumen and establish a biofilm. Several antiseptic caps are available, which are applied to the hubs of the intravenous tubing and are not removed until medication is administered. Although "before and after" studies have shown a significant reduction in the rate of CLABSI, the baseline rates in these studies were higher than 1.0 per 1000 catheter-days. Consequently, if the baseline rate is low, the caps may not provide any additional benefits (Voor In 't Holt et al., 2017).

In summary, use of a checklist and bundled approach to insertion and care of central venous catheters will result in a reduction in CLABSIs.

ANNOTATED REFERENCES FOR PREVENTION OF CENTRAL LINE–ASSOCIATED BLOODSTREAM INFECTIONS

1. Sherertz RJ, Ely EW, Westbrook DM et al. Education of physicians-in-training can decrease the risk for vascular catheter infection. *Ann Intern Med.* 2000;132(8):641–648.

A simple education program given to interns during the first week of their residency resulted in a decrease in catheter infections compared to historical infection rates.

2. Raad II, Hohn DC, Gilbreath BJ et al. Prevention of central venous catheter-related infections by using maximal sterile barrier precautions during insertion. *Infect Control Hosp Epidemiol.* 1994;15(4 Pt 1):231–238.

Catheter infection rates were reduced when the proceduralist used cap, mask, sterile gloves and gown, and a sterile drape covering the entire patient when inserting a central venous catheter.

3. Maki DG, Ringer M, Alvarado CJ. Prospective randomised trial of povidone-iodine, alcohol, and chlorhexidine for prevention of infection associated with central venous and arterial catheters. *Lancet.* 1991;338(8763):339–343.

Skin preparation with chlorhexidine was found to be superior to povidone-iodine in preventing catheter infections.

4. Raad I, Darouiche R, Dupuis J et al. Central venous catheters coated with minocycline and rifampin for the prevention of catheter-related colonization and bloodstream infections. A randomized, double-blind trial. The Texas Medical Center Catheter Study Group. *Ann Intern Med.* 1997;127(4):267–274.

One of two seminal investigations demonstrating how the use of an antibiotic impregnated catheter reduces CLABSIs.

5. Maki DG, Stolz SM, Wheeler S, Mermel LA. Prevention of central venous catheter-related bloodstream infection by use of an antiseptic-impregnated catheter. A randomized, controlled trial. *Ann Intern Med.* 1997;127(4):257–266.

The second of two seminal investigations demonstrating how the use of antiseptic catheters reduces CLABSIs.

6. Darouiche RO, Raad II, Heard SO et al. A comparison of two antimicrobial-impregnated central venous catheters. Catheter Study Group. *N Engl J Med.* 1999;340(1):1–8.

Central venous catheters impregnated with minocycline and rifampin (external surface and lumen) were found to be superior in preventing CLABSIs compared to catheters impregnated with chlorhexidine and silver-sulfadiazine on the external surface.

7. Parienti J-J, Mongardon N, Mégarbane B et al. Intravascular complications of central venous catheterization by insertion site. *N Engl J Med.* 2015;373(13):1220–1229.

The subclavian insertion site was associated with lower risk of infection compared to internal jugular and femoral sites. However, mechanical complications were higher.

8. Mermel LA. Prevention of intravascular catheter-related infections. *Ann Intern Med.* 2000;132(5):391–402.

A review of the state of the art in preventing catheter infections. Subsequent reviews a decade later (MMWR) demonstrated a significant decline in CLABSIs nationwide.

9. Berenholtz SM, Pronovost PJ, Lipsett PA et al. Eliminating catheter-related bloodstream infections in the intensive care unit. *Crit Care Med.* 2004;32(10):2014–2020.

Use of a checklist and bundled approach to insertion of central venous catheters resulted in a sustained decrease in CLABSIs.

10. Pronovost P, Needham D, Berenholtz S et al. An intervention to decrease catheter-related bloodstream infections in the ICU. *N Engl J Med.* 2006;355(26):2725–2732.

Use of the protocol outline in reference 9 was successfully implemented in Michigan ICUs.

11. Walz JM, Ellison RT 3rd, Mack DA et al. The bundle plus: The effect of a multidis-ciplinary team approach to eradicate central line-associated bloodstream infections. *Anesth Analg.* 2015;120(4):868–876.

   Adding antimicrobial impregnated catheters and chlorhexidine dressings to the bundle and treating every CLABSI as a sentinel event resulted in sustained reductions in CLASBIs to 0.5–0.8/1000 catheter-days.

12. Cartier V, Haenny A, Inan C, Walder B, Zingg W. No association between ultrasound-guided insertion of central venous catheters and bloodstream infection: A prospective observational study. *J Hosp Infect.* 2014;87(2):103–108.

   Although use of the ultrasound during insertion of central venous catheters may prevent complications, CLABSIs do not appear to be reduced.

13. Zacharioudakis IM, Zervou FN, Arvanitis M, Ziakas PD, Mermel LA, Mylonakis E. Antimicrobial lock solutions as a method to prevent central line-associated blood-stream infections: A meta-analysis of randomized controlled trials. *Clin Infect Dis.* 2014;59(12):1741–1749.

   Antimicrobial locks appear to be useful in preventing CLABSIs but the data are heavily weighted toward hemodialysis catheters.

14. Voor In 't Holt AF, Helder OK, Vos MC et al. Antiseptic barrier cap effective in reducing central line-associated bloodstream infections: A systematic review and meta-analysis. *Int J Nurs Stud.* 2017;69:34–40.

   Antiseptic barrier caps may be useful in preventing CLABSIs if the baseline rate is high.

AN INTERVENTION TO DECREASE CATHETER-RELATED BLOODSTREAM INFECTIONS IN THE ICU

Pronovost P, Needham D, Berenholtz S, Sinopoli D, Chu H, Cosgrove S, Sexton B, Hyzy R, Welsh R, Roth G, Bander J, Kepros J, and Goeschel C, *N Engl J Med* 2006;355(26):2725–2732

ABSTRACT

Background   Catheter-related bloodstream infections occurring in the intensive care unit (ICU) are common, costly, and potentially lethal.

Methods   We conducted a collaborative cohort study predominantly in ICUs in Michigan. An evidence-based intervention was used to reduce the incidence of catheter-related bloodstream infections. Multilevel Poisson regression modeling was used to compare infection rates before, during, and up to 18 months after implementation of the study intervention. Rates of infection per 1000 catheter-days were measured at 3-month intervals, according to the guidelines of the National Nosocomial Infections Surveillance System.

Results   A total of 108 ICUs agreed to participate in the study, and 103 reported data. The analysis included 1981 ICU-months of data and 375,757 catheter-days. The median rate of catheter-related bloodstream infections per 1000 catheter-days decreased from 2.7 infections at baseline to 0 at 3 months after implementation of the study intervention (P ≤ 0.002), and the mean rate per 1000 catheter-days decreased from 7.7 at baseline to 1.4 at 16−18 months of follow-up (P < 0.002). The regression model showed a significant decrease in infection rates from baseline, with incidence-rate ratios continually decreasing from 0.62 (95% confidence interval [CI], 0.47−0.81) at 0 to 3 months after implementation of the intervention to 0.34 (95% CI, 0.23−0.50) at 16 to 18 months.

Conclusions An evidence-based intervention resulted in a large and sustained reduction (up to 66%) in rates of catheter-related bloodstream infections that was maintained throughout the 18-month study period.

Editor Notes

Assessment: This was a large collaborative cohort study of 103 ICUs. An evidence-based intervention was used to reduce the incidence of catheter-related bloodstream infections. The median rate of catheter-related bloodstream infections per 1000 catheter-days decreased from 2.7 infections at baseline to 0 at 3 months after implementation of the intervention (p < 0.002). The mean rate per 1000 catheter-days decreased from 7.7 at baseline to 1.4 at 16−18 months of follow-up. In addition to the intervention to reduce the rate of catheter-related bloodstream infections, the ICUs implemented other changes including the use of a daily goals sheet to improve clinician-to-clinician communication, intervention to reduce the incidence of ventilator-associated pneumonia, and a comprehensive unit-based safety program to improve the safety culture. The study intervention was hand-washing, taking full-barrier precautions during the insertion of central venous catheters, cleaning the skin with chlorhexidine, avoiding the femoral site if possible, and removing unnecessary catheters. Strategies to increase the use of the intervention were education, central line cart with necessary supplies, and a checklist. If procedures were not followed removal of the line was discussed during the next-day rounds.

Limitations: The data was from 67 hospitals, of which 52% were teaching facilities, and the types of ICU included medical, surgical, cardiac, neurologic, trauma, and one pediatric unit. There were multiple interventions and when the ICU implemented them was varied. The number of ICUs reporting the data decreased over time. Compliance was not evaluated.

Conclusions: The implementation of a simple and inexpensive intervention to reduce central line infections, as well as other infections, was associated with a reduction in catheter-related infections that was sustained over time. The specific intervention or cause is unknown.

CHAPTER 46

A Comparison of Low-Dose Heparin with Low-Molecular Weight Heparin (LMWH) as Prophylaxis against Venous Thromboembolism after Major Trauma

Review by Contributor: Ara Feinstein

The advent of thromboprophylaxis in trauma patients really came to the forefront when Geerts and colleagues published this article in 1996. This publication has led to a plethora of studies with variable levels of evidence in the last two decades, making venous thromboembolism (VTE) in trauma one of the most controversial topics in trauma literature (Velmahos, 2006).

Prior to this landmark study, the primary focus of traumatic VTE was prevention of pulmonary embolus (PE), with numerous investigators advocating the use of vena caval filters (VCF) (Rogers et al., 1995; Greenfield et al., 1997). Recent investigations have demonstrated that ultrasound surveillance of high-risk trauma patients results in low PE rates of 1.7% compared to rates of 7.0% when patients were not routinely evaluated ($p = 0.014$). In light of the costs and complications associated with filters, it appears that ultrasound surveillance with early VTE prophylaxis is a better approach than routine VCF for prevention of PE in high-risk trauma patients (Allen et al., 2016).

In 2003, a large randomized study in 442 high-risk trauma patients that found no significant difference between mechanical and chemical prophylaxis. While inconclusive, this trial led the way to more investigations into the value of a combination of mechanical and chemical prophylaxis of VTE (Ginzburg et al., 2003). The 611 Enoxaparin multicenter spinal cord injury trial demonstrated that a combination of mechanical and chemical prophylaxis with unfractionated heparin (UFH) three times a day (TID) resulted in no difference in VTE outcome compared to low-molecular weight heparin (LMWH) twice daily (BID). However, when patients went to rehabilitation where mechanical modality was not used, LMWH BID was superior to UFH. These two studies suggest the utilization of mechanical prophylaxis together with chemical prophylaxis may be the best approach for the injured patient (Spinal Cord Injury Thromboprophylaxis Investigators, 2003a,b).

Critics have argued that one reason Geerts' study showed better efficacy of LMWH over UFH is explained by the UFH's twice-daily dosing. In light of this, Jacobs et al. (2017) recently demonstrated that LMWH was superior to UFH in reducing the VTE rates in 18,010 patients. Due to the small incidence of PE, we may never get a large enough randomized trial to understand the optimal method for preventing this devastating complication.

In the last decade, studies comparing various anticoagulants, use of guiding anti-Xa levels, and currently the role of aspirin in venous thrombosis prophylaxis have added promising perspectives to this controversial topic.

In summary, the current best evidence-based approach to managing VTE prophylaxis is using ultrasound surveillance of high-risk trauma patients and using a combination of mechanical and chemical prophylaxis (preferably LMWH BID) for all trauma patients not at risk for significant bleeding.

ANNOTATED REFERENCES FOR A COMPARISON OF LOW-DOSE HEPARIN WITH LOW-MOLECULAR WEIGHT HEPARIN (LMWH) AS PROPHYLAXIS AGAINST VENOUS THROMBOEMBOLISM AFTER MAJOR TRAUMA

1. Velmahos GC. The current status of thromboprophylaxis after trauma: A story of confusion and uncertainty. *Am Surg*. 2006;72(9):757–763.

   There is no convincing research that any of the currently used methods is consistently effective. The rates of deep venous thrombosis and pulmonary embolism are widely different even among similar trauma populations. The UFH, LMWH, and calf compression methods fail to show a reproducible effect in decreasing venous thromboembolic events.

2. Rogers FB, Shackford SR, Ricci MA, Wilson JT, Parsons S. Routine prophylactic vena cava filter insertion in severely injured trauma patients decreases the incidence of pulmonary embolism. *J Am Coll Surg*. 1995;180(6):641–647.

   Five-year retrospective review of 63 patients' vena cava filters in one center. The rate of pulmonary embolism was low compared to historical controls. They concluded that prophylactic vena cava filters are efficacious in decreasing the risk of pulmonary embolism in high-risk trauma patients.

3. Greenfield LJ, Proctor MC, Rodriguez JL, Luchette FA, Cipolle MD, Cho J. Posttrauma thromboembolism prophylaxis. *J Trauma*. 1997;42(1):100–103.

   Study of 54 patients who had a DVT rate of 43%. Suggested advantage of low molecular weight heparin.

4. Allen CJ, Murray CR, Meizoso JP et al. Surveillance and early management of deep vein thrombosis decreases rate of pulmonary embolism in high-risk trauma patients. *J Am Coll Surg*. 2016;222(1):65–72.

   Screening of 1282 trauma ICU admissions with Greenfield's Risk Assessment Profile. Trauma patients at high risk for VTE and who received VDU surveillance and early management of deep vein thrombosis have decreased rates of pulmonary embolism.

5. Ginzburg E, Cohn SM, Lopez J, Jackowski J, Brown M, Hameed SM. Randomized clinical trial of intermittent pneumatic compression and low molecular weight heparin in trauma. *Br J Surg.* 2003;90(11):1338–1344.

A prospective randomized trial was performed of 442 patients who received thromboprophylaxis using either an IPC device or low-molecular weight heparin (LMWH). DVT was detected in 2.7% in the IPC group and 0.5% in the LMWH group (p = 0.122). Pulmonary embolism occurred in one patient in each group. The low rate of thromboembolic complications and the cost savings suggested that IPC might be used safely and effectively for thromboprophylaxis in trauma patients.

6. Spinal Cord Injury Thromboprophylaxis Investigators. Prevention of venous thromboembolism in the acute treatment phase after spinal cord injury: A randomized, multicenter trial comparing low-dose heparin plus intermittent pneumatic compression with enoxaparin. *J Trauma.* 2003a;54(6):1116–1124; discussion 1125–1126.

The risk of venous thromboembolism is high after spinal cord injury (SCI). This prospective, multicenter study on 107 patients compared unfractionated heparin (UFH) plus intermittent pneumatic compression (IPC) to enoxaparin alone as thromboprophylaxis after SCI. In the acute treatment phase after SCI, safety and thromboprophylactic efficacy were generally similar with UFH-IPC and enoxaparin.

7. Spinal Cord Injury Thromboprophylaxis Investigators. Prevention of venous thromboembolism in the rehabilitation phase after spinal cord injury: Prophylaxis with low-dose heparin or enoxaparin. *J Trauma.* 2003b;54(6):1111–1115.

This prospective, multicenter study compared low-dose unfractionated heparin (UFH) with enoxaparin for prophylaxis against venous thromboembolism (VTE) during the rehabilitation phase after spinal cord injury in 119 patients. In this nonrandomized comparison, enoxaparin appeared more effective than heparin in the prevention of thromboembolic complications during rehabilitation after spinal cord injury. Both interventions were safe in this population.

8. Jacobs BN, Cain-Nielsen AH, Jakubus JL et al. Unfractionated heparin versus low-molecular-weight heparin for venous thromboembolism prophylaxis in trauma. *J Trauma Acute Care Surg.* 2017;83(1):151–158.

TQIP database study on 18,010 patients. LMWH was found to be superior to UFH in reducing the incidence of mortality and VTE events among trauma patients. Recommendation was therefore that LMWH should be the preferred VTE prophylaxis agent for use in hospitalized trauma patients.

9. Olson EJ, Bandle J, Calvo RY et al. Heparin versus enoxaparin for prevention of venous thromboembolism after trauma: A randomized noninferiority trial. *J Trauma Acute Care Surg.* 2015;79(6):961–969.

A regimen of UFH every 8 hours was found to be noninferior to enoxaparin every 12 hours for the prevention of VTE following trauma. Given UFH's cost advantage, the use of UFH for VTE prophylaxis may offer greater value.

A COMPARISON OF LOW-DOSE HEPARIN WITH LOW-MOLECULAR WEIGHT HEPARIN AS PROPHYLAXIS AGAINST VENOUS THROMBOEMBOLISM AFTER MAJOR TRAUMA

Geerts WH, Jay RM, Code KI, Chen E, Szalai JP, Saibil EA, and Hamilton PA, *N Engl J Med.* 1996;335(10):701–707

ABSTRACT

Background Patients who have had major trauma are at very high risk for venous thromboembolism if they do not receive thromboprophylaxis. We compared low-dose heparin and a low-molecular weight heparin with regard to efficacy and safety in a randomized clinical trial in patients with trauma.

Methods Consecutive adult patients admitted to a trauma center who had Injury Severity Scores of at least 9 and no intracranial bleeding were randomly assigned to heparin (5000 units) or enoxaprin (30 mg), each given subcutaneously every 12 hours in a double-blind manner, beginning within 36 hours after the injury. The primary outcome was deep vein thrombosis (DVT) as assessed by contrast venography performed on or before day 14 after randomization.

Results Among 344 randomized patients, 136 who received low-dose heparin and 129 who received enoxaparin had venograms adequate for analysis. Sixty patients given heparin (44%) and 40 patients given enoxaparin (31%) had DVT ($p = 0.014$). The rates of proximal-vein thrombosis were 15% and 6%, respectively ($p = 0.012$). The reductions in risk with enoxaparin as compared to heparin were 30% (95% confidence interval, 4%–50%) for all DVT and 58% (95% confidence interval, 12%–87%) for proximal-vein thrombosis. Only six patients (1.7%) had major bleeding (one in the heparin group and five in the enoxaparin group, $p = 0.12$).

Conclusions Low-molecular weight heparin was more effective than low-dose heparin in preventing venous thromboembolism after major trauma. Both interventions were safe.

Editor Notes

Assessment: This study was an open-label, randomized controlled trial of patients recruited from 20 hospitals in Norway. The two primary outcomes were frequency of post-thrombotic syndrome and iliofemoral patency after 6 months of treatment. The treatment was a catheter-directed thrombolysis using alteplase; if the patient was 18–75 years of age, the onset of symptoms was within the past 21 days and the clot was in the upper half of the thigh, the common iliac vein, or the combined iliofemoral segment. Post-thrombotic syndrome was significantly lower in the treatment group compared to the controls (41% vs. 56%, $p < 0.05$). This is a 14.4% absolute risk reduction, and the number of patients needed to treat was seven. Post-thrombotic syndrome was measured using Villalta score at 24 months. The iliofemoral patency was significantly higher in the treatment group compared to controls (66% vs. 47%, $p < 0.012$). There were 20 bleeding complications related to catheter-directed thrombolysis out of 101; three were major and five clinically relevant.

Limitations: Patients with increased risk of bleeding were excluded.

Conclusions: A previous systematic review showed that systemic treatment can prevent vein dysfunction and post-thrombotic syndrome but was associated with unacceptable risk of bleeding. The risk of bleeding in this study was interpreted as being low. Therefore, additional catheter-directed thrombolysis should be considered in patients with a high proximal DVT and low risk of bleeding.

CHAPTER 47

Pulmonary Embolism

Review by Contributor: Mary Condron

Venous thromboembolic disease and pulmonary embolism remain relatively common, potentially fatal events for trauma and acute care surgical patients. Here we discuss some of the most influential studies that have guided our understanding of risk factors, methods used to detect, and management strategies for pulmonary embolism (PE).

German physician Rudolf Virchow was one of the first to describe risk factors for venous thrombosis, and therefore thromboembolic disease. He postulated that stasis, endothelial damage, and hypercoagulable states promote thrombus formation. Additional nuance has developed over the centuries. It is now thought that estrogen, obesity, immobility, cancer, and traumatic injury increase the risk of venous thromboembolism (VTE). A reasonable estimate for the rate of PE in hospitalized patients is approximately 0.5%, depending on the patient population.

The classic clinical picture of a patient with PE is the sudden onset of pleuritic chest pain, tachypnea, dyspnea, hemoptysis, and in severe cases, cardiovascular collapse. As patients often have a subset of these relatively common symptoms, additional diagnostics beyond clinical acumen are frequently needed. Electrocardiogram and chest radiograph are routinely employed to evaluate for other pathologies with similar presentations. Arterial blood gas analysis is often utilized in the evaluation of these patients, however the classic association of PE with hypoxia and hypocapnia is suggestive at best. While tempting to rule out PE in patients with a normal $(A-a)DO_2$ gradient, a well-designed study from Ottawa Hospital (Rodger et al., 2000) showed that these values were not significantly different in patients with and without PE. These limitations have made imaging the standard (in patients not suffering hemodynamic compromise) for the diagnosis of PE.

Ventilation/perfusion (V/Q) scan was the historically preferred imaging modality to screen for PE because it is (1) noninvasive, (2) highly sensitive and specific in "high risk" patients, and (3) less likely to cause kidney damage. Unfortunately, in patients suspected of PE, approximately 40% of V/Q scans result in low and moderate risk scans. The meaning of these scans is much more difficult to discern, and true PE would be missed in 10%–40% of these patients if they are treated as negative. Because of these major limitations, CT angiograms have become the modality of choice and have replaced angiography. A practice-changing study by Anderson et al. in 2007 demonstrated that CT scanning was more sensitive for PE, with the added benefits of being able to diagnose non-PE causes for symptoms in patients that are ruled out for PE. In addition, it can be completed more quickly than V/Q scan, which can be critically important in a tenuous patient. Use of screening a duplex ultrasound remains controversial. In an elegant study examining adult patients admitted to a trauma/surgical intensive care unit, Azarbal et al. (2011) demonstrated that screening duplex found deep vein thrombosis (DVT) in >15% of asymptomatic patients, and even in patients without high risk features (long bone fractures, inability to be anticoagulated), the rates remained >10%. Questions remain about the clinical importance of DVT found on screening and their relationship to PE.

Determining the pre-test risk of PE is a key step in evaluation of a suspected PE, as interpretation of imaging results is dependent on the pre-test probability. It can also identify patients for whom you may decide to initiate aggressive treatment, without confirming the diagnosis with imaging. The Wells Score (Wells et al., 1995) is the most commonly employed tool used to perform this risk stratification. This scoring system incorporates risk factors for venous thromboembolic disease as well as clinical findings. The highest risk group (score >6) is associated with a nearly 60% rate of PE. D-dimer level is part of most risk-stratification algorithms as well; however, it is generally elevated after surgery or trauma.

Management of patients at risk for venous thromboembolism has evolved as well. Perioperative use of heparin derivatives has become standard of care, thanks to now classic studies (Collins et al., 1988), showing that the practice decreases DVT and possibly even PE rates. More recent work has shown that preventing PE with prophylactic vena cava filters may be possible (Rodriguez et al., 1996). At this point, however, filter use is generally reserved for those in whom anticoagulation is contraindicated, or in whom even a small PE would be expected to cause catastrophic decompensation. This is because filter use has not been shown to be more effective than anticoagulation alone and is not without complications (Mismetti et al., 2015). This randomized, open-label, blinded study (PREPIC2) showed no difference in recurrent symptomatic PE at 3 months in patients with severe acute PE receiving anticoagulation, whether they received a temporary filter or not. Disadvantages of filters include propagation of clot above the filter, and removal of these theoretically temporary devices does not always occur. In addition, placement of a caval filter does nothing to manage or prevent the other sequelae of DVT, such as post-phlebitis syndrome. This chronic condition predisposes patients to pain, poor wound healing, and ulcers which can be debilitating. Fortunately, the severe manifestations of this condition are uncommon. Finally, local trauma to the chest may result in primary pulmonary artery thrombosis which is not improved by filter placement.

Patients with DVT were routinely immobilized in hopes of avoiding disrupting a clot and causing PE. Junger et al. (2006) put this idea to rest with a randomized controlled trial demonstrating that patients with DVT who were immobilized and those who were encouraged to be out of bed walking had similar rates of PE and that those who were immobilized had higher rates of clot propagation. A similar concept still encountered on the surgical wards today is that of avoiding sequential compression devices (SCDs) on extremities with DVT to avoid clot migration. Review of the current medical literature does not provide data to support this theory.

Systemic therapeutic anticoagulation is the cornerstone of preventing future PE, but as an acute treatment for PE, anticoagulation is imperfect. In cases with hemodynamic instability secondary to PE, lytic therapy or embolectomy may be used. Extracorporeal membrane oxygenation (ECMO) support may be needed in severe cases and can be considered when there is right-sided heart failure.

ANNOTATED REFERENCES FOR PULMONARY EMBOLISM

1. Anderson DR, Kahn SR, Rodger MA et al. Computed tomographic pulmonary angiography vs. ventilation-perfusion lung scanning in patients with suspected pulmonary embolism: A randomized controlled trial. *JAMA.* 2007;298(23):2743–2753.

   Important study in validating the use of CT instead of V/Q scan for diagnosing PE: Randomized 1417 consecutive patients thought likely to have PE based on D-dimer, Wells criteria, or clinical assessment to undergo either V/Q or CTPA. Managing physicians were given generic reports of positive, nondiagnostic, or negative. PE rate on initial imaging was higher with CT than V/Q (19.2% vs. 14.2%, p = 0.01). Their primary outcome was development of symptomatic PE or DVT in the following 3 months for patients who initially had negative imaging—CT scan performed better (0.4% vs. 1%) in this regard.

2. Azarbal A, Rowell S, Lewis J et al. Duplex ultrasound screening detects high rates of deep vein thromboses in critically ill trauma patients. *J Vasc Surg.* 2011;54(3):743–747; discussion 747–748.

   Best paper on screening ultrasound in asymptomatic but severely injured patients: One year of trauma/surgical ICU admissions was evaluated at a level I trauma center with analysis of the 264 patients who underwent lower extremity Doppler ultrasound (DUS). During the study, routine screening DUS was done weekly for all patients. These screening DUS were positive in 15.2% (40/264), most of which were calf vein DVTs (60%). Patient groups with higher rates were older patients, longer ICU stay, lower GCS, and higher ISS. High-risk patients (based on injury pattern [e.g., long bone fractures] and not on pharmacologic VTE prophylaxis) did not actually have a different rate. There was no subpopulation of trauma surgery intensive care unit (TSICU) patients with a rate <10%.

3. Collins R, Scrimgeour A, Yusuf S, Peto R. Reduction in fatal pulmonary embolism and venous thrombosis by perioperative administration of subcutaneous heparin. Overview of results of randomized trials in general, orthopedic, and urologic surgery. *N Engl J Med.* 1988;318(18):1162–1173.

   Classic study showing that perioperative heparin prophylaxis against VTE is effective. The authors performed a meta-analysis regarding perioperative use of low-dose heparin for VTE prophylaxis. They demonstrated a decreased rate of DVT, PE (fatal and nonfatal), and death. There was, however, an increased rate of bleeding events in patients receiving heparin.

4. Junger M, Diehm C, Störiko H et al. Mobilization versus immobilization in the treatment of acute proximal deep venous thrombosis: A prospective, randomized, open, multicentre trial. *Curr Med Res Opin.* 2006;22(3):593–602.

This study helped end the belief that patients with proximal DVT should be kept immobile to prevent embolic events such as PE. With more movement toward outpatient management, physicians started to question the utility of immobilization. The study randomized 402 inpatients with DVT to bed rest for 5 days or up ad lib for 5 days, with standardized anticoagulation regimen being the same across both groups. No differences were seen in serious adverse events or death. A higher rate of DVT progression (28% vs. 13.5%) was found in immobilized patients, who also had more back pain and more difficulty toileting.

5. Koehler DM, Shipman J, Davidson MA, Guillamondegui O. Is early venous thromboembolism prophylaxis safe in trauma patients with intracranial hemorrhage? *J Trauma.* 2011;70(2):324–329.

Demonstrated evidence that pharmaceutical VTE prophylaxis can be started early in patients with TBI. This is a retrospective cohort study over 4 years which includes the 2 years before and after initiating a practice management guideline recommending Lovenox prophylaxis to start 48 hours after stable head CT in patients with traumatic intracranial hemorrhage. All patients received Lovenox 30 q12. In the 699 patients studied, those with progression of their bleed prior to starting Lovenox often had Lovenox initiation delayed, however, rates of progression were the same after starting prophylaxis (1.46% and 1.54%) and no patients required craniotomy after Lovenox was initiated.

6. Mismetti P, Laporte S, Pellerin O et al.; PREPIC2 Study Group. Effect of a retrievable inferior vena cava filter plus anticoagulation vs. anticoagulation alone on risk of recurrent pulmonary embolism: A randomized clinical trial. *JAMA.* 2015;313(16):1627–1635.

Further evidence that inferior vena cava (IVC) filter use should be judicious: 399 consecutive adult patients who were hospitalized for symptomatic PE associated with lower extremity venous thrombosis were randomized to filter + anticoagulation versus anticoagulation alone. Their primary outcome was PE recurrence at 3 months. Those with filters had six (3%) recurrences versus anticoagulation alone, which had three (1.5%). They observed no difference in DVT, major bleeding, or all-cause death. The authors note that anticoagulation was less reliable at the time of many older studies and conclude that filter use is not supported in patients who can have anticoagulation.

7. Rodger MA, Carrier M, Jones GN et al. Diagnostic value of arterial blood gas measurement in suspected pulmonary embolism. *Am J Respir Crit Care Med.* 2000;162(6):2105–2108.

Prospectively evaluated all inpatients and outpatients (not on a ventilator) suspected of having PE over the course of 30 months. Obtained D-dimer, ABG, V/Q scan, and pulmonary angiogram and tested if pO_2, pCO_2, and $(A\text{-}a)DO_2$ were significantly different between those who did and did not have PE on imaging. Found that only D-dimer was predictive (83% vs. 42.4%).

8. Rodriguez JL, Lopez JM, Proctor MC et al. Early placement of prophylactic vena caval filters in injured patients at high risk for pulmonary embolism. *J Trauma.* 1996;40(5):797–802; discussion 802–804.

Evaluation of prophylactic IVC filters showing the importance of pharmacologic treatment whenever able. This study compares a prospective group with historical controls of injured patients deemed as high risk of PE from 1991–1993. The authors evaluated PE rate, PE-related mortality, and morbidity from filter placement before and after a practice change where they started placing prophylactic filters in patients even when they could receive pharmacologic prophylaxis as well. They did observe lower PE rates and lower PE-related and overall mortality in patients with venocaval filters; however, using comparison to historical controls weakens the persuasiveness of this finding. They also describe venocaval thrombosis causing lower extremity edema in several patients as well as cavograms revealing thrombus extending above the filter. They report a practice of placing a second filter higher in the IVC above the thrombus in these cases.

9. Stein PD, Beemath A, Olson RE. Obesity as a risk factor in venous thromboembolism. *Am J Med.* 2005;118(9):978–980.

   Large study demonstrating the role of obesity in VTE. The authors use the National Hospital Discharge Survey (NHDS) from 1979–1999 and looked at patients with PE or DVT based on the ICD9 code VTE. Their main finding was that 0.76% of patients with obesity had PE whereas only 0.34% of those without obesity (RR 2.2) had PE. They found the same discrepancy in DVT rates (2.02% with and 0.8% without [RR 2.5]). They also did an analysis by age group, and this showed that obesity had the biggest impact on those <40 years old. The effect was seen in both men and women.

10. Wells PS, Hirsh J, Anderson DR et al. Accuracy of clinical assessment of deep vein thrombosis. *Lancet.* 1995;345(8961):1326–1330.

    Initial description of the Wells scoring tool for risk-stratifying patients suspected of having a PE.

Landmark Article of 21st Century

EFFECT OF A RETRIEVABLE INFERIOR VENA CAVA FILTER PLUS ANTICOAGULATION VS. ANTICOAGULATION ALONE ON RISK OF RECURRENT PULMONARY EMBOLISM: A RANDOMIZED CLINICAL TRIAL

Mismetti P, Laporte S, Pellerin O, Ennezat PV, Couturaud F, Elias A, Falvo N, Meneveau N, Quere I, Roy PM, Sanchez O, Schmidt J, Seinturier C, Sevestre MA, Beregi JP, Tardy B, Lacroix P, Presles E, Leizorovicz A, Decousus H, Barral FG, and Meyer G; PREPIC2 Study Group, *JAMA.* 2015;313(16):1627–1635

ABSTRACT

Importance   Although retrievable inferior vena cava filters are frequently used in addition to anticoagulation in patients with acute venous thromboembolism, their benefit–risk ratio is unclear.

Objective   To evaluate the efficacy and safety of retrievable vena cava filters plus anticoagulation versus anticoagulation alone for preventing pulmonary embolism recurrence in patients presenting with acute pulmonary embolism and a high risk of recurrence.

Design, Setting, and Participants   Randomized, open-label, blinded endpoint trial (PREPIC2) with 6-month follow-up conducted from August 2006 to January 2013. Hospitalized patients with acute, symptomatic pulmonary embolism associated with lower-limb vein thrombosis and at least one criterion for severity were assigned to retrievable inferior vena cava filter implantation plus anticoagulation (filter group; n = 200) or anticoagulation alone with no filter implantation (control group; n = 199). Initial hospitalization with ambulatory follow-up occurred in 17 centers in France.

Interventions   Full-dose anticoagulation for at least 6 months in all patients. Insertion of a retrievable inferior vena cava filter in patients randomized to the filter group. Filter retrieval was planned at 3 months from placement.

Main Outcomes and Measures   Primary efficacy outcome was symptomatic recurrent pulmonary embolism at 3 months. Secondary outcomes were recurrent pulmonary embolism at 6 months, symptomatic deep vein thrombosis, major bleeding, death at 3 and 6 months, and filter complications.

Results   In the filter group, the filter was successfully inserted in 193 patients and was retrieved as planned in 153 of the 164 patients in whom retrieval was attempted. By 3 months, recurrent pulmonary embolism had occurred in six patients (3.0%; all fatal) in the filter group and in three patients (1.5%; two fatal) in the control group (relative risk with filter, 2.00 [95% CI, 0.51–7.89]; P = .50). Results were similar at 6 months. No difference was observed between the two groups regarding the other outcomes. Filter thrombosis occurred in three patients.

Conclusions and Relevance   Among hospitalized patients with severe acute pulmonary embolism, the use of a retrievable inferior vena cava filter plus anticoagulation compared with anticoagulation alone did not reduce the risk of symptomatic recurrent pulmonary embolism at 3 months. These findings do not support the use of this type of filter in patients who can be treated with anticoagulation.

Editor Notes

Assessment: This was a large (n = 399) 7-year multicenter randomized open-label study in 17 centers in France, comparing temporary IVC filter (3 months) versus no filter in anticoagulated patients with acute symptomatic pulmonary embolism (PE). About two-thirds of patients had right ventricular dysfunction. Primary endpoint of PE at 3-month follow-up was not different between groups (3% all fatal in filter group vs. 1.5%, 2 fatal in control group). There was no difference in secondary outcomes of fatal or nonfatal symptomatic PE at 6 months, or recurrent symptomatic DVT.

Limitations: The sample size may have been small considering the lower-than-expected incidence of PE recurrence. The authors of this study excluded patients with an acute PE who had a contraindication to anticoagulation, as filter is the only option in this group of patients. The long recruitment time period (7 years) is a potential limitation. The extremely high retrieval rate of the filters (79%) in this study is probably not achievable in the general community.

The primary endpoint which was recurrence of PE at 3 months is by design short, thus does not permit assessment of long-term benefit. Finally, this study does not necessarily negate the possible long-term benefit of *permanent* inferior vena cava filters for acute PE.

Conclusions: Removable inferior vena cava filters do not reduce the risk of recurrent pulmonary embolism in patients with acute symptomatic pulmonary embolism at 3 months.

CHAPTER 48

Abdominal Compartment Syndrome

Review by Contributor: Keneeshia Williams

The deleterious effects of intra-abdominal hypertension (IAH) in critically ill patients was first described in the mid-nineteenth century. Marey (1863) was the first to document the impact of IAH on pulmonary function. This was later re-demonstrated by Burt (1870) and Henricius (1890). The impact of IAH on renal function was first described by Wendt in 1876. The cardiovascular collapse associated with IAH was demonstrated by Emerson in 1911. By 1923, Thorington and Schmidt were able to show an improvement in renal function following abdominal decompression in an animal model. The concept of bladder pressure measurements for identification of IAH was later introduced by Kron in 1984. The true incidence and prevalence of abdominal compartment syndrome (ACS) remained unclear during the following two decades; however, the medical community became increasingly aware of the profound effect that ACS had on outcomes in critically ill patients. In 2004, a study comprising 265 patients from 14 ICUs in 6 countries found that the occurrence of IAH during an ICU admission was an independent predictor of mortality in critically ill patients (Malbrain, 2004; Malbrain et al., 2004, 2005, 2006). In that same year, a group of international physicians formed the World Society of the Abdominal Compartment Syndrome (WSACS). The WSACS soon published evidence-based consensus definitions and guidelines for the treatment of IAH and ACS in 2007. These were the first evidence-based guidelines for ACS published—nearly 150 years after IAH was first described. Updated definitions and guidelines followed in 2013 and 2017.

Today, it is recognized that IAH affects every organ system within the body. Intra-abdominal effects include (but are not limited to) decreased renal function, decreased celiac blood flow, and decreased portal blood flow. As IAH worsens, pulmonary function is disrupted by multiple mechanisms, including decreased chest and abdominal wall compliance, cephalad displacement of the diaphragms, and elevation in intra-thoracic pressure. Decreased IVC blood flow and cardiac output leads to cardiovascular collapse. Additionally, elevated intracranial pressure (ICP) and decreased cerebral perfusion pressure are noted with IAH.

IAH is defined as a repeated or sustained intra-abdominal pressure (IAP) of ≥12 mmHg. Normal IAP is approximately 5–7 in critically ill patients. IAH has been categorized into a grading system based on the range of IAP; Grade I: 12–15 mmHg, Grade II: 16–20 mmHg, Grade III: 21–25 mmHg, and Grade IV: >25 mmHg. As with any compartment with elevated pressure, it is important to consider the perfusion pressure within that compartment. Abdominal perfusion pressure (APP) is the mean arterial pressure

(MAP)-(IAP). Sustained APP less than 60 mmHg has been shown to decrease survival from IAH and ACS (Cheatham et al., 2007; Cheatham, 2009a,b). ACS is defined by sustained IAP >20 mmHg associated with new-onset organ dysfunction. ACS is divided into primary, secondary, and tertiary (previously termed recurrent). Primary ACS occurs in the presence of intra-abdominal injury or disease. Secondary ACS refers to processes not originating within the intra-abdominal cavity. Tertiary ACS occurs when ACS redevelops following medical or surgical treatment.

ACS occurs in a mixed population of critically ill patients, most commonly occurring in surgical, trauma, medical (i.e., severe acute pancreatitis and sepsis), and burn patients who require aggressive resuscitation. ACS most commonly results from reduced abdominal wall compliance, increased intraluminal contents, increased extraluminal contents, or capillary leak/fluid resuscitation. Large-volume resuscitation, increased disease severity score, abdominal surgery, liver disease, obesity, sepsis, and ileus have been shown to be risk factors for the development of IAH (Malbrain, 2004; Malbrain et al., 2004, 2005, 2006; Holodinski et al., 2013).

A high index of suspicion is required to identify and treat IAH and ACS early. Signs of ACS include abdominal distension, oliguria refractory to volume resuscitation, elevated ICP, hypoxia refractory to escalated ventilatory support, and refractory metabolic acidosis. Bladder pressure measurement is a reliable technique for measuring intra-abdominal pressure and should be performed expeditiously in any patient suspected of having IAH or ACS. Proper technique for measuring bladder pressure must be used to ensure accurate measurement. A standard three-way foley bladder catheter is used. Measurements are performed using the irrigation port, sterile normal saline irrigation, and a pressure transducer placed at the level of the iliac crest at the mid-axillary line.

ACS can be treated medically and/or surgically. The course of treatment depends on the underlying cause or ACS and the patient's clinical status. Medical treatment options for reducing intra-abdominal pressure include increased sedation and analgesia and use of neuromuscular blockades to improve abdominal wall compliance, evacuation of intraluminal contents via nasogastric tube or rectal decompression, evacuation of abdominal fluid (ascites/hematoma) via paracentesis or percutaneous drainage, correcting positive fluid balance with the use of diuretics, colloids, hemodialysis, and last, organ support with optimized mechanical ventilation (Cheatham et al., 2007; Cheatham, 2009a,b).

Early surgical decompression should be considered in patients with continued elevated IAP after medical treatment and in those patients with rapid progression of organ dysfunction secondary to IAH. Surgical decompression can be performed at bedside in the ICU in patients too unstable for transport to the operating room. Following surgical decompression, medical treatment options to reduce IAP should be continued (Kirkpatrick et al., 2013).

An increase in awareness and interest in abdominal compartment syndrome has led to evidence-based practices and guidelines in the twenty-first century. There is a collective appreciation for the impact that IAH and ACS has on the outcomes of critically ill patients. Both IAH and ACS occur in a comprehensive cohort of patients, and the true prevalence remains largely unknown. Any suspicion of ACS should prompt immediate efforts to reduce IAP. Although the number of references for ACS have increased over the last 20 years, the need for high-quality intervention trials persists.

ANNOTATED REFERENCES FOR ABDOMINAL COMPARTMENT SYNDROME

1. Balogh Z, McKinley BA, Cocanour CS et al. Supranormal trauma resuscitation causes more cases of abdominal compartment syndrome. *Arch Surg.* 2003;138(6):637–643.

   A retrospective analysis of a prospective database at a 20-bed ICU in a level I trauma center. This study included 156 patients with injury severity score >15. Patients with supranormal resuscitation were found to have decreased intestinal perfusion and increased incidence of IAH (42% vs. 20%; p <.05), ACS (16% vs. 8%; p <.05), multiple organ failure, and death. This study provided further evidence that a positive fluid balance increased the incidence of IAH, organ failure, and death.

2. Malbrain M. Different techniques to measure intra-abdominal pressure (IAP): Time for critical re-appraisal. *Intensive Care Med.* 2004;30:357–371.

   A review of indirect IAP measurement techniques and revised methods of IVP measurement. This is an essential read as it provides reliable techniques for measuring bladder pressure and addresses the problem of user error in bladder pressure measurement.

3. Malbrain ML, Chiumello D, Pelosi P et al. Prevalence of intra-abdominal hypertension in critically ill patients: A multicentre epidemiological study. *Intensive Care Med.* 2004;30:822–829.

   A multicenter study on the prevalence of intra-abdominal hypertension in critically ill patients. Ninety-seven patients from 13 ICUs across 6 countries were included. BMI was found to be an independent predictor of IAH.

4. Balogh Z, Jones F, D'Amours S et al. Continuous intra-abdominal pressure technique - a new gold standard. *Am J Surg.* 2004;188:679–684.

   This study validated the use of continuous IAP measurement using a standard three-way foley bladder catheter. Measurements are performed using the irrigation port, continuous sterile normal saline irrigation, and a pressure transducer placed at the level of the iliac crest at the mid-axillary line.

5. Malbrain ML, Chiumello D, Pelosi P et al. Incidence and prognosis of intraabdominal hypertension in a mixed population of critically ill patients: A multiple-center epidemiological study. *Crit Care Med.* 2005;33:315–322.

   The first multicenter epidemiological study on the incidence of IAH. The study included 265 patients. The presence of IAH during an ICU admission was an independent outcome predictor.

6. Malbrain ML, Cheatham ML, Kirkpatrick A et al. Results from the international conference of experts on intra-abdominal hypertension and abdominal compartment syndrome. I. Definitions. *Intensive Care Med.* 2006;32:1722–1732.

   ACS was redefined as an IAP above 20 mmHg with evidence of organ dysfunction/failure. ACS was further classified as primary, secondary, or recurrent based on duration and cause of the IAH-induced organ failure.

7. Cheatham ML, Malbrain ML, Kirkpatrick A et al. Results from the international confer-ence of experts on intra-abdominal hypertension and abdominal compartment syn-drome. II. Recommendations. *Intensive Care Med.* 2007;33:951–962.

   A review of the prevalence and etiology of IAH and ACS. Evidence-based treatment guide-lines described for the diagnosis and management of IAH and ACS.

8. Cheatham ML. Nonoperative management of intraabdominal hypertension and abdominal compartment syndrome. *World J Surg.* 2009a;33:1116–1122.

   A review of nonoperative management of IAH and ACS including evacuating intraluminal con-tents, evacuating intra-abdominal space-occupying lesions, improving abdominal wall compli-ance, optimizing fluid administration, and optimizing systemic and regional tissue perfusion.

9. Cheatham ML. Abdominal compartment syndrome: Pathophysiology and definitions. *Scand J Trauma Resusc Emerg Med.* 2009b;17:10.

   An in-depth review of the history and pathophysiologic implications of elevated IAP. Illustrates the multisystem impact of ACS. Defines IAH and ACS.

10. Kirkpatrick AW, Roberts DJ, De Waele J et al. Intra-abdominal hypertension and the abdominal compartment syndrome: Updated consensus definitions and clinical practice guidelines from the World Society of the Abdominal Compartment Syndrome. *Intensive Care Med.* 2013;39:1190–1206.

    An update on the consensus definitions and clinical practice guidelines from the WSACS. The WSACS defined the open abdomen and abdominal compliance, and proposed an open-abdomen classification system. Recommendations included IAP measurement, avoidance of sustained IAH, protocolized IAP monitoring and management, and decom-pressive laparotomy for overt ACS.

11. Holodinski KJ, Roberts DJ, Ball CG et al. Risk factors for intra-abdominal hyperten-sion and abdominal compartment syndrome among adult intensive care unit patients: A systemic review and meta-analysis. *Critical Care.* 2013;17:R249.

    A systemic review and meta-analysis which included 14 studies and a total of 2500 patients. Obesity, abdominal surgery, and large-volume fluid resuscitation were found to be increased risk factors for IAH in mixed ICU patients.

Landmark Article of 21st Century

IS THE EVOLVING MANAGEMENT OF INTRA-ABDOMINAL HYPERTENSION AND ABDOMINAL COMPARTMENT SYNDROME IMPROVING SURVIVAL?

Cheatham ML and Safcsak K, *Crit Care Med.* 2010;38(2):402–407

ABSTRACT

Objective   The diagnosis and management of intra-abdominal hypertension and abdominal compartment syndrome have changed significantly over the past decade with improved understanding of the pathophysiology and appropriate treatment of these disease processes. Serial intra-abdominal pressure measurements, nonoperative pressure-reducing interventions, and early abdominal decompression for refractory intra-abdominal hypertension or abdominal compartment syndrome are all key elements of this evolving strategy.

Design   Prospective, observational study.

Setting   Tertiary referral/level I trauma center.

Patients   Four hundred seventy-eight consecutive patients requiring an open abdomen for the management of intra-abdominal hypertension or abdominal compartment syndrome.

Interventions   Patients were managed by a defined group of surgical intensivists using established definitions and an evidence-based management algorithm. Both univariate and multivariate analyses were performed to identify patient and management factors associated with improved survival.

Measurements and Main Results   Whereas patient demographics and severity of illness remained unchanged over the 6-year study period, the use of a continually revised intra-abdominal hypertension/abdominal compartment syndrome management algorithm significantly increased patient survival to hospital discharge from 50% to 72% (p = .015). Clinically significant decreases in resource utilization and an increase in same-admission primary fascial closure from 59% to 81% were recognized. Development of abdominal compartment syndrome, prophylactic use of an open abdomen to prevent development of intra-abdominal hypertension/abdominal compartment syndrome, and use of a multimodality surgical/medical management algorithm were identified as independent predictors of survival.

Conclusions   A comprehensive evidence-based management strategy that includes early use of an open abdomen in patients at risk significantly improves survival from intra-abdominal hypertension/abdominal compartment syndrome. This improvement is not achieved at the cost of increased resource utilization and is associated with an increased rate of primary fascial closure.

Original Author Commentary: Michael L. Cheatham and Karen Safcsak

Young surgeons unfamiliar with the history of intra-abdominal hypertension (IAH) and abdominal compartment syndrome (ACS) management may take for granted damage control laparotomy as a valuable tool in the acute care surgeon's armamentarium. Just over two decades ago, IAH and ACS were essentially unrecognized causes of morbidity and mortality among the critically ill. Abdominal decompression was regarded with skepticism and reserved as a highly morbid last resort for patients who had failed contemporary resuscitation. ACS mortality was exceedingly high, with some surgeons arguing that abdominal decompression was futile. As the new millennium approached, however, surgeon attitudes toward decompression softened as studies demonstrated improved survival through *preventing* rather than *reacting to* IAH/ACS.

We began prospectively studying our open abdomen patients in 1997, ultimately creating the largest single-center IAH/ACS database in the world. Our survival rate was initially a dismal 35%. By employing an evidence-based management algorithm that included serial intra-abdominal pressure (IAP) measurements, goal-directed resuscitation using judicious crystalloid volumes and massive transfusion protocols, multimodality medical IAP management, and especially prophylactic abdominal decompression, we increased our survival rate to 72% a decade later with an enviable primary fascial closure rate of 81%. We found ACS to be independently associated with a five-fold increase in mortality and prophylactic decompression to have a three-fold increase in survival compared to a reactive decompression strategy.

Thankfully, IAH/ACS is not seen with the frequency it once was. The evolution of IAH/ACS management serves to remind us of the value of constantly pursuing better strategies for patient survival.

CHAPTER 49

End-of-Life Issues

Review by Contributor: Christine S. Cocanour

END-OF-LIFE ISSUES IN ACUTE CARE SURGERY

End-of-life decision making has become increasingly important as more people are aging, and they are living longer. In addition, end-of-life care is shifting from survival at all costs to a focus on functional outcome and quality of life.

The Patient Self-Determination Act (PDSA) of 1991 required that health care providers give patients information about their right to make advance directives. In 2015, the Institute of Medicine (IOM) released its report "Dying in America" and concluded that "a person-centered, family-oriented approach that honors individual preferences and promotes quality of life through the end of life should be a national priority" (IOM, 2015). Yet, 25 years after the PDSA, only a third of the US population has executed an advance directive. The exception is La Crosse, Wisconsin. They achieved this through communication. In the 1990s, local medical leaders led a systematic campaign ("Respecting Choices Advance Care Planning") to get medical personnel and patients to discuss end-of-life wishes. Within 2 years, advance directives in La Crosse rose from 2% to 45%. By 1995, 85% that died had advance directives in their hospital chart, and by 2008, that number had risen to 96% (Hammes et al., 2010).

Cooper's article "Pitfalls in Communication" illustrates the many factors that contribute to communication breakdown and include surgeon, patient, surrogate, and systemic factors (Cooper et al., 2014). Surgeons face time constraints, inadequate communication training, and a belief that patients do not want to talk about death and dying. Surgeons are often at a loss because of the uncertainty of the prognosis. They generally tend to overestimate the prognosis and focus on a curative approach. Because of a lack of training in talking about death or in providing a palliative approach to care, surgeons are less likely to respond to the patient's emotional cues. Instead, as a defense, surgeons focus on medical details, offer reassurance or problem solving and avoidance. There are multiple patient variables that come into play at the end of life. Race, religiosity, functional ability, and availability of family support all affect the intensity of treatment at the end of life. Surrogate decision makers are often unprepared to use substituted judgement. They must make decisions based on what the patient would want, or when unclear, decide what is in the patient's best interests.

Atul Gawande's *Being Mortal* made many pertinent observations on physicians' relationships with patients and even their own family members at the end of life (Gawande, 2014). Gawande notes that our reluctance to honestly examine the experience of aging and dying has increased the harm that we inflict on patients and deny them the basic comforts that they most need. Although Temel et al. (2010) found that less aggressive interventions are associated with better quality of life at the end of life, there appears to be an increasing intensity in interventions. Medicare patients had increased ICU use in 2009 compared to 2000 (Teno). Nearly one in ten Medicare patients have surgery during their last week of life (Kwok). Despite trends toward more aggressive care at the end of life, Barnato et al. found that fewer than 10% of patients want to spend their last days hospitalized, and they do not want potentially lifesaving drugs if these drugs would worsen their quality of life (Barnato et al.).

Most end-of-life discussions center around the patient with either chronic illness or cancer. These patients' course toward death is slower, often with ups and downs. Patients and their families have more time to acknowledge the disease and the alterations in health and daily activities that come with chronic illness. However, trauma and emergency general surgery are abrupt disruptions in patients' lives which are much harder for patients and their families to deal with.

A structured approach using shared decision-making concepts between the surgeon and patient can enable the surgeon to better recommend treatments that will best match the patient's goals. It is critical that this approach include the following: clarifying the patient's understanding of the diagnosis, the prognosis and expectations for recovery, identifying the patient's priorities and goals, determining the health states that the patient would find unacceptable, and affirming the physician's commitment to the patient's well-being. Kruser et al. (2017) developed a tool called "Best Case/Worst Case," based on an established shared decision-making model. It allows physicians, patients, and caregivers to better deliberate difficult decisions and make informed choices that reflect the patient's values and goals. An illustrative video, available on the internet, clearly shows the process.

Although palliative care is often thought of as for only end of life, it is an approach that improves the quality of life of patients and their families when facing life-threatening illness through the prevention, assessment, and treatment of pain and other physical, psychosocial, and spiritual problems. Mosenthal et al. (2008) found that when a structured, interdisciplinary model for palliative care was integrated into standard ICU care, the rates of mortality, do-not-resuscitate (DNR) orders, and withdrawal of life support were unchanged, but DNR and withdrawal of life support occurred earlier in the hospital course. Her model led to the development of the ACS Trauma Quality Improvement Program (TQIP) Palliative Care Best Practice Guidelines.

Respect for autonomy, a fundamental tenet of medical ethics, forms the ethical basis for many of the issues that arise at end of life, such as the patient's decision to forego further therapy, or for a patient or their surrogate to withdraw a life-sustaining treatment.

Another is the doctrine of double effect. This may occur when a treatment is intended to relieve pain, such as a palliative operation for malignant bowel obstruction, but instead hastens death through unintended complications. Withdrawal of support (never withdrawal of care) requires careful vigilance and communication between the care team, patient, and family in order that pain, anxiety, dyspnea, nausea, and vomiting are adequately controlled. A guideline for withdrawal of life-sustaining measures was published in 2016 (Downar et al., 2016). Peschman and Brasel (2015) provide a comprehensive review of how to approach end-of-life care in the geriatric surgical patient.

Communication is one of the hardest things for physicians to do, but quality end-of-life care demands that we provide good communication and compassionate, culturally competent care.

ANNOTATED REFERENCES FOR END-OF-LIFE ISSUES IN ACUTE CARE SURGERY

1. IOM (Institute of Medicine). *Dying in America: Improving Quality and Honoring Individual Preferences near the End of Life.* Washington, DC: National Academies Press; 2015.

   This is a consensus report from the Institute of Medicine that studied the current state of health care for persons of all ages who are nearing the end of life. The committee of experts concluded that improving the quality and availability of medical and social services for patients and their families could not only enhance the quality of life through the end of life but may also contribute to a more sustainable care system.

2. Hammes BJ, Rooney BL, Gundrum JD. A comparative, retrospective, observational study of the prevalence, availability, and specificity of advance care plans in a county that implemented an advance care planning microsystem. *J Am Geriatr Soc.* 2010;58(7):1249–1255.

   This paper looks at the outcomes of a managed, systematic approach to advance care planning over time. The authors proved that it is possible to achieve a high prevalence of advance care plans that are specific enough to assist with clinical decisions. Creating such a system requires a sustained commitment of resources and leadership that results in a health care culture in which knowing and honoring patient preferences is a high priority.

Author to Provide

1. Gawande A. *Being Mortal: Medicine and What Matters in the End.* New York: Metropolitan Books Henry Holt & Company; 2014.

   The author provides a personal perspective on age-related frailty, serious illness, and approaching death as he follows his father and grandmother-in-law through their own end-of-life journeys. He compares and contrasts the Western medical reality with more traditional societies as he explores aging and dying. The book emphasizes the need for better communication between patients, families, and their caregivers at the end of life.

2. Temel JS, Greer JA, Muzikansky A et al. Early palliative care for patients with metastatic non-small-cell lung cancer. *N Engl J Med.* 2010;363(8):733–742.

These authors randomized 151 patients with metastatic non-small-cell lung cancer to receive either early palliative care integrated with standard oncologic care or standard oncologic care alone. They found that early palliative care led to significant improvements in both quality of life and mood. They also found that when compared to patients receiving standard care, patients receiving early palliative care had less aggressive care at the end of life but longer survival.

3. Kruser JM, Taylor LJ, Campbell TC et al. Best case/worst case: Training surgeons to use a novel communication tool for high-risk acute surgical problems. *J Pain Symptom Manage.* 2017;53(4):711–719.e5.

   This group of authors developed a communication tool, "Best Case/Worst Case," that is based on an established conceptual model of shared decision making that helps facilitate difficult decision making. This paper showed that surgeons trained in its use found it to help establish patient expectations, provide clarity, and facilitate deliberation. They created the Best Case/Worst Case Communication Tool—Whiteboard Video, this training tool can be found on YouTube: https://www.youtube.com/watch?v=FnS3K44sbu0.

4. Mosenthal AC, Murphy PA, Barker LK, Lavery R, Retano A, Livingston DH. Changing the culture around end-of-life care in the trauma intensive care unit. *J Trauma.* 2008;64(6):1587–1593.

   The authors describe the implementation of a structured, palliative care intervention that was integrated into standard ICU care. Although there was no difference in rates of mortality, DNR orders, and withdrawal of life support, DNR and withdrawal of life support were instituted earlier in the hospital course. They showed that structured communication between physicians and families resulted in earlier consensus around goals of care for dying trauma patients.

5. American College of Surgeons, Committee on Trauma (COT), Trauma Quality Improvement Program (TQIP) Best Practice Guideline for Palliative Care. https://www.facs.org/-/media/files/quality-programs/trauma/tqip/palliative_guidelines.ashx?la=en.

   The COT developed these guidelines to focus on the delivery of primary palliative care for trauma patients and their families. Since specialist palliative care is delivered by an interdisciplinary team and not all trauma centers may have the luxury of having a board-certified palliative care provider, these guidelines provide a framework for incorporating the most essential aspects of palliative care into the trauma setting. This guideline's focus is on performing a palliative care assessment and triage of patients and management of the trauma patient near the end of life.

6. Downar J, Delaney JW, Hawryluck L, Kenny L. Guidelines for the withdrawal of life-sustaining measures. *Intensive Care Med.* 2016;42(6):1003–1017.

   These authors convened an interdisciplinary group of ICU providers and using a modified Delphi process to develop guidelines for the process of withdrawing life-sustaining measures in the clinical setting.

7. Peschman J, Brasel KJ. End-of-life care of the geriatric surgical patient. *Surg Clin North Am.* 2015;95(1):191–202.

   The authors review important aspects of end-of-life care, including how to discuss goals of care, or running a family care conference. They go over the definitions of terminology used in end-of-life care such as various forms of advanced care directives, who is authorized to make decisions when the patient is medically unable, and DNR orders including in the perioperative period. They review symptom management for the dying patient. They also briefly discuss the ethical issues that arise at the end of life.

Landmark Article of 21st Century

PITFALLS IN COMMUNICATION THAT LEAD TO NONBENEFICIAL EMERGENCY SURGERY IN ELDERLY PATIENTS WITH SERIOUS ILLNESS: DESCRIPTION OF THE PROBLEM AND ELEMENTS OF A SOLUTION

Cooper Z, Courtwright A, Karlage A, Gawande A, and Block S. *Ann Surg.* 2014;260(6):949–957

ABSTRACT

Objective To provide a description of communication breakdowns and to identify interventions to improve surgical decision making for elderly patients with serious illness and acute, life-threatening surgical conditions.

Background Communication between surgeons, patients, and surrogates about goals of treatment plays an important and understudied role in determining the surgical interventions elderly patients with serious illness receive. Communication breakdowns may lead to nonbeneficial procedures in acute events near the end of life.

Methods We review the available literature on factors that lead to communication challenges and nonbeneficial surgery at the end of life. We use this review to identify solutions for navigating surgical decision making for seriously ill elderly patients with acute surgical conditions.

Results Surgeon, patient, surrogate, and systemic factors—including time constraints, inadequate provider communication skills and training, uncertainty about prognosis, patient and surrogate anxiety and fear of inaction, and limitations in advance care planning—contribute to communication challenges and nonbeneficial surgery at the end of life. Surgeons could accomplish more effective communication with seriously ill elderly patients if they had a structured, standardized approach to exploring patients' preferences and to integrating those preferences into surgical decisions in the acute setting.

Conclusions Improved communication among surgeons, patients, and surrogates is necessary to ensure that patients receive the care that they want and to avoid nonbeneficial treatment. Further research is needed to learn how to best structure these conversations in the emergency surgical setting.

Original Author Commentary: Zara Cooper

Although potentially lifesaving, major surgery in frail and seriously ill patients may worsen functional disability and exacerbate chronic symptoms, leading to institutionalization and worse quality of life. For patients who die in the weeks to months after surgery, final days are frequently spent in the hospital characterized by anxiety, pain, and burdensome medical care. The benefits of surgery must be weighed against the uncertainty of other poor outcomes that may be unacceptable to patients. The evidence about longer-term patient outcomes to inform clinical decisions is sparse and decisions are marked by emotional distress on the part of patients, family members, and clinicians alike. As we describe in this article, the epicenter of each decision is a conversation between surgeons and patients or surrogates that is heavily influenced by factors that are frequently out of the control of either party.

Ideally, clinical decisions are guided by the patient's priorities, treatment is aligned with the patient's goals and values, and the most likely outcome is one that the patient and family would find acceptable. However, too frequently, clinical momentum and inadequate communication leads to patients receiving surgery that cannot achieve their clinical goals. Understanding factors leading to discordant care helps us to address them. Surgeons must actively formulate and share prognosis, elicit patients' priorities, goals, and values for health care, and develop processes of care to document such conversations. Surgeons must also embrace palliative adjuncts or alternatives to surgery that can alleviate suffering and help patients better reach their goals near the end of life.

CHAPTER 50

Alcohol Withdrawal

Review by Contributor: Gary A. Vercruysse

Alcohol in various forms has been made, traded, sold and used by humans for millennia. Beer and wine were noted to be safe alternatives to the relatively unsafe sources of available polluted water found in most cities during the middle ages and was and still is produced by monks for personal use and trade. Physicians encouraged the consumption of these beverages by both adults and children. Alcohol was also used as an early anesthetic; its stupefying effects were relied on for hundreds of years until better anesthetic alternatives were developed in the mid-nineteenth century. Along the same timeframe, it can be assumed that people began to self-treat with various forms of alcohol for chronic pain, psychological disorders, depression, and other maladies, which continues to date, with no end in sight. Alcohol-related surgical research, which really began during the last century, relates mainly to the identification of those suffering from alcohol abuse, as well as those with withdrawal potential, the treatment of withdrawal, and diminishing preventable death from trauma as related to alcohol use and abuse.

A number of screening tools have been created, validated, and are routinely used to both identify those engaging in alcohol abuse and to recognize those who are the most prone to withdrawal and delirium tremens after admission to the hospital for pre-, intra-, and postoperative care. Perhaps the simplest and most recognized tool is the CAGE questionnaire developed by John Ewing in 1968. It is easy to use, consisting of only four simple questions. While a positive response to the CAGE interview is not diagnostic of alcoholism, it should alert the interviewer to the possibility of the presence of alcoholism and trigger a more thorough evaluation. Another well-used instrument for detection of the possibility of withdrawal is the Clinical Institute Withdrawal Assessment for Alcohol (CIWA) Scale, which is validated and has high inter-rater reliability. The CIWA scale's goal is to provide an efficient and objective means of assessing the need for treatment for alcohol withdrawal. Studies have shown that use of the scale in management of alcohol withdrawal leads to decreased frequency of over-sedation with benzodiazepines in patients with milder alcohol withdrawal than would otherwise be detected without use of the scale, and decreased frequency of undertreatment in patients with greater severity of withdrawal than would otherwise be determined without the scale. Perhaps a flaw in the CIWA scale is the requirement for the answering of subjective questions, which is not possible in many ICU patients who are sedated and ventilated due to injuries, or because they have developed severe symptoms consistent with delirium tremens.

Treatment for alcohol withdrawal and delirium tremens with regard to acute care surgery is mainly concerned with identifying withdrawal potential, and the prevention of delirium tremens seen in patients who are in the hospital for other treatment related to emergency general surgery or trauma. Early works touted oral or intravenous alcohol empirically for the prevention of withdrawal, while later research focused on accurately determining who might go through withdrawal using validated questionnaires, and then deriving treatment regiments that promoted the use of non-alcohol GABA receptor agonists, such as paraldehyde, chloral hydrate, barbiturates, and later benzodiazepines, as well as B and multivitamin supplementation, as these treatments are thought to have a better safety profile and are more efficacious and morally sound as compared to alcohol, which, when prescribed as treatment by physicians, is construed by some to be interpreted as the act of health care providers reinforcing behaviors that lead to alcoholism by treating the problem with the agent causing the problem.

Since the development of regionalized trauma systems 45 years ago, preventable death rates due to trauma have been reduced from about 40% to approximately 3%. Demographic studies of trauma and alcohol use have shown that approximately 1 in 8 inpatient beds in the United States are occupied by trauma patients, and of those, half are the result of trauma related to alcohol intoxication. Therefore, logic would dictate that reducing the rate of alcohol use and dangerous behavior associated with its use would have greater impact on the remaining trauma-related mortality than any other means. Gentilello et al. (1989) in their landmark study showed that by employing a brief intervention as a part of the hospital course of treatment in mild to moderate drinkers resulted in sustained and repeated reduction in alcohol consumption, a 47% reduction in trauma recidivism a year, and a 48% reduction at 3 years as compared to matched controls not offered this brief intervention. Unfortunately, this same benefit was not seen in heavy drinkers, as explained by Dr. Gentilello during his presentation at the American Surgical Association meeting, "Most patients who are cirrhotic have been seen by doctors dozens and dozens of times without receiving any form of screening, intervention, and counseling. To step in after their disease has become end-stage and expect to easily turn it around is quite unrealistic. It is like treating metastatic cancer at that point." To date, this description of a simple intervention has no rival in its effect on the prevention of trauma. This study should be studied by all trainees and used as an example by all attending surgeons.

ANNOTATED REFERENCES FOR ALCOHOL WITHDRAWAL

1. Ewing JA. Detecting alcoholism: The CAGE questionnaire. *JAMA*. 1984;252:1905–1907.

   The CAGE questionnaire, consisting of four clinical interview questions, has proved useful in helping to alert the clinician to the possibility of alcoholism. The questions focus on Cutting down, Annoyance by criticism, Guilty feeling, and Eye-openers. The acronym "CAGE" helps the physician to recall the questions. This article describes how these questions were identified, and their use in clinical and research studies is described.

2. Saitz M, Mayo-Smith MF, Redmond HA, Bernard DR, Calkins DR. Individualized treatment for alcohol withdrawal. A randomized double-blind controlled trial. *JAMA.* 1994;272:519–523.

   This randomized, double-blind trial showed that management for alcohol withdrawal that was guided by the CIWA scale resulted in decreased treatment duration and total use of benzodiazepines.

3. Chapman CB. Delirium tremens. *N Engl J Med.* 1944;231(7):249–255.

   This is an excellent description of the definition, incidence, precipitating factors, diagnosis, clinical features, treatment, and mortality of delirium tremens in the first half of the twentieth century.

4. Ntais C, Pakos E, Kyzas P, Ioannidis JP. Benzodiazepines for alcohol withdrawal. *Cochrane Database Syst Rev.* 2005;20(3).

   An analysis of all randomized controlled trials examining the effectiveness and safety of a benzodiazepine in comparison with a placebo or other pharmacological intervention were considered. The authors concluded that benzodiazepines are effective against alcohol withdrawal symptoms when compared to placebo. In addition, compared to other agents, except anticonvulsants, benzodiazepines were more effective in preventing seizures due to alcohol withdrawal.

5. Dunn CW, Donovan DM, Gentilello LM. Practical guidelines for performing alcohol interventions in trauma centers. *J Trauma.* 1997;42(2):299–304.

   This nuts-and-bolts paper provides practical guidelines for the administration of alcohol interventions that are suitable for trauma center use and that have documented efficacy in reducing alcohol consumption. It is a good guide for the practitioner who is learning about how to talk with patients about their alcohol consumption, to determine whether or not they are at risk for withdrawal, and need further intervention or treatment.

Landmark Article of 21st Century

ALCOHOL INTERVENTIONS IN A TRAUMA CENTER AS A MEANS OF REDUCING THE RISK OF INJURY RECURRENCE

Gentilello LM, Rivara FP, Donovan DM, Jurkovich GJ, Daranciang E, Dunn CW, Villaveces A, Copass M, and Ries RR, *Ann Sur.* 1999;230(4):473–483

ABSTRACT

Objective Alcoholism is the leading risk factor for injury. The authors hypothesized that providing brief alcohol interventions as a routine component of trauma care would significantly reduce alcohol consumption and would decrease the rate of trauma recidivism.

Methods This study was a randomized, prospective controlled trial in a level I trauma center. Patients were screened using a blood alcohol concentration, gamma glutamyl transpeptidase level, and Short Michigan Alcoholism Screening Test (SMAST). Those with positive results were randomized to a brief intervention or control group. Reinjury was detected by a computerized search of emergency department and statewide hospital discharge records, and 6- and 12-month interviews were conducted to assess alcohol use.

Results   A total of 2524 patients were screened; 1153 screened positive (46%). There were 366 randomized to the intervention group and 396 to controls. At 12 months, the intervention group decreased alcohol consumption by 21.8+/−3.7 drinks per week; in the control group, the decrease was 6.7+/−5.8 (p = 0.03). The reduction was most apparent in patients with mild to moderate alcohol problems (SMAST score 3–8); they had 21.6+/−4.2 fewer drinks per week, compared to an increase of 2.3+/−8.3 drinks per week in controls (p < 0.01). There was a 47% reduction in injuries requiring either emergency department or trauma center admission (hazard ratio 0.53, 95% confidence interval 0.26–1.07, p = 0.07) and a 48% reduction in injuries requiring hospital admission (3 years follow-up).

Conclusion   Alcohol interventions are associated with a reduction in alcohol intake and a reduced risk of trauma recidivism. Given the prevalence of alcohol problems in trauma centers, screening, intervention, and counseling for alcohol problems should be routine.

Original Author Commentary: Larry M. Gentilello

Fifty-four illnesses are attributable to excessive alcohol use. Thirty-six are the result of chronic diseases, 15 of which result in admission to a surgical service. The remaining 18 are due to acute causes (mainly injuries). Overall, 88,000 deaths and 2.4 million hospital discharges per year are attributable to excess consumption, and many of these patients are frequently on a surgical service.

Given these extraordinary statistics, clinicians should be familiar with how to screen, counsel, and provide an intervention, or to arrange the availability of such services in their practice. In November 2018, the US Preventive Services Task Force acknowledged this and formally recommended it. However, trauma centers were 13 years ahead of this time. In 2005, the American College of Surgeons Committee on Trauma (COT) required trauma centers to provide such services as criteria for verification.

The first publication on alcohol screening and interventions on any hospital service occurred in 1988, when as a resident this author noted that half of the patients admitted to the trauma center were intoxicated. The Chief of Trauma conducting rounds was asked, "Where do these patients go for treatment?" The response was, "This is a trauma center. We are not in the business of addressing alcohol problems."

This sparked creation of liaisons with multiple treatment centers to send interventionists to the trauma center whenever an intoxicated patient was ready for discharge. Eighty four percent of patients agreed to treatment.

This led to this NIH-funded trial comparing screening and brief interventions on a trauma service with standard care. The result was over a 50% reduction in returns to the ER or hospital readmission for treatment of another injury in the intervention group, with up to 5 years follow-up.

The subsequent COT mandate requiring trauma centers to implement this practice resulted in the Centers for Disease Control granting them the Injury Control and Health Impact Award in recognition that this was the first time in the history of medicine that any requirement had ever been passed requiring physicians to address substance misuse.

References

Gentilello LM, Duggan P, Drummon D et al. Major injury as a unique opportunity to initiate treatment in the alcoholic. *Am J Surg.* 1988;156:558–561.

Gentilello LM, Rivara FP, Donovan DM et al. Alcohol interventions in a trauma center as a means of reducing the risk of injury recurrence. *Ann Surg.* 1999;230:473–480.

US Preventive Services Task Force. Screening and behavioral counseling interventions to reduce unhealthy alcohol use in adults and adolescents. US Preventive Services Task Force Recommendation Statement. *JAMA.* 2018;320(18):1899–1909.

Index

322   Index

Printed in the United States
by Baker & Taylor Publisher Services